Nurses' Aids Series

MEDICAL NURSING

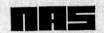

NURSES' AIDS SERIES

Nurses' Aids Series

Medical
Nursing

NINTH EDITION REVISED BY
Christine M. Chapman
B.Sc.(Soc.), M.Phil., S.R.N., S.C.M., R.N.T.
Director of Advanced Nursing Studies,
Welsh National School of Medicine

BAILLIÈRE TINDALL · LONDON

A BAILLIÈRE TINDALL book published by
Cassell Ltd.
35 Red Lion Square, London WC1R 4SG
and at Sydney, Auckland, Toronto, Johannesburg
an affiliate of
Macmillan Publishing Co. Inc.
New York

First published 1941
Eighth edition
    Reprinted 1973
Ninth edition 1977
    Reprinted 1979
    Reprinted 1981
Spanish translation, eighth edition (CECSA, Mexico)
Portuguese translation, eighth edition (Publicacoes
    Europa-America, Mira-Sintra)
Turkish edition (Turkish Government)

Margaret Hitch wrote the first edition of *Medical Nursing* and
subsequent editions were prepared by Marjorie Houghton, the
seventh in collaboration with Mary Whittow. The eighth and
ninth were prepared by Christine M. Chapman.

ISBN 0 7020 0616 5

Printed in Great Britain by
Spottiswoode Ballantyne Ltd.

Contents

Preface

It is five years since I first revised *Medical Nursing*. At that time the major change made was one of format. This has been retained in this edition and the main changes are those required due to progress in diagnosis and treatment. One of the major changes since 1975 has been the introduction of Systèmes International, or S.I. units and these have been incorporated in the text.

From the preface in the first edition (by the late Miss Margaret Hitch) onwards, successive authors have stated that a book of this size must be selective and this remains true. It cannot, and does not, attempt to cover all aspects of nursing care nor can it mention every medical condition that may be met with in varying parts of the world. It does, however, attempt to develop a reasoning approach to nursing care so that new and unexpected conditions may be dealt with adequately.

Many people have given me help and advice during the preparation of this book; in particular I would like to thank Mrs M. Thomas, University Hospital of Wales for her help in revising 'Psychological Aspects of Illness and Mental Disease'.

I gratefully acknowledge permission to reproduce illustrations as follows: Fig. 7 from Vickers Ltd, Medical Group; Figs 17, 19, 30, 38 and 40 from the Department of Medical Illustration, St Bartholomew's Hospital, London; Fig. 21 from the *Nursing Times*; Figs 22 and 42 from the Medical Illustration Department, Institute of Child Health, Great Ormond Street, London; Fig. 23 from Avon Medicals Ltd; Fig. 24 from Dr G. S. Crockett, Department of Pathology, General Hospital, Kettering; Figs 27–29 from E. Lipman Cohen and J. S. Pegum *Dermatology* (C.M.T.) published by Baillière Tindall; Fig. 43 from Dr D. N. Cardew, Department of Audio-Visual Communication, St Mary's Hospital Medical School, London; Fig. 44 from Dr. A. D. Evans, The Virology Unit, University Hospital of Wales, Cardiff, and Fig. 45 from

H. G. East & Co Ltd, Oxford. Finally I would like to express my appreciation of the help and encouragement that I have received from the publishers during the time this edition was being prepared.

August 1976   CHRISTINE M. CHAPMAN

Introduction

TRADITION and convenience have resulted in the care of sick people being divided into classes, based largely on either the part of the body affected or on the type of treatment involved, thus we have ophthalmology, gynaecology, medicine and surgery. While the possible logic of such decisions cannot be denied, it has had the unfortunate effect of producing an aura of mystery about the different types of care and has often made nurses feel inadequate when transferring from one area to another. It is important to realize that all sick people, whatever the cause or site of their illness, require the same basic nursing care to provide for their comfort and hygiene, and to meet their needs for food, fluid support and protection. However, it is also true to say that there may be some specific care or treatment to be added to the patients' basic requirements and it is in this context that medical nursing should be seen.

Medical wards contain patients whose illness is largely that of disordered function, such as cardiac and respiratory disease, endocrine disorders and degenerative changes, although there is no sharp line drawn between those requiring medical or surgical treatment and often both may be employed at different stages of a disease.

When talking to nurses about the care of patients a tutor is constantly told, 'but I've never nursed a patient with that', and this is meant to exclude all possibility of knowledge of the care of such a patient. While not wishing to minimize the value of experience in any field of life, nevertheless the intelligent student should be able, to a great extent, to 'work out' the care such a patient would require, by using knowledge already possessed of basic human requirements, physiology, function of the part affected and basic nursing techniques.

It is with this in mind that this textbook is produced. It is meant to be a guide to the main principles involved in medical nursing and needs to be supplemented by class teaching and practical experience. Medical science moves so quickly it can never be a completely up to date account of all a nurse needs to know.

The way in which this book is divided and classified has been based on more or less arbitrary decisions which have been adhered to throughout. The first chapter deals with some basic medical and nursing concepts which are relevant in many diseases. Once dealt with fully they can then be referred to briefly in subsequent chapters.

Classification within chapters is based on the prime cause of the breakdown in health. This itself is not an easy concept, as causation may be a result of a combination of factors in which man's inherited physical and mental make up interact with his environment. Dr Clark-Kennedy in *Human Disease* sums up this concept by saying: 'Diseases are not entities, each with an independent existence, which can be neatly labelled, like birds and flowers ... they are really alterations for the worse in individuals; essentially reactions, some common, others rare, many complicated and little understood, between the inborn constitution of a man and his environment.'

Heredity gives each one of us those unique characteristics of body and mind which are transmitted by the genes in the particular ovum and spermatozoon which came together to produce the new individual. No two people are ever, or have ever been, identical, not even 'identical' twins, and this is an important fact for the nurse to bear in mind. It is convenient to have a number of measuring sticks in deciding what is normal and what is abnormal and therefore certain measurements are described as 'average', such as average weight, or average body temperature, representing the mean figure obtained by taking a large number of recordings, but it is a complete misconception to say that an individual is abnormal who does not completely fit in with the average. Later in this book there is a statement that on average men are larger than women; all who read this sentence, which is quite true, will immediately call to mind at least one very large woman and one very small man amongst their acquaintances. If to this factor of inborn uniqueness we add the effect of varying environment, it should be easy to understand that, while all human beings share certain characteristics and certain experiences in life, no two patients will react to illness, physically or mentally, in quite the same way.

Heredity

Some diseases are transmitted from parent to child in the genes, such as haemophilia, a defect in the blood clotting mechanism. In others such as asthma or diabetes there may be an inherited tendency but whether the disease develops or not depends on other factors.

Congenital Abnormalities

These are not inherited but develop in the intra-uterine life of the child or are caused by some abnormality at the time of birth. These may be traced to such things as deficiency in the diet of the mother, for example calcium. Bacteria or toxins can pass from the maternal to the foetal circulation, syphilis in the mother can infect and kill the foetus, and a trivial infection, German measles in the early months of pregnancy for example, can produce congenital defects. Apparently harmless drugs can cause abnormalities of fetal development if given to pregnant women. The tragedy of the 'thalidomide babies' a few years ago is an outstanding example. This sedative drug given to women in the early months of pregnancy arrested the development of the long bones of the foetus and babies were born with only rudimentary arms or legs.

Infection

Infection is one of the more clear-cut factors in producing disease, and one which is more amenable to control than most, as has been shown by the virtual disappearance of such infectious diseases as smallpox and diphtheria in countries where preventive medicine is highly developed. However, if the public fails to cooperate, these controls can readily break down, and in countries where health services are as yet only beginning to be developed, infection, including parasitic infections, are major causes of preventable disease and death.

Allergy

In certain sensitive subjects there may be an inflammatory reaction to specific substances such as foreign protein (e.g. vaccines), food stuffs, pollen, dust and even bacteria (this is quite different to infection by the organism and often occurs in a different part of the body, e.g. acute nephritis as an allergic reaction to a streptococcal infection of the throat). Such a reaction may be local as in hay fever or generalized as in urticaria.

Injury

Injuries due to a variety of physical and chemical agents are common causes of illness and disability. Serious accidents constitute one of the major problems in this age of motor vehicles and industrial machinery. In recent years the increasing use of various sources of radioactivity both in medical practice and in industry has given prominence to the hazards of exposure to gamma rays and to ionizing radiations from radioactive elements. The use of such sources demands strict control and the enforcement of safety measures. Large doses of radiation are destructive to all types of tissue, including the superficial tissues, the bone marrow and lymphatic tissue. Repeated exposure to small amounts of radiation from X-rays and other radioactive sources can produce malignant changes in the blood (leukaemia) and also affect the germ cells in the testes and ovaries, with possible genetic effects, that is to say the children of parents who have undergone such exposure may have physical or mental defects.

Other physical agents which can damage the body include exposure to excessive heat or cold or to variation in the pressure on the surface of the body at great heights or depths. These factors become increasingly important as technical advances enable man to explore the space above the earth and depths of the oceans beneath him. Chemical agents represent another hazard; the toxic effects of certain drugs, and of chemicals used in industry, arsenic, cyanides and carbon monoxide gas, are examples of these. Alcohol and tobacco are potentially toxic substances, and social customs and fashions may possibly enhance the dangers from these sources in certain sections of the community.

Deficiency

Deficiency disorders are dealt with in some detail later in the book. In many parts of the world lack of sufficient food for the body's needs for growth, repair and energy is a major cause of ill-health, but dietary deficiencies may also be due to ignorance, to customs and taboos relating to certain foods, or to lack of health education and of provision for preventive medical and nursing care.

Degeneration

We are all aware that 'growing old' is at present inevitable, but this may occur at different rates in different individuals and even within one individual certain parts of the body may 'degenerate' more quickly than others. Catastrophes such as myocardial infarction and cerebral haemorrhage may be due to this process as may some rheumatic disorders and endocrine disfunctions. The cause of 'ageing' is still little understood and is the area of much research and interest as the population of aged persons in the community increases.

New Growths

These may be benign or malignant. If the former they may produce symptoms due to pressure on surrounding tissues, by obstruction of tubes or cavities or by over-production of substances such as hormones. If malignant then their effect may be similar plus general constitutional disturbance and the probability of spread by metastasis, resulting in the abnormal tissue replacing normal tissue at such a rate that body functions are distorted or arrested and eventually death will occur.

Idiopathic Disease

There remains a large group of diseases whose cause is not yet understood and which do not easily fall into classified groups. Medical science may eventually bring these and many other common conditions under control, but although the actual cause of disease may not be completely known, it can truly be said that the great advances in medical science, aided by the contributions of such sciences as biology, biochemistry and electronics, which have been made in the present century, have vastly improved the outlook for many patients. If, for example, we look back to the days before the discovery of insulin, we find that many diabetic patients, particularly young people, died of this disease or its complications. The discovery that the pancreas secreted insulin, a substance controlling metabolic processes, and that the patient's condition responded in a remarkable way to the injection of insulin, was a great advance in the treatment of this common disorder. Yet, to say that diabetes is due to failure of the pancreas to secrete sufficient insulin is in fact only a half-truth, since the reason why the body either fails to produce this material or fails to use it effectively is still not completely understood.

Stress

Finally account must be taken of physical and emotional stress, both of which are recognized as factors in the production of ill-health under modern conditions of life. Emotional strain will often produce physical symptoms and this makes it impossible to separate the mind from the body when considering the cause of ill-health in an individual.

Nurses themselves are not exempt from this phenomenon of stress and uncongenial work or surroundings; frustration, feelings of inadequacy and anxiety may produce symptoms such as headaches, faintness and excessive fatigue to name but a few. It is important that this 'cry for help' from the individual is not regarded as malingering but recognized and the basic problem uncovered. The care of the sick is a responsibility which frequently produces great anxiety much of which can be relieved by adequate understanding and support from both superiors and peers. No nurse should be ashamed of her feelings of stress in whatever sphere they occur but should seek to 'talk them over' with a sympathetic listener; she will often be surprised to find that they have been experienced by many of her colleagues even those who appear most competent and controlled.

The influence of social factors on health is increasingly recognized. The World Health Organization defines health as a state of physical, mental and social well-being. This 'social well-being' implies that the individual fits in with the society in which he lives and is able to establish satisfying relationships not only within his own family, but with the network of social groups with which he is involved in his work and in his leisure-time pursuits and activities.

The pattern of disease in any country reflects its social and economic development. In the economically developed countries infectious diseases are, on the whole, controlled but with the increased life span there are many more old people suffering from chronic illness. In the emergent countries of the world diseases which are largely preventable are major causes of ill health and death, particularly amongst the young population.

Both birth rates and death rates are high and the expectation of life is considerably below that of Western societies. The situation is, however, a dynamic one and in many African countries, for example, changes are rapidly taking place.

This brief account of the present concept of disease may help the student nurse to appreciate the complexity of the problem and also, perhaps, to arouse her interest in the subject of research, since every unsolved problem is a challenge. Research is not confined to the laboratory; every day in the wards of hospitals new drugs are on trial and clinical investigations are being carried out, not only for the benefit of the individual patient, but also to add to the body of knowledge on which future progress depends. Therefore the nurse is also a member of the clinical research team; much depends on her observation of the patient, her ability to keep clear and accurate records and reports, her meticulous attention to the instruction from the physician and the laboratory and, not least, on her sympathetic encouragement of the patient which helps him to cooperate readily in what must sometimes appear to him to be somewhat alarming or tedious forms of treatment.

While of necessity a textbook tends to concentrate on the scientific and technical aspects of care it must never be forgotten that the patient is an individual human being who needs all the skill, comfort, support and understanding that the nurse can give him. This is the essence of good nursing practice.

1
Basic principles in medical nursing care

THE definition of the unique function of the nurse has been most succinctly expressed by Virginia Henderson when she states, 'The unique function of the nurse is to assist the individual, sick or well, in the performance of those activities contributing to health or its recovery (or to a peaceful death) that he would perform unaided if he had the necessary strength, will or knowledge. And to do this in such a way as to help him gain independence as rapidly as possible.' It is increasingly realized that nursing has its roots in fundamental human needs, such as the desire for food, shelter, clothing, love and/or approval; a sense of being 'wanted' and useful in society, and an ability to act independently showing initiative. These needs are common to all human beings although their importance may vary with age and culture but they exist regardless of the patient's diagnosis although they may be modified by it. There is therefore a common core of care required by all patients whether they be confined to bed or able to move freely about the ward. It is this latter group that may suffer a degree of neglect as the nurse perceives them as caring for themselves, yet they may still need help, encouragement and praise. Alternatively it is possible for the nurse to perpetuate the dependency of the patient when they should be encouraged to revert to self-sufficiency, i.e. their need has changed from one of requiring help to that of showing independence.

These points must be borne in mind by the nurse and each patient be seen as an individual despite the possession of a common core of needs and a similar diagnostic label.

One of the ways in which the onset of illness can be recognized is by observation of disturbances in normal bodily functions. These may be classed as symptoms, that is how the patient feels, or as signs, things that can be seen with the eye or measured clinically. For example one of the first things that most people do when they feel unwell is to take their temperature: on this they base their next move—to go to bed, to call the doctor, or to carry on with their work.

Unfortunately, such behaviour may be less sensible than it appears as although 37°C (98·4°F) is considered a 'normal' temperature it is only an average and there may be great variations, some people showing a raised temperature very easily, while others never seem to produce a reading that is above 'normal'. A more realistic approach therefore, is to take account of all signs and symptoms rather than one, and it is on such a pattern of evidence that the doctor makes his clinical diagnosis.

The following manifestations of constitutional disturbances are common in most cases of illness due to infection although they will naturally vary in degree according to its type and severity.

Pyrexia

Pyrexia, or a rise in body temperature. This is a constant feature of all but very mild infections and can be regarded as one of the body's defence mechanisms against invading organisms. 'Fever' has the same meaning as pyrexia, but is often used in a wider sense to describe any illness which is marked by a high temperature, as for example scarlet fever and glandular fever.

As stated, the normal body temperature in health varies with the individual and shows a slight daily variation, within a limited range, being higher in the evening than in the early morning, but is between 36° and 37·5°C (97° and 99°F). A temperature above 37°C (99°F) is usually accepted as pyrexial; a temperature above 40·5°C (105°F) is regarded as excessively high or hyperpyrexial. Hypothermia, shown by a temperature below 36°C (97°F) is usually a manifestation of a degree of myxoedema and is dealt with in Chapter 13. The degree of fever and its duration are now usually reduced by the use of chemotherapeutic drugs and the typical patterns on temperature charts, which were formerly often diagnostic in certain diseases, are now seldom seen.

When the onset of infection is abrupt the temperature rises rapidly in the course of an hour or so and may reach hyper-pyrexial levels. This rapid rise is often accompanied by a violent shivering attack, known as a 'rigor', during which the patient feels cold, although his temperature is steadily climbing. The term rigor is also used to describe the condition which is typical of malarial infection and some other conditions such as reactions to the injection of foreign protein in which the shivering stage is followed in about $\frac{1}{2}$ to 1 hr by the 'hot stage'; the patient's skin is hot and dry and he complains of being 'burning hot'. This stage which may only last for 1 or 2 hr, is followed by profuse sweating and a fall of temperature.

In the majority of febrile stages the temperature subsides gradually, taking 24 to 48 hr or more to return to normal; this gradual abatement of fever is sometimes described as 'lysis'. A dramatic drop in temperature from pyrexial or hyperpyrexial levels to normal within a few hours is known as a 'crisis' and was the typical termination of continuous fever in pneumococcal pneumonia before the introduction of chemotherapeutic drugs made it possible to cut short this infection and reduce the high temperature within 48 hr of the onset of the illness.

Although infection is the commonest cause of pyrexia, other conditions can produce a rise of body temperature. These include the injection of foreign protein, as for example TAB vaccine (typhoid–paratyphoid A and B vaccine), disorders of the central nervous system affecting the heat-regulating centre and the absorption of the products of damaged tissues following injury or destruction of tissue, as in myocardial infarction or necrosis due to malignant disease.

General Malaise

This term applies to the state of 'feeling ill', which is often accompanied by aching muscles and joints. It is characteristic of most acute infections.

Increased Heart Rate

The systolic blood pressure rises, the pulse is rapid and full, sometimes described as bounding. There is a definite ratio between the rise of temperature and the increased heart rate in most infections, the pulse rate being increased by approximately 10 beats per min for every 0·5°C (1°F) that the temperature rises. Thus if the temperature rises 2°C (4°F) above the normal then the pulse rate may be expected to increase to 40 beats per min faster than normal. There are exceptions to this general rule; for example in typhoid and paratyphoid fever the pulse rate is usually relatively slow, and in scarlet fever it may be faster than would be expected from the temperature (see p. 327).

Respiratory Signs

The respiration rate increases in proportion to the rise in pulse rate, but maintains the normal ratio of 4 : 1, therefore if the pulse rate increases to 120, a respiration rate of 30 may be expected. A disproportionate rise in the respiratory rate is, however, often seen in acute infections of the lungs and respiratory tract.

Disturbances of the Digestive Functions

These are shown by a dry mouth, furred tongue, loss of appetite. Nausea and vomiting, particularly at the onset of infection and either constipation or diarrhoea are common symptoms.

Disturbances of the Excretory Functions

These are shown by a diminished output of urine, and proteinuria (albuminuria), which, however, disappears when the fever abates. While the temperature remains raised the skin is hot and dry; sweating occurs when the temperature is falling. In some infectious diseases the bacterial toxins produce a typical rash.

Disturbances of the Nervous System

These are shown by headache, drowsiness in some cases and restlessness and insomnia in others. Severe infections may be accompanied by delirium which may end in coma.

It is the doctor's responsibility to find the cause for these signs and symptoms. Meanwhile the nurse must observe and record her findings accurately and keep the patient as comfortable as possible.

General Nursing Treatment

The nursing treatment for any patient with fever includes bed rest, liberal fluids and adequate sleep. The bowels should be regulated; the view once held that toxins were eliminated by the bowel which led to the free use of aperients is not now upheld, but constipation will add to the patient's discomfort.

If the patient is able to drink freely this is of great assistance in keeping the mouth moist and clean, and the usual care of the mouth and teeth will be sufficient. In cases where the patient is not taking sufficient fluids by mouth and intravenous therapy is used, his mouth needs special care. Some drugs, such as those containing belladonna, will also cause the patient to have a dry mouth. The nurse should use her judgment as to the frequency with which the mouth should be cleaned in order to keep it moist and in good condition. In most cases it is advisable to attend to it before and after taking food, but if the patient is not taking food or fluids by mouth, then attention should be given 4-hourly, or if the mouth is very dirty at 2-hourly intervals. If an unconscious patient or a very ill patient has dentures, these are removed, placed in a container and labelled with his name.

For regular attention to the mouth a tray may be kept at the patient's bedside, and should contain the requirements needed for the individual patient:

(1) A small bowl containing wool swabs.

(2) Mouth sticks or a pair of fine clip forceps and a pair of dissecting forceps, in a dish.

(3) Gallipots containing hydrogen peroxide or sodium bicarbonate solution; glycothymoline, or other suitable antiseptic; an emollient such as glycerin and borax.

(4) A small receiver for soiled swabs.

(5) A mouthwash such as sodium bicarbonate solution (5 ml sodium bicarbonate to 300 ml water), or normal or half normal sodium chloride solution.

The swabs are secured on the mouth sticks or on the clip forceps, dipped in the peroxide or sodium bicarbonate solution and then applied systematically to all surfaces of the mouth and teeth. This is followed by similar swabbing with the glycothymoline solution. If the patient is able to use a mouthwash this may take the place of the second swabbing. Glycerin and borax is applied as necessary if the lips are dry. Hydrogen peroxide in 2-volume strength is particularly useful when dried mucus and epithelial debris form crusts, or sordes; hydrogen peroxide should be followed by a saline or other mild mouthwash to remove the froth that forms. Where fruit juices are allowed these, being acid, stimulate the flow of saliva and mucus, and thus help to keep the mouth clean and moist.

Chewing gum is helpful in some cases as it also stimulates the salivary glands.

Apart from the discomfort of a dry and dirty mouth, serious complications may result from neglect of its care in ill patients. Food will be taken less readily and this in itself retards recovery; parotitis may occur from spread of infection from the mouth to the parotid gland and this is a special danger when the patient is unable to take either food or fluids by the mouth. Spread of infection from the mouth or teeth may cause cellulitis, most often in the submaxillary area, a condition known as Ludwig's angina; inhalation of septic material may give rise to broncho-pneumonia (aspiration pneumonia).

As a rule there are no restrictions on diet, but most febrile patients will prefer fluids, such as sweetened fruit juices and tea or milk and semi-solid foods, egg custard, ice-cream and fruit or milk jelly. The increase in metabolism, which accompanies fever, necessitates a high calorie diet if this condition continues for more than a few days.

Measures to minimize the patient's discomfort include light bedclothes and personal clothing; a bed cradle is useful to take the weight of the bedclothes and to allow free circulation of air. Aspirin is often ordered for the relief of headache and aching joints. In all cases where the patient is suffering from a severe infection a daily fluid intake and output record should be kept and a specimen of urine tested daily for specific gravity, albumin, sugar and acetone.

If the patient's temperature is high, 40°C (104°F) or over, and the skin is dry, or if he is feeling very hot and uncomfortable although the temperature is only moderately raised, sponging will often give relief and reduce the temperature by one or two degrees.

Method of Sponging

To be effective sponging must be carried out with the least possible exertion on the part of the patient, as every movement increases heat production. It is not a very drastic treatment and signs of collapse are unlikely to occur if it is done skilfully. The object is to increase the heat loss by evaporation from the body and a successful 'sponge' will reduce the temperature about one degree Centigrade (two degrees Fahrenheit).

Several sponges are needed, and marine ones are best, but

pieces of lint or soft towelling can be used. The temperature of the water may be ordered, e.g. 37·5°C (100°F) reduced to 26·5°C (80°F), although it is not materially important. Most patients will not appreciate sponging with cold water except, perhaps, in the tropics. The body is sponged in sections and long, smooth, rhythmic strokes are used which always go in the same direction. Each sponge is used for two strokes only, first one side and then it is turned and the other side brought into contact with the skin. No drying is required, as the value of the treatment lies in the cooling resulting from evaporation of the moisture from the hot dry skin. The sponge should be wet enough to leave small beads of water on the skin. The whole procedure should not take longer than 15 to 20 min and should depend on the fall in the temperature; this should be taken after 10 min and again in 5 to 10 min, according to the rate of fall. A fall of about 1°C (2°F) only during the treatment is aimed at, as the temperature continues to fall for $\frac{1}{2}$ to 1 hr afterwards, usually by another one to two degrees. The lowest point to which the temperature falls after sponging should be charted to show the effect of treatment.

More drastic measures for reducing the body temperature, such as cold or ice packs, or immersion in a bath of cold or iced water, are seldom required in the care of patients suffering from infectious disease. They may be employed to reduce a hyperpyrexial temperature in such conditions as heat stroke or to bring about a deliberate lowering of the temperature to subnormal levels. This form of treatment is known as hypothermia and it is used to slow metabolism and decrease cellular activity in some cases of severe damage to the brain, or in conjunction with anaesthesia in cardiac and brain surgery. If so used, drugs are required to prevent shivering which will produce heat.

Care of the Patient During a Rigor

During the shivering stage the patient requires warmth, as although his temperature is rising the surface of the body is cold. At this stage of violent shivering the axilla is a safer place for the clinical thermometer than the mouth when taking the patient's temperature. Warmth is provided by additional blankets; hot water bottles are not advisable as the patient may not feel the heat and in his desire for warmth may move the

bottle from the safe position in which it was first placed in the
bed to one of danger. Hot drinks are usually acceptable.

In the hot stage blankets are removed and a large bed cradle
covered over with a sheet will help to circulate air and cool the
skin. Warm blankets, towels, bed gowns and bed linen will be
needed in the sweating stage, during which the patient and his
bed will be soaked with sweat. A quick sponge all over with hot
water and drying with a warm towel is refreshing and comforting. The damp bedclothes should be replaced by fresh ones
as quickly as possible and the patient dressed in a clean warm
bed gown or pyjamas.

Salt and Water Balance

One of the problems of a high temperature, accompanied by
excessive sweating is that the patient may become dehydrated
and the delicate balance of water and salts in the body upset.

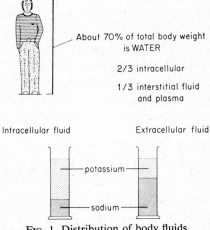

About 70% of total body weight
is WATER

2/3 intracellular

1/3 interstitial fluid
and plasma

Intracellular fluid   Extracellular fluid

—— potassium ——

—— sodium ——

FIG. 1. Distribution of body fluids.

This balance is essential to life and its mechanism needs to be
understood as it tends to be affected in all disease.

Water accounts for about 70 per cent of the total weight of
the adult human body (Fig. 1). Two-thirds of this water is

inside the cells and is referred to as the intracellular fluid. One-third, the extracellular fluid, lies outside the cells, mainly in the blood plasma and the lymph which bathes the cells. An adult weighing 70 kg contains in his body approximately 49 litres of water, of which about 31·5 litres will be intracellular and about 17·5 litres extracellular fluid. The water content of the blood is approximately 3·5 litres, weighing 3·5 kg, or about 5 per cent of the total body weight.

The body fluids contain some substances in solution, such as glucose and urea, which bear no electric charge and other substances known as electrolytes because they dissociate in water into electrically charged particles called ions. The chief positively charged ions (cations) in body fluids are sodium (Na^+), potassium (K^+), calcium (Ca^{++}) and magnesium (Mg^{++}); the chief negatively charged ions (anions) are chloride (Cl^-), bicarbonate (HCO_3^-) and phosphate (PO_4^-).

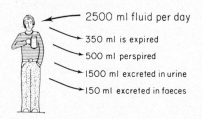

2500 ml fluid per day

350 ml is expired

500 ml perspired

1500 ml excreted in urine

150 ml excreted in faeces

FIG. 2. Passage of fluids through body tissues, variations in intake and output.

Interstitial fluid and plasma have virtually the same ionic composition, so that extracellular fluid can be considered as a whole; in it the main ions are sodium and chloride, with some bicarbonate. By contrast the intracellular fluid has a very different composition, with much less sodium and much more potassium with phosphate rather than chloride, providing most of the anions.

The normal balance of body fluids is maintained by variations of both intake and output.

Intake is normally by mouth, but intravenous, rectal or subcutaneous routes can also be used in treatment.

Output is normally by:

(1) *Kidneys:* about 1 litre per 24 hr is the minimum volume of urine which enables the kidneys to excrete the metabolic products which have accumulated in that time.

(2) *Skin:* the body loses about 500 ml of water per day by insensible perspiration, but this will be more in hot weather.

(3) *Lungs:* the body loses about 500 ml a day as water vapour in the expired air.

(4) *Faeces:* normally only a small amount is lost by this route (Fig. 2).

The normal fluid requirement of the body is thus 2 to 3 litres daily, together with 3 to 4 g of sodium chloride to replace losses of salt in urine and sweat. If normal intake is disturbed for long periods, additional substances such as potassium salts may have to be given. Normal intake of fluid and salts is deficient in conditions of great weakness, in coma, when the patient has a painful mouth or difficulty in swallowing, or if nursing care is inadequate. Although it is often necessary to remedy these deficiencies of intake by intravenous therapy, it is essential that the fluid given should not be excessive, since the body may suffer from a surfeit of water and salts as well as from a deficiency. Excessive administration of saline may lead to pulmonary oedema or congestive heart failure, and excessive administration of water (in the form of glucose solutions) may lead to mental confusion and fits.

More commonly, however, the fluid balance of the body is altered by disturbances of output rather than by deficient or excessive intake and the causes of this are as follows:

(1) Excessive urinary loss of water and salts, even when the body is deficient in these materials. This process occurs in diabetic ketosis, when the large amount of sugar in the urine leads to a diuresis, while the excreted keto-acids carry with them a base in the form of sodium ions, thus leading to a deficiency of sodium also. Other ions are also lost in excessive amounts in diabetic ketosis. An excessive renal loss of water and salts may also occur in various kidney diseases.

(2) Vomiting.

(3) Diarrhoea.

(4) Drainage from gastro-intestinal suction, or from an artificial opening such as an ileostomy.

(5) Excessive sweating in fever or hot climates.

(6) Oozing from burns or severe skin disorders.

(7) Bleeding.

The composition of the fluid lost depends on its source and for correct treatment it is necessary to know the nature of the electrolytes lost from these various sources. For example, gastro-intestinal fluid losses lead to potassium depletion and it is essential to correct this if the serum potassium is low.

Another feature of electrolytes is that they may be either acid or alkaline (basic). Cations are basic and anions are acid and together they maintain the acid-base balance of the body as indicated by a measurement called pH. On the pH scale 7·0 is neutral, a figure below 7·0 indicates acidity and above 7·0 an alkaline (basic) reaction. Apart from the stomach which is frequently acid, tissues of the body have a pH of 7·4, that is they are slightly alkaline. In persistent vomiting with loss of much hydrochloric acid from the stomach, the body fluids will tend to become more alkaline than normal (alkalosis). By contrast acidosis occurs when alkali is lost from the body through severe diarrhoea, or when acid metabolites are not excreted normally in renal failure or in diabetic ketosis.

The body maintains its acid–base balance by the kidneys where acid substances may be excreted in the urine; via the lungs which remove carbon dioxide which is carbonic acid when in solution in the plasma; and by the use of 'buffers', these are substances such as protein which resist changes in pH.

The diagnosis of a deficiency or excess of the various substances depends on a combination of clinical signs and biochemical investigation of the blood levels.

When the body is deficient in water the main features are thirst and a dry tongue. When salt is also deficient the classic signs of dehydration are found, inelastic skin, sunken eyes and, in severe degrees, a low blood pressure and rapid thready pulse.

A severe deficiency of potassium is shown by electrocardiographic changes, muscular weakness and even paralysis. An excess of potassium in the serum (which may, however, occur when there is a cellular deficiency of this ion) is dangerous in that it may cause cardiac arrhythmias and even cardiac arrest; electrocardiographic changes may be seen before the clinical signs appear.

The clinical sign of severe acidosis is overbreathing, some-times with mental confusion, while alkalosis is characterized by tetany. All these clinical features may occur only with serious alterations from the normal levels and laboratory estimations play an essential part in assessing such disorders.

Treatment of fluid and electrolyte disorders is based on:

(1) Correcting existing disturbances, using the clinical and biochemical criteria which have just been discussed together with a knowledge of the particular deficiencies resulting from various types of fluid loss.

(2) Maintaining fluid balance after the initial disturbances have been corrected. This depends on an accurate fluid balance chart (Fig. 3), on which is recorded all the sources of intake and output, the volumes of each, the type of fluids given orally or parentally, together with a daily summary showing the total balance over the preceeding 24 hr.

Also associated with abnormal distribution of fluid in the body is the condition known as oedema. In this condition there is an excessive amount of fluid in the interstitial spaces and this goes to the most dependent part of the body, i.e. ankles if standing, or sacrum if sitting, and causes swelling. Characteris-tically if the swollen area is pressed with the fingers the indentation takes some time to disappear and this 'pitting' is diagnostic of oedema.

Oedema may be caused by any mechanism which upsets the free passage of fluid through the body tissues (Fig. 2, p. 17) such as changes in blood pressure due to injury, obstruction on the venous side of the capillary loop, or of the lymphatics; or may be due to excessive ions (usually sodium) holding fluid in the interstitial spaces by altering the osmotic pressure.

The main nursing concern is that oedematous tissues tend to be deprived of adequate oxygen and nutrients and therefore very easily become damaged by pressure and are difficult to heal. A patient with oedema of the sacrum is very liable to develop pressure sores and all appropriate steps must be taken to prevent them occurring.

Blood Pressure

The blood pressure has been mentioned several times and this is a reading the nurse may be asked to make. By blood pressure

INTAKE AND OUTPUT CHART

NAME *M. D. Brown*
DATE *10-1-76* WARD *XX* CASE No _____

TIME	IN		OUT				NOTES
	ORAL	INTRAVENOUS	ASPIRATION	URINE	VOMIT	DRAINAGE	
1 a.m.	— ml (cc)	*1000 Dextrose/Saline* ml (cc)	30 ml (cc)	ml (cc)	ml (cc)	ml (cc)	Clear fluid aspirated
2 a.m.	Water 30 ml	ml	24 ml	200 ml	ml	ml	"
3 a.m.	— ml	ml	20 ml	ml	ml	ml	"
4 a.m.	— ml	ml	15 ml	ml	ml	ml	"
5 a.m.	— ml	ml	10 ml	ml	ml	ml	"
6 a.m.	Water 30 ml	ml	20 ml	250 ml	ml	ml	"
7 a.m.	ml	ml	36 ml	ml	ml	ml	"
8 a.m.	Water 30 ml	ml	30 ml	ml	ml	ml	"
9 a.m.	Water 30 ml	ml	36 ml	150 ml	ml	ml	"
10 a.m.	Water 30 ml	*1000 Dextrose 5%* ml	24 ml	ml	ml	ml	"
11 a.m.	Water 30 ml	ml	16 ml	ml	ml	ml	"
12 noon	Water 60 ml	ml	18 ml	360 ml	ml	ml	"
1 p.m.	Water 60 ml	ml	20 ml	ml	ml	ml	"
2 p.m.	Water 60 ml	ml	10 ml	ml	ml	ml	"
3 p.m.	Water 60 ml	ml	24 ml	ml	ml	ml	"
4 p.m.	Water 60 ml	ml	16 ml	500 ml	ml	ml	"
5 p.m.	Water 60 ml	ml	18 ml	ml	ml	ml	"
6 p.m.	Water 60 ml	ml	14 ml	ml	ml	ml	"
7 p.m.	Water 60 ml	*1000 Dextrose/Saline* ml	10 ml	ml	ml	ml	"
8 p.m.	Water 60 ml	ml	10 ml	160 ml	ml	ml	"
9 p.m.	Water 60 ml	ml	12 ml	ml	ml	ml	"
10 p.m.	— ml	ml	— ml	ml	ml	ml	"
11 p.m.	— ml	ml	10 ml	ml	ml	ml	Bile stained fluid
12 midn't	— ml	ml	— ml	ml	ml	ml	—
24 Hour Totals	780 ml	3000 ml	423 ml	1920 ml	ml	ml	

Na	K	Cl	HCO₃	Hb			
							TOTAL IN 3780 ml
							TOTAL OUT 2343 ml
133-142 mmol/l	3·4-5·2 mmol/l	95-105 mmol/l	22-30 mmol/l				BALANCE 1437 ml

FIG. 3. Fluid intake and output chart.

is meant the pressure of the blood on the arterial wall. This is dependent upon several factors:

(1) The force of the ventricular contraction.

(2) The volume of blood in circulation.

(3) The condition of the arterial wall.

(4) The resistance in the arterioles to the passage of the blood into the capillaries.

(5) The viscosity of the blood.

The pressure is higher when the ventricles are contracting, in the period of systole, than during the diastolic or resting phase of the cardiac cycle. The normal systolic pressure in an adult is between 110 and 130 mmHg (millimetres of mercury), that is a column of mercury will be raised to this height by the force of the blood pressure as the ventricles contract; the diastolic pressure is about 40 mmHg lower than the systolic. The apparatus used for estimating blood pressure is the sphygmomanometer; it consists of a glass manometer, containing mercury and graduated in millimetres, to this a cuff is attached by a piece of rubber tubing. The cuff is a cotton bag, in the shape of a band, inside which is an inflatable rubber bag. The cuff is fixed round the patient's upper arm and the rubber bag inflated, the pressure rises in the cuff as air is pumped in and at a certain height will obliterate the radial pulse. The operator then slowly deflates the cuff, at the same time listening with a stethoscope over the brachial artery at the bend of the elbow for the first sound of the returning pulse beat. The level of the mercury column is noted at this point; this is the systolic pressure. Further reduction of the cuff pressure to the level at which all sounds disappear gives the diastolic pressure. The difference between these two is known as the pulse pressure; for example, if the systolic pressure is 120 mmHg and the diastolic pressure is 80 mmHg then the pulse pressure is 40 mmHg.

Raised blood pressure may cause no symptoms until or unless cardiac, cerebral or renal complications ensue; sometimes it gives rise to frequent headaches. Treatment is dealt with in a later chapter.

Low blood pressure may be unrelated to obvious organic disease. It may occur in conditions of shock—when lying the patient down and raising the feet will ensure adequate cerebral circulation—or may be related to specific physiological conditions which are described later in the book.

Nutrition

One of the most important aspects of life whether in health or disease is food. Adequate nutrition is essential to health and may play a big part both in the treatment and prevention of disease. Nutrition quite simply means the supplying of nutriment or food, but only in comparatively recent years has nutrition become a scientific study. The *Manual of Nutrition* (Ministry of Agriculture, Fisheries and Food, United Kingdom) defines it as 'a science which entails the study of all the processes of growth, maintenance and repair of the living body which depend on the intake of food'. Good nutrition means the supply in adequate quantities of all the constituent foods that make up a balanced diet; proteins, carbohydrates, fats, with the mineral salts, vitamins and water which are necessary for the body fluids and the regulation of the body chemistry.

Proteins are necessary for growth and repair of tissue, for the production of enzymes and hormones and antibodies, for the plasma proteins in the blood which maintain its osmotic pressure, and to a certain extent for energy. Proteins are obtained from animal foods such as meat, fish, eggs, milk, cheese and from vegetable sources, cereals, peas and beans and nuts. Proteins from animal sources are described as 'complete' (first class) proteins, as the amino acids resulting from their oxidation supply all those necessary to the human body. The proteins of vegetables (second class) contain less of the essential amino acids for growth and repair and therefore need to be taken in larger quantities. In a mixed diet as ordinarily eaten we obtain it from both these sources. A daily intake of about 1 g of protein per kg of body weight is usually regarded as an ample allowance for the average adult but since protein is essential for growth, the proportion needs to be increased in the diet of children, pregnant and nursing women.

Carbohydrates, the starches and sugars, are the main source of heat and energy. They are also necessary for the complete oxidation of fats; in their absence fats are not completely broken down and ketone substances are produced which disturb the acid–base balance of the blood. Many of the foods in the daily diet have a high carbohydrate content, for example bread, potatoes, root vegetables, biscuits, jam, sugar and fruits.

Carbohydrates also act as 'protein sparers'; if they are taken in sufficient quantities to provide most of the energy requirements of the body, protein need not be used for this purpose. In a reducing diet carbohydrates are deliberately restricted in order that the body may burn its own tissues and the protein eaten in the food provides energy and heat. Vegetables and fruits contain a substance, cellulose, which is not digested in the human alimentary tract and therefore has no food value; it does however add bulk to the intestinal contents as 'roughage', which stimulates the intestinal muscle and helps in the elimination of faeces. In some disorders, such as peptic ulcer and ulcerative colitis, this roughage must be omitted from the diet, which should contain as little residue as possible.

Fats are needed for heat and energy and also to provide the materials for some of the essential constituents of the body, such as cholesterol, and for protective tissues such as the nerve sheaths. Good sources of fat are butter, cream, cheese, fat meat, fish liver oils and fatty fish such as herrings and salmon, vegetable oils, ground nut and palm oil, used in the manufacture of margarine and also in cooking. Fat is a very rich source of energy.

The energy value resulting from the metabolism of proteins, carbohydrates and fats is calculated in units of heat production, or joules. Until recently heat production in dietetics was calculated in 'large calories' = kilocalories (kcal). This was the amount of heat required to raise the temperature of 1000 ml of water 1°C (2°F). The new 'Système International' or SI units are the kilojoule (kJ) and the megajoule (MJ).

100 kJ = 1 MJ.
To convert kcal to kJ and MJ:
               1 kcal   = 4·2 kJ
               1000 kcal = 4200 kJ = 4·2 MJ

To calculate the energy value of food. Oxidation in the body of:
1 gram protein yields approximately 4 kcal   = 17 kJ
1 gram carbohydrate yields approximately 3·8 kcal = 16 kJ
1 gram fat yields approximately 9 kcal   = 30 kJ

Energy derived from food is needed to maintain the fundamental processes of living, breathing, circulation of the blood and maintenance of body temperature; these needs represent the body's basal metabolic requirements. Further energy has to be found for such everyday physical activities as eating, talking, moving about and maintaining body posture and still more for such activities as the muscular work involved in whatever occupation the individual follows, playing games, running, walking and other muscular efforts which our daily life demands. The joule requirements are also related to the size of the individual and the surface area of the body. Men are, on average, larger than women and therefore need a higher joule intake; children although smaller have a relatively larger surface area and their needs are greater than might be expected if size alone counted. The average daily requirements for a moderately active man are commonly said to be about 12 600 kJ or 12·6 MJ (3000 kcal), for a woman 10 080 kJ or 10·08 MJ (2400 kcal). A child of 10 years needs at least as much as an average adult woman.

Nutritive Values of Some Common Foodstuffs
Values are given for 30 g (1 oz approximately)

	Carbo-hydrate	Protein	Fat	Calories (approximate)	Joules (approximate)
Bacon, raw (average)	0·3	2·7	19·1	184	773
Barley, pearl (raw)	22·8	3·0	0·5	108	454
Bengers food	24·0	3·0	0·3	111	466
Biscuits:					
cream crackers	16·3	2·6	9·4	158	664
Ryvita	22·4	2·1	0·6	98	412
rusks	20·8	1·9	2·4	108	454
Bread:					
wholemeal	14·5	2·4	0·2	69	290
white	15·2	2·1	0·2	71	332
Butter	–	–	24·3	219	920
Cheese:					
Cheddar type	0·5	6·8	9·2	112	470
skimmed milk	1·2	5·5	0·2	29	122
Chicken (average, cooked)	–	6·0	1·4	38	160
Cocoa	7·8	2·7	5·4	91	382
Cornflakes	22·9	2·3	0·2	107	450
Cornflour	22·9	2·4	0·2	103	433
Cream (average, as purchased)	0·7	0·5	11·9	115	483

	Carbohydrate	Protein	Fat	Calories (approximate)	Joules (approximate)
Egg (average, 60 g)	–	6·6	7·0	90	378
Fish, white (steamed)	–	5·1	0·3	23	97
Flour:					
standard wholemeal	19·6	3·8	0·5	98	412
white	20·9	3·4	0·4	100	420
Ice-cream (average)	5·0	1·1	3·8	58	244
Jam	21·0	–	–	84	353
Malted milk powder	20·1	4·1	2·4	114	479
Meat, lean (average, cooked)	–	7·3	3·5	74	311
Milk:					
whole, per 30 g	1·5	1·0	1·0	19	80
skimmed	1·4	1·0	0·1	10	42
dried (whole)	11·0	7·5	8·4	150	965
dried (skimmed)	15·6	10·6	0·3	107	450
Oats, rolled or oatmeal	20·1	4·2	2·2	117	491
Orange juice, per 30 g	2·7	0·2	–	11	46
Ovaltine, or Milo	17·4	3·7	2·2	101	424
Potato (boiled)	5·6	0·4	–	23	97
Rice (uncooked)	23·7	2·3	0·1	105	441
Sugar	29·8	–	–	119	500
Syrup	22·0	–	–	88	370

Where ample food is available and the majority of people are able to buy what they like the average daily diet contains protein in the proportion of from 10 to 15 per cent of the total intake, carbohydrate 50 to 60 per cent and fat 30 to 35 per cent. These proportions depend, however, on the economic situation of the individual as well as personal tastes; protein foods such as meat, eggs and fish are expensive, while carbohydrates, bread, potatoes, sugar, are comparatively cheap. In some poor communities carbohydrate foods may form as much as 80 per cent of the daily diet (i.e. old age pensioners). In the feeding of sick people variations in the diet are often required to meet the particular circumstances; proportions may be altered, as in a low fat or a high protein diet, the joule value may have to be restricted as in a reducing diet, or raised as in thyrotoxicosis, the texture of the diet may need to be considered, as in the bland, low residue diet often ordered in gastro-intestinal disorders. In every case where a restricted diet is necessary for more than a few days it is important to see that deficiency of any essential food or accessory factor such as minerals and vitamins, does not occur. Such a situation may have to be met by supplementing the food intake, as for example by vitamin preparations, by intravenous therapy, or by adding concentrated protein to a fluid diet.

Where reference is made in the text to a high joule, low protein, or other variation in the diet, resource to the table given on page 25 will afford some guidance to the content and joule value of some of the commoner foods. A summary of the more important mineral and vitamin substances and their sources follows later in the text.

The following foods contain little or no carbohydrate and therefore need not be restricted in diets:

Vegetables	Beverages
Cabbage	Clear soup
Cauliflower	Lemon juice (unsweetened)
Celery	Meat extracts
Cucumber	Soda water
Lettuce	Tea and coffee without milk or sugar
Mushrooms	
Mustard and cress	
Spinach	
Watercress	

More protein can be supplied without greatly increasing either the fat content of the diet or its bulk by adding dried skimmed milk; this can be added to other foods such as milk drinks, puddings or cereals. Complan, a proprietary preparation containing predigested protein, is also useful where a high protein diet is needed or if the diet is restricted to fluids. One pound (453 g) of Complan powder mixed with water only will provide 140 g of protein, 200 g of carbohydrate, 74 g of fat and all necessary vitamins and mineral salts. This quantity of Complan gives 8400 kJ (2000 kcal).

Mineral, or inorganic, elements are present in almost all of the foods that we usually eat, or are supplied, as in the case of sodium and chloride, by the addition of salt in cooking or at the table. The most important minerals are calcium, phosphorus, sodium, potassium, iron, copper and iodine.

(1) Calcium is required for growth of bones and teeth, for normal muscle function and is also one of the factors in the clotting process which arrests bleeding. The average daily requirement for an adult is 1 g; more is required during the growth period and during pregnancy and lactation and it is usually accepted that 1·5 g will meet these additional needs satisfactorily. Milk and milk products, cheese and dried milk are the richest sources of calcium, although flour and bread contain considerable amounts and also some vegetables, such as cabbage and turnips. In Britain calcium carbonate is added by Regulation to all flour except wholemeal. Calcium eaten in the food may not be available to the body unless vitamin D in sufficient amounts is also present.

(2) Phosphorus is required with calcium for bones and teeth and also for the normal functioning of all types of tissue cells. It is present in all the foods which contain calcium.

(3) Sodium is a constituent of tissue cells and body fluids. It is present in many ordinary foods including meat. In the form of common salt or sodium chloride it is almost universally added to food for flavouring so that serious shortage seldom happens. A daily intake of 5 g is a liberal allowance, but in hot climates excessive amounts may be lost by sweating and extra salt is needed.

(4) Potassium is an essential constituent of tissue cells and is unlikely to be deficient in any average diet. It is present in most common foods such as meat, fish, milk and eggs.

(5) Iron is a constituent of the red blood cells, and between 10 and 15 mg represents the average daily requirement. The body is very economical in its use of iron because, although red blood cells are constantly being destroyed and renewed, much of it is salvaged from the break-up of red cells and used again. If, however, so little iron is eaten in the daily food that the small loss is not replaced, anaemia eventually results. Good sources of iron are meat, especially liver, wholemeal bread, eggs and vegetables, such as green peas and cabbage.

(6) Copper is needed for the formation of haemoglobin, but only in very small quantities, and if the diet is sufficient in other respects there will be no lack of copper.

(7) Iodine is needed for the manufacture of thyroxine by the thyroid gland; again only very small amounts are needed and are commonly supplied by fish and other sea foods and vegetables. Where the soil in which vegetables are grown is known to be deficient in iodine and sea fish is not often eaten, iodine must be supplemented in the diet, usually by supplying iodized table salt.

Vitamins are substances which are essential for life and health, which the body is unable, in whole or in part, to manufacture itself and must obtain from the daily food intake. This fact was not realized until the beginning of this century when research into problems of nutrition first showed that a diet which was adequate in calorie value and in protein, fat and carbohydrate did not necessarily supply these accessory factors. Since the early work on vitamins and their functions, research has continued and more and more of these factors controlling body chemistry have been identified, although the exact role of some of these substances is still obscure.

Some vitamins are found in fatty foods and are classed as fat-soluble vitamins; these are vitamins A, D, E and K. Others form the water-soluble group, which includes the many substances of the vitamin B complex and vitamin C.

Vitamin A is needed for growth and for the protection of surface tissues and certain parts of the eye. It is present in animal tissues such as liver, cod- and halibut-liver oils, butter and cheese. In a partly formed state, carotene, it is found in the orange pigment of such vegetables as carrots, tomatoes and dried apricots. Vitamin A or carotene is also added to margarine. The human body is able to form vitamin A from vegetable carotene, but needs greater amounts of this substance than of pure vitamin A; 5000 units, some of which may be taken in the form of carotene, represent the average daily requirement, 6000 during the later months of pregnancy and 8000 during lactation.

Vitamin B complex includes B_1, thiamine or aneurine, B_2, riboflavine, nicotinic acid and B_{12} or cyanocobalamin, folic acid and a number of other substances, pyroxidine, biotin and pantothenic acid. There is not at present any evidence that human beings may suffer from deficiency of the last two substances in this group. Although the various components of the vitamin B complex are not related chemically, they are grouped together because they are all found in the same types of food, meat, liver, eggs, whole grain cereals. Brewer's yeast is a rich source of all these vitamins.

Thiamine is necessary for the proper use of the products of carbohydrate metabolism, riboflavine and nicotinic acid are also concerned in the processes of utilizing food for the provision of energy. Folic acid and cyanocobalamin prevent the development of certain types of anaemia and assist metabolism; cyanocobalamin is also necessary for the preservation of the health of nerve cells. As little as 1 to 2 mg of thiamine and riboflavine and 10 to 15 mg of nicotinic acid meet the daily requirements.

Vitamin C or ascorbic acid, occurs almost entirely in vegetable foods and is easily destroyed by the process of cooking, therefore in certain circumstances, where no fresh vegetables or raw fruits are eaten, deficiency can readily happen. It is necessary for normal growth of teeth and bones and for the material which holds the cells together, such as the 'cement' in the walls of the capillary blood-vessels. Good sources of vitamin C are citrus fruits, blackcurrants, green vegetables, and potatoes, especially when new. Daily requirements are estimated as being from 20 to 50 mg, the largest amounts being needed by women during pregnancy and lactation.

Vitamin D regulates the metabolism of calcium and phosphorus which are essential for the growth of bone and teeth and for the repair of bone; it is therefore particularly needed during the growth period of life and in the diet during pregnancy and lactation. The main dietary sources of vitamin D are milk, butter, fats including margarine to which vitamin D (calciferol) has been added, fish and fish-liver oils such as halibut- and cod-liver oils. The amount of this vitamin needed by adults is small, but during the later half of pregnancy 600 international units is the recommended daily allowance, 800 during lactation, and 400 for children and adolescents. Vitamin D can be produced by the body if the skin is exposed to sunlight, and the need for vitamin D in the food is then reduced.

Vitamin E has been found experimentally to influence fertility in rats, but there is little evidence that it plays any such part in human beings. It is found in milk, wheat germ and green vegetables.

Vitamin K is an essential factor in the normal clotting of blood and is found in many green vegetables. The presence of bile in the small intestine is necessary for the absorption of vitamin K, and therefore, in cases of obstructive jaundice lack of bile and consequent lack of available vitamin K delays the clotting of blood. In the normal individual lack of vitamin K is a very unlikely event.

Some vitamins can be built up in the intestinal canal by the action of the normal bacterial flora in quantities sufficient to have some importance. This is particularly true in the case of vitamin K, nicotinic acid, riboflavine and cyanocobalamin. The giving of antibiotics may sterilize the intestine to such an extent that this synthesis of vitamins within the body ceases and leads to deficiency. On the other hand, in some circumstances, the presence of abnormal bacteria may lead to destruction of vitamins in the intestine and in such cases antibiotics may be given with good effect.

However it is not enough to provide all the correct foodstuffs and vitamins if the presentation of the meal is poor. Sick people more than most need to be tempted to eat and a skilful nurse will use all means in her power to make a meal attractive when serving it, ensuring adequate and clean cutlery and china; hot foods served hot and vice versa; small portions with the possibility of second helpings rather than a large amount which may discourage the patient and most of all an atmosphere of calm so that the patient does not feel hurried.

Occupation

Although rest is an essential requirement for the sick person it is important to realize that the normal person's day contains some form of meaningful activity. Most patients once they begin to feel better occupy themselves with knitting, reading, card-playing or other activities. However some may need stimulation by the nurse in order to recommence these pursuits and in the case of prolonged hospitalization the occupational therapist should be contacted in order to provide some form of diversional therapy or possibly to allow the patient to develop a skill which may assist in his rehabilitation.

Sleep

Finally sleep, this is often disturbed in illness and once again much can be done by a thoughtful nurse to ensure that the patient has adequate sleep. Position, number of pillows, weight of bedclothes, warmth of room, amount of air circulating, lack of noise, shaded lights if essential, the provision of a warm drink are all elementary factors which may hinder or aid sleep. Anxiety is one of the commonest causes of sleeplessness and the nurse should be prepared to talk to the sleepless patient and in this way may be able to identify his fears and possibly relieve them.

2
Infection

THIS chapter deals with the nature of infection, its prevention and control, including the use of vaccines, sera and chemotherapeutic drugs, the general signs and symptoms of infection and the general nursing care of the febrile patient. In a later chapter the commoner infectious diseases and their treatment are discussed.

'Infection' is the term used to describe the invasion of the body by pathogenic, i.e. disease-producing bacteria, viruses and protozoa. Infection is not synonymous with disease, since conditions may not be suitable for the infecting organisms or they may not invade in sufficient numbers and be rapidly overcome by the body's defences with no ill-effects of the host. In some cases the invasion is unsuccessful because the individual has had a previous attack and in the process of overcoming this has produced antibodies in sufficient quantities to prevent a second attack from developing, in other words the individual is now immune. Strictly speaking, any disease which is caused by micro-organisms is infectious, since the infecting agent can be transmitted to another person. In a number of such conditions, however, the infectivity is of a very low order and widespread outbreaks are unlikely. The term 'infective' is used to describe those diseases which are not readily communicable or contagious. The diseases commonly referred to as 'the specific fevers' or 'infectious diseases' are those communicable diseases which are readily transmitted from person to person and can cause epidemics. Well-known examples of these are the illnesses usually encountered in childhood such as measles, whooping cough and chickenpox; influenza is another example of a highly infectious illness.

How infection is spread. The mode of spread will depend upon the site of the infection; if for example it is in the upper air passages the pathogenic organisms are likely to be expelled into the surrounding air in droplets of moisture from the patient's mouth when he breathes, and still more when he coughs. If the intestine is the site of the infection as in typhoid fever or dysentery, then it will be spread by contamination from faecal matter. The reservoir of infection is usually a human or animal host, but some organisms can live for a considerable period outside living tissues, and therefore dissemination by dust or by infected articles such as clothes is possible, while other organisms cannot survive for more than a few hours.

Prevention of spread of infection. Many diseases which we now tend to consider as tropical, or possibly confined to under-developed countries where the living conditions are in general of a low standard, were prevalent in this country not so long ago, for example cholera, typhoid fever and typhus fever. The fact that these are now rare diseases is in large measure due to the improvement in living conditions and to the control exercised by the health authorities, the Department of Health and Social Security, and Local Health Authorities, over such matters as sewage disposal, purification of water, and the production and sale of milk and other foods. Decrease in epidemic diseases also goes hand-in-hand with slum clearance, since overcrowding and poor sanitation are associated with the spread of many diseases. While it certainly cannot be said that in both town and country the position with regard to enviromental hygiene is completely satisfactory, great improvements have been and are being carried out.

This century has seen advances in medical knowledge which have brought many diseases under control by giving individual protection by means of vaccination or inoculation. As a result of massive worldwide vaccination programmes, smallpox has almost been eradicated and other diseases such as diphtheria are now rare in the United Kingdom although they still occur elsewhere. However as long as a disease exists anywhere in the world it remains a potential hazard to non-immunized persons in the population. Immunization is not compulsory and is largely a matter of health education, as indeed are most preventive measures, for without individual co-operation no health programme can command complete success. Few members of the community have better opportunities than the health visitor, the community nurse and the midwife for health teaching in the home, and, in the world of commerce and industry, health teaching is recognized as part of the occupational health nurse's responsibilities. It is perhaps not always appreciated that the nurse in hospital has a golden opportunity for such teaching at a time when patients or their relatives are likely to be particularly receptive.

Control of Infection

Most infectious diseases are notifiable to the Medical Officer of Health of the Local Health Authority. One of the main reasons for this requirement is that immediate steps can be taken to investigate the source of the infection and to trace persons who have been in contact with patients. Prompt action in tracing and immunizing contacts, will limit the infection and an epidemic may be avoided. Equally important in some instances, notably intestinal infections and diphtheria, is the search for carriers of the disease, i.e. persons who have at some time been infected but have not developed symptoms of the disease, or who have had the disease and recovered from it. In both cases such persons may continue to harbour the infecting organisms in the intestinal tract, or in the throat or nose in the case of diphtheria organisms, and are therefore potential sources of infection.

Isolation of those persons who have already contracted the disease is an obvious precaution. Quarantine, i.e. segregating susceptible contacts from persons who have not had the infection for a period slightly longer than the usual incubation period (the time elapsing between exposure to infection and the appearance of the first symptoms) for the disease, was at one time widely practised. While it may still be a necessary precaution in some serious infections strict enforcement of quarantine is not now regarded as of great importance in many infectious diseases, and 'surveillance', or keeping contacts under observation, is a more usual practice.

The discovery of substances able to counteract the activities of pathogenic organisms or to prevent their multiplication, first in the form of antitoxic or antibacterial sera and later the chemotherapeutic drugs, provided specific remedies for many infectious diseases, which by reducing the period of illness also lessen the period of infectivity.

Immunity and Immunization

The fact that some individuals, although exposed to infection do not develop the disease because they already possess effective

antibodies has already been mentioned. Such immunity may be
inherited as part of the genetic pattern of the species, race or
family, or it may be acquired as the result of the production of
antibodies, immunoglobulins, during a previous attack. The
other way in which immunity can be acquired is by deliberately
provoking the production of antibodies. The principle that
small doses of organisms, or their products, could stimulate the
body tissues to produce the specific antibodies and could be
used without danger provided that they were first made harmless, or relatively harmless, was established by Edward Jenner
who introduced vaccination against smallpox at the end of the
eighteenth century. As knowledge of the nature of infectious
disease grew and bacteriologists were able to demonstrate the
causal organism in some, though not all, infections, so immunization against typhoid fever, diphtheria and more recently
whooping cough, tuberculosis and poliomyelitis has come to
play a major role in controlling these diseases.

Vaccines

A vaccine is prepared from dead organisms, living organisms
which have been altered to reduce their virulence (attenuated),
or from the toxins which the bacteria produce. A toxin which
has been treated in such a way as to make it safe to use for this
purpose is known as a toxoid.

Smallpox vaccination is carried out by inoculating the skin
with material, referred to as 'lymph' although it is in fact the
fluid from a vesicle, which contains vaccinia virus and produces
a local lesion. The lymph is obtained from healthy calves whose
skin has been inoculated with vaccinia virus, which is similar
to smallpox virus. The passage of the virus from a human to an
animal host and back again to the human, attenuates the virus,
so that it has a low virulence but still has the power to provoke
the production of antibodies in the human host.

Vaccination depends on circumstances, but it may be noted
that travellers to some countries are required to hold an
International Certificate of Vaccination and that such a certificate is valid for only 3 years from the date of issue.

Diphtheria immunization is carried out with diphtheria toxoid
and the three injections are given at intervals of one month,
usually starting about the age of 6 months; for the first few
months of life the infant is protected by antibodies obtained

from his mother. A 'booster' dose should be given when the child reaches school age.

Combined immunization is now a common practice: the infant receives protective doses of pertussis (whooping cough) vaccine, tetanus toxoid with diphtheria toxoid.

Tuberculosis immunization with the bacillus Calmette-Guérin (BCG), is used as a means of protecting those persons who are likely to be at considerable risk of tuberculous infection, such as children with parents suffering from tuberculosis. Nurses, doctors, medical students and other persons likely to come in close contact with active cases of tuberculosis are immunized if necessary following a tuberculin (Mantoux or Héaf) test. A positive reaction is evidence that the individual already possesses a degree of immunity to tuberculosis; negative reactors are regarded as susceptible to the infection and are offered immunization.

Poliomyelitis immunization has resulted in the control of a very serious epidemic disease. The first type of vaccine used was the Salk vaccine prepared from killed poliomyelitis vaccine. More recently the Sabin oral vaccine, containing live but attenuated virus, has been widely adopted. It is given in three successive doses at 4 to 6 weeks interval, the dosage being 3 drops of the vaccine on a lump of sugar or, in the case of infants, dropped into the back of the mouth.

Measles immunization has been available since 1968 using a live attenuated vaccine which is given at 12 to 15 months of age. A live attenuated vaccine against German measles (rubella) is also used. The value of this is to immunize young married women who have not had the disease to reduce the risk of them contracting it while pregnant, when it may result in a deformed child.

Antitoxic and Antiviral Sera

Antitoxic and antiviral sera can be considered as a gift of additional antibodies to patients already ill as a result of infection, or as a means of affording a temporary protection to particularly susceptible persons who have been exposed to infection. The immunity conferred is passive; it is not the result of a stimulation of the patient's own antibody production, which is the aim of an immunizing vaccine.

Antitoxic serum is obtained from an animal, usually the

horse, which has been given increasingly large doses of a specific organism and in consequence has developed large quantities of antitoxin in its blood. The blood serum, obtained by bleeding the animal, is prepared for injection and standardized in units. Two infections in which large doses of the specific antitoxin are life-saving measures are tetanus and diphtheria.

Antiviral serum, obtained from human blood, can be used to give temporary protection where the individual exposed to the infection is at special risk. The antibodies, globulins, are obtained from the blood plasma of a convalescent who has had a recent attack of the particular disease or from pooled human plasma.

Examples of the use of human globulins are:

(1) To protect a debilitated or sick infant known to have been exposed to measles infection and whose life might be endangered by this disease.

(2) To protect a woman in the first 3 months of pregnancy who has not had rubella (German measles) and is exposed to this infection. In such patients this mild disease can cause abnormalities of fetal development.

(3) To give short-lived passive immunity to poliomyelitis. Active immunity acquired by vaccination is, of course, the type of protection universally used, but there may be occasional special instances where passive immunity is of value.

Since sensitivity to foreign protein is readily produced in some individuals it is essential to ask about any previous injections of sera and their effect before giving a large dose of antitoxic horse serum. An additional precaution is the administration of a test dose before giving the full dose. Desensitization can be carried out by giving the dose in fractions, beginning with a small dose, at 30-min intervals.

An immediate reaction to the injection of foreign protein is known as anaphylactic shock and is shown by pallor, dyspnoea and collapse. The treatment of this condition is the intramuscular injection of adrenaline (epinephrine) 0·5 to 1 ml of a 1 : 1000 solution, which should always be ready for immediate injection when antitoxic serum is being given. Serum sickness is a condition that sometimes develops about 7 to 10 days after the serum injection. The patient has a rise of temperature, joint pains and an urticarial rash. These symptoms usually subside in a few days, but meanwhile discomfort can be relieved by aspirin for the pain and applications of calamine lotion, or sodium bicarbonate solution to the irritating rash, which, however, generally responds quickly to the administration of an antihistamine drug, such as promethazine (Phenergan) or diphenhydramine (Benadryl).

Chemotherapy

Chemotherapy is the term used to describe the oral or parenteral, i.e. hypodermic, intramuscular or intravenous, administration of chemical substances which will destroy pathogenic organisms or inhibit their growth with the minimum of harm to the living tissues of the host. The administration of organic arsenical compounds as the first really effective treatment for syphilis, and the use of quinine to control malaria infection, are examples of early successes in chemotherapy.

The spectacular advances in this form of treatment, however, began in Germany in 1935 with the discovery of the first sulphonamide preparation, Prontosil, and received a still greater impetus when the first antibiotic, penicillin, was produced in this country in 1940. In 1928 Professor Fleming had observed the destructive effect of a mould *Penicillium notatum* which had accidentally contaminated a culture plate inoculated with staphylococci. The subsequent work of extracting and concentrating penicillin from this mould was carried out by Professor Florey and his team in Oxford. In 1944 streptomycin was discovered in the United States and first used for the treatment of tuberculosis. These two discoveries led to the introduction of a wide range of antibiotics.

The chemotherapeutic group of drugs also includes para-aminosalicylic acid (PAS) and isoniazid (isonicotinic acid hydrazide), both widely used in the treatment of tuberculosis (see p. 65), and sulphone compounds, of which dapsone is an example, used in the treatment of leprosy.

The Sulphonamides

The sulphonamide preparations are bacteriostatic and are effective against streptococci, meningococci, pneumococci, and *Escherichia* (*Bacterium*) *coli*. They are considered the best therapeutic agents in meningococcal infections and urinary tract infections due to *Escherichia coli*. In many other infections they have been replaced by antibiotics, although they may be used if the particular strain of the micro-organism has proved resistant to antibiotics, or in combination with antibiotics. The sulphonamides have the disadvantage of producing toxic side-effects, some of them serious; these include haematuria and anuria, resulting from the deposition in the kidney of an insoluble crystalline substance, and blood changes, anaemia and leucopenia, from the effect of the drug on the bone marrow. Drug sensitivity is another danger and there is evidence that this is particularly likely to happen if sulphonamides are used as local applications; they are now seldom used for this purpose. Other less serious, although unpleasant, side-effects are depression, nausea, vomiting and headache. However, measures can be taken to prevent these complications. All patients taking sulphonamides should drink at least 3 litres (5 pints) of fluid daily, and since the deposit of crystalline products in the kidneys is less likely if the urine is made alkaline, sodium bicarbonate is given for this purpose. An accurate fluid intake and output record should be kept, and the urine should be tested daily for the reaction and presence of red blood cells. Careful observation of the patient's condition and the immediate reporting of such symptoms as a rise in temperature, the appearance of a rash, nausea and vomiting, will enable an early decision to be made on the advisability of discontinuing the treatment. A daily blood count may be required. Sulphonamides also tend to produce drug-resistant strains of organisms. They are also inhibited by the presence of pus so are only used if a suppurating lesion is draining freely.

Treatment with the sulphonamides is not usually continued for longer than one week. The adult initial dose is from 2 to 4 g with a maintenance dose of from 4 to 6 g in 24 hr. Some preparations are more slowly excreted than others and therefore a smaller dose may be given. Sulphadiazine, sulphamerazine, sulphadimidine and sulphafurazole are examples of sulphonamides that are readily absorbed from the intestinal tract into the bloodstream and other body fluids. Trisulphonamide, containing sulphadiazine, sulphamerazine and sulphathiazole, may be prescribed, because it is held that a combination of these drugs is less toxic than the single drug. Sulphonamides which are not readily absorbed from the intestinal tract may be used in the treatment of enteritis and bacillary dysentery; examples of these are phthalylsulphathiazole (Thalazole) and sulpha-guanidine.

Co-trimoxazole (Bactrim or Septrin) has a wider spectrum than sulphonamides alone and is bacteriocidal. It is given by mouth and is effective in many acute urinary and respiratory infections.

The Nitrofurans

The nitrofuran compounds are effective against a wide range of both Gram-positive and Gram-negative organisms. They may be prescribed in cases where the infecting organism has proved resistant to other chemotherapeutic agents, but their use is restricted by their liability to produce side effects such as nausea, vomiting and skin reactions.

An example of this group is nitrofurantoin (Furadantin) which is excreted in the urine and therefore effective in the treatment of urinary infections which have not responded to treatment by sulphonamides or antibiotics. It may be given in the following dosage: 50 to 100 mg, three times a day, in tablet form, in a suspension (25 mg in 2·5 ml), or by injection. Cases of megaloblastic anaemia and peripheral nerve damage have been reported following the administration of nitrofurantoin and therefore it is only given to patients who can be under close medical supervision.

Antibiotics

The antibiotics are substances either derived from living organisms or produced synthetically which are bacteriocidal. As has already been mentioned, the first of this now very large group was penicillin, derived from the mould *Penicillium notatum*. This was followed by streptomycin, chloramphenicol, and the tetracyclines. These were first produced from organisms in soil, but chloramphenicol and others have been successfully synthesized.

Penicillin. Forms of penicillin commonly in use are:
(1) Benzyl penicillin or penicillin G is a crystalline, readily soluble form which is quickly absorbed when given by intramuscular injection.
(2) Procaine penicillin is a preparation of benzyl penicillin and procaine which is insoluble and therefore slowly absorbed, so that the effect of the injection is prolonged.

(3) Phenoxymethylpenicillin (penicillin V), phenethicillin (Broxil) and other forms of penicillin are preparations suitable for oral administration as they are not inactivated by the acid gastric juice.

(4) Methicillin (Celbenin) and cloxacillin (Orbenin) are synthetic preparations, which are active against penicillin-resistant strains, since they are not broken down by the enzyme penicillase which destroys other forms of penicillin.

(5) Ampicillin (Penbritin) is active against Gram-negative bacilli, such as the *Shigella* group, *Salmonella* and *Escherichia coli* infections. Ampicillin can be given by mouth in capsule form, or by parenteral injection.

Cephalosporins are a group of penicillin-like antibiotics with a similar action to ampicillin and are active against Gram-positive cocci and Gram-negative bacilli. An example of this group is cephaloridine which is given by intramuscular injection.

New forms of broad spectrum penicillin-like antibiotics are constantly being added to this list. Preparations (1) and (2) are frequently given together, the first for quick action and the second to carry on the effect so that injections need only be given every 12 hr instead of every 3 hr.

Although penicillin in its various forms is effective against a number of common organisms, including streptococci, staphylococci, pneumococci and gonococci, and in the majority of patients produces no untoward reactions, there has been a progressive development of penicillin-resistant strains, particularly of the *Staphylococcus aureus*. Furthermore some persons readily become sensitive to penicillin, and allergic reactions, such as urticaria or even anaphylactic shock, can occur in such individuals. Therefore penicillin, or indeed any antibiotic, should not be given indiscriminately for every minor infection.

In order to maintain the required level of penicillin in the blood, substances which hinder its excretion may be given at the same time; an example of these substances is probenecid (Benemid).

Streptomycin comes from a mould *Streptomyces griseus*. Its influence on bacteria was first discovered by Waksman in America in 1943. At first it was in limited supply in this country and its use was reserved solely for cases of miliary tuberculosis and tuberculosus meningitis, two diseases that were invariably fatal before the discovery of streptomycin.

The introduction of streptomycin has greatly improved the outlook in all its forms of tuberculosis, but it has one main disadvantage in that it produces drug-resistant strains of *Mycobacterium tuberculosis*. The discovery of two drugs, para-aminosalicylic acid and isoniazid, which are also used in the treatment of tuberculosis, has helped to reduce this tendency when they are used in combination with streptomycin.

Tetracyclines comprise a group of antibiotics, derived from types of *Streptomyces*, which are bacteriostatic against a wide range of micro-organisms and are therefore known as broad spectrum antibiotics. They have the advantage of being effective when given by mouth. The tetracyclines are: (1) chlortetracycline (Aureomycin), (2) tetracycline (Achromycin), (3) oxytetracycline (Terramycin), and (4) demthychlortetracycline (Ledermycin).

Tetracyclines are very similar in their chemistry and in their effects, being useful against Gram-negative and Gram-positive organisms, a few viruses and also the rickettsiae which cause typhus fever. They may all give rise to resistant strains of these organisms and they are all liable to produce such side-effects as nausea, vomiting and intestinal upsets; diarrhoea so produced may in turn be associated with acute pruritus ani. Special care is necessary to prevent 'thrush' and other fungal infections of the mouth. Acid mouthwashes, acid drinks and acid drops to suck are used freely during the treatment (which usually lasts 5 days); these provoke a free flow of saliva, the natural mouth-wash, erythromycin or spiromycin may be used to treat enteritis if it occurs and nystatin for the mouth condition. A vitamin B preparation and Empac, a preparation containing *Lactobaccillus acidophilus*, may be ordered.

Chloramphenicol, also known as Chloromycetin, was originally derived from *Streptomyces venezuelae*, but is now prepared synthetically. It is especially effective in the treatment of typhoid and paratyphoid fever and of meningitis caused by *Haemophilus influenzae*. Like the tetracyclines it is given by mouth. Its use is restricted because of its liability to produce a toxic effect on the bone marrow with resulting aplastic anaemia.

Erythromycin, lincomycin and clindamycin are a narrow group of antibiotics derived from a type of streptomyces. They are given orally and are effective against Gram-positive organisms.

Non-Absorbable Antibiotics

Under this classification are grouped a number of antibiotics which are either non-absorbable or only slightly absorbed from the alimentary tract when given by mouth. Examples of these are neomycin, paramomycin and colistin. They are prescribed in the treatment of certain intestinal infections, e.g. amoebic dysentery, and prior to operations on the intestines in order to reduce the number of intestinal micro-organisms. It may also be used as ear or eye drops.

Nystatin, also derived from streptomyces, is used as a local application for fungal infections of the skin and mucous surfaces.

Griseofulvin (Fulcin) is a fungicide and is given by mouth in the treatment of ringworm.

Cycloserine and **viomycin** are antibiotics effective against strains of *Mycobacterium tuberculosis* which are resistant to streptomycin.

Polymixins are derived from cultures of *Bacillus polymyax*. Polymixin B and E are the only members of this group used in medical practice. Polymixin B is effective against infections due to *Pseudomonas pyocyanea*. Both B and E can have injurious effects on the kidneys.

The range of antibiotic drugs is constantly increasing, and there seems little doubt that the immense amount of research now being carried out in this field will continue to produce drugs with a wide range of effectiveness and having low toxicity.

3
Disorders of the respiratory system

THE main features of disorders of the respiratory system are cough, sputum, pain in the chest and alterations in the rate and type of respiration. Some of these manifestations are, however, not confined to respiratory disease; pain in the chest may be a symptom of cardiac disease and disturbances of respiration are seen in diseases primarily affecting other body functions.

The following terms are used to describe various types of respiration:

Dyspnoea, difficulty in breathing.

Orthopnoea, inability to breathe comfortably except in the upright position.

Hyperpnoea, deep and quickened breathing.

Apnoea, temporary cessation of breathing.

Shallow breathing occurs when the breathing movements cause pain, as for example in pleurisy or fracture of the ribs. It may also be caused by cerebral depression and is one of the effects of large doses of morphine when the rate is also reduced.

Acidotic, deep sighing breathing may be seen in diabetic coma and in uraemia.

Cheyne–Stokes breathing shows characteristic alternation of periods of quick deep breathing followed by decreasing depth and rate and a period of apnoea before the cycle begins again. It may be noted particularly at night in patients with long-standing cardiovascular or renal disease.

Obstructed breathing may be due to lack of tone of the tongue and palate muscles in an unconscious patient and is then often stertorous. Retained secretions produce a rattling sound in pharynx or trachea. The harsh sound heard when air is inspired through a partly closed larynx is known as stridor. Obstruction may be due to a number of causes and occur at any level of the respiratory tract. When it happens, movement of the accessory muscles of respiration in the shoulders and neck can be seen, and also movements of the alae nasi. The lower chest wall may be sucked in instead of expanding with respiration. It is essential to remove the cause of the obstruction whatever it may be.

Cough

Coughing is a reflex action resulting from stimulation of the vagus nerve branches in the respiratory passages, pleura or stomach; it is brought about by a spasmodic expiration in which the abdominal and chest muscles contract and force the closed glotti to open.

The object of the cough is to expel an irritant, such as excess mucus, from the air passages. The cough is said to be 'productive' when sputum is expectorated as a result of the effort, and 'non-productive' when there is no sputum. A non-productive cough is often persistent and exhausting.

Sputum

Sputum consists of the secretion from the mucous membrane of the respiratory tract combined with epithelial cells, foreign bodies such as dust or soot and micro-organisms. The actual cause of its production is usually a foreign body of some kind, around which mucus becomes deposited. Bacteria may be the exciting cause, or they may infect the material produced by other irritants.

Note should be made of the type and amount of sputum expectorated, and of the effort required to produce it.

Sputum is classified according to its appearance:

Mucoid sputum. The sputum is clear and slightly sticky, as is seen in the early stages of respiratory catarrh.

Muco-purulent sputum. The sputum is a mixture of mucus and pus.

Purulent sputum. The sputum consists mainly of pus, and occurs in lung abscess and bronchiectasis.

Frothy sputum, which may be blood-tinged, occurs in acute pulmonary oedema.

Sputum containing blood. The sputum may be:

(1) Streaked only, in some cases the blood is from the larynx, pharynx or mouth, and it may come from the lungs.

(2) The rusty sputum of pneumonia, containing altered blood.

(3) Diffusely red sputum, true haemoptysis. Blood which is

coughed up is bright red in colour due to the oxygen in it and tends to be frothy unless it is in very large quantities, which is rare.

The commonest causes of haemoptysis are:

Pulmonary tuberculosis.

Carcinoma of the lung.

Pulmonary infarction (embolism).

Pulmonary congestion from disease of the mitral valve of the heart.

Bronchiectasis.

To obtain a specimen of sputum for pathological investigation. It is best to get the patient to cough the sputum into a specially sterilized and correctly labelled container on waking, when it is likely that the sputum will have accumulated. It should be collected before taking food, and no antiseptic mouthwash should have been given for some hours beforehand. No antiseptic should be added, but a little sterile water keeps the sputum moist. The container is then sent to the laboratory.

Hygiene in Relation to Diseases of the Respiratory System

Sputum and expired air (which contains droplets of moisture) are liable to be infected by micro-organisms. Sputum should on no account be allowed to contaminate the fingers. Containers made of cardboard may be used, or metal containers with a cardboard lining, the whole cardboard container should be burnt.

The nurse should always avoid inhaling the breath of a patient and should be especially careful not to do so if he is coughing, as the micro-organisms are forcibly expelled in fine droplets of moisture with exhaled air. It is safest to stand rather behind the patient than directly in front of him and should nursing duties, e.g. lifting, demand a closer contact, it is nearly always possible to hold the breath for the short time needed. In very virulent infections a mask should be worn.

Good ventilation lessens the risks to the nurse and to other persons in the vicinity of the patient. Adequate air and floor space is of first importance.

Experiments have proved that cross-infection can occur in hospital wards from the pollution of the air with infected particles during the activities of bed-making and sweeping. Such infection is especially dangerous to open wounds, and is also a possible source of spread of respiratory diseases. Various practices have been introduced to reduce the dust content of the air, as for example special treatment of the ward floor with oil and the use of vacuum suction in place of sweeping. Cotton cellular blankets are now often used in place of woollen ones, mainly because they can be frequently laundered without damage and they also have the advantage of being less fluffy. Bed-making should always be done quietly without shaking and flapping the bedclothes; brushing mattresses in the ward should not be permitted.

The use of paper handkerchiefs which can be burnt should be encouraged. If linen handkerchiefs are used they must be disinfected before being laundered and should be kept in a paper bag which can be burnt.

The nurse must always wash her hands if there has been any possible contamination before attending other patients and always before going to her own meals.

Feeding utensils should be kept separately for the use of the infected person, and this also applies to articles used for the patient's toilet and for cleaning the mouth.

Investigations Used in Respiratory Diseases

Respiratory Function Tests

Vital capacity: this is estimated by measuring the amount of air that the patient expires into a container linked to a scale, following a full inspiration.

Blood tests carried out on arterial blood measure: normal oxygen saturation of the blood is 97, normal carbon dioxide tension is 40 mmHg; pH normal, 7·4.

Bacteriological Tests

Sputum and pleural fluid: in both cases malignant cells may also be sought.

Tuberculin Tests

Mantoux and Héaf tests: in both cases a small amount of old Tuberculin (0·1 ml in 1 : 10 000 dilution) is given intradermally. The result is positive if a raised area of inflammatory oedema occurs after 2 to 4 days.

Laryngoscopy

Indirect: the larynx can be seen by use of a small mirror placed in the back of the mouth. Direct: a laryngoscope with a light is passed into the larynx; the patient is anaesthetized.

Bronchoscopy

A similar tube with a light in is passed into the bronchus. This can be carried out under a general or local anaesthetic.

Thoracoscopy

A telescopic type instrument is inserted through an intercostal space into the pleural cavity which has been distended with a small amount of air. In all these endoscopies it is possible to take a biopsy as well as to inspect the area.

Radiography

Plain X-ray of the chest.

Screening, which demonstrates the position and function of the diaphragm.

Tomography, to illustrate the depth of cavities in lung tissue.

Bronchogram.

RESPIRATORY TRACT INFECTIONS

The Common Cold—Acute Tracheobronchitis

Respiratory tract infections are extremely common and are particularly prevalent in the winter months. The mildest infection is the common cold, which is probably a virus infection causing inflammation of the mucous membrane of the nose and pharynx. The general symptoms are headache, malaise, sometimes generalized aches and pains and a mild degree of fever.

Spread of infection and more severe symptoms are usually due to secondary bacterial or viral invaders and the bacteria are often found to be normal inhabitants of the nose and mouth which do not, however, attack healthy mucous membranes. The inflammation may then involve the accessory nasal sinuses, causing acute sinusitis and the whole of the respiratory tract, with laryngitis, tracheitis and bronchitis. The symptoms of a more severe infection include local pain if the nasal sinuses are infected, hoarseness, pain on swallowing and in the chest, persistent cough, which is at first dry and later produces mucoid and mucopurulent sputum. The temperature is raised and the patient feels ill. In infants infection is likely to spread to the middle ear, causing otitis media and if unrecognized and untreated the infection may spread to the mastoid air cells. Infants with tracheitis may develop signs of respiratory obstruction. Owing to the small size of the respiratory passages in infancy, blocking by swollen mucous membrane and by secretions can readily occur. The condition known as croup, i.e. acute attacks of dyspnoea with stridor in infants, is often due to this cause.

In those cases where the infection spreads down the bronchial tree causing acute bronchitis, the general symptoms are more severe. The patient's temperature rises to $37 \cdot 7°$ to $39 \cdot 4°C$ ($100°$ to $103°F$) and sometimes higher, with headache, malaise and pain in the chest behind the sternum. This pain is aggravated by the constant coughing which in the early stages is unproductive. The patient has difficulty in expelling the sticky, mucoid sputum. Generally the illness is not serious and the patient is well on the way to recovery by the end of a week. In young children and old people particularly, however, there is always some danger of the infection spreading to the lungs and causing bronchopneumonia.

Treatment

An uncomplicated and limited infection, the 'cold in the head', often receives little attention because of its prevalence, but it is very desirable that the person suffering from a cold should rest, preferably in bed, for 24 hr. This will usually shorten the attack and diminish the likelihood of further more severe spread and of secondary infections. Such a measure also helps to protect others from infection. Infants and old people are particularly liable to succumb to serious respiratory infections as a complication of a cold. There is no need to restrict food, although if the patient is febrile he may be disinclined to eat, in any case liberal intake of fluids should be encouraged. Steam inhalations often relieve congestion of the nasal mucous membrane and also the hoarseness and dry cough. Aspirin is useful for the relief of headache and muscular pains. The value of cough lozenges or linctus in combating the inflammation is doubtful, but most people find them soothing. If the cough is severe codeine phosphate may be prescribed.

Tracheobronchitis and sinusitis are treated by rest in bed at least during the febrile period. Steam inhalations may be given; a steam kettle, if available, is probably the best method if the patient is a young child. In some cases, particularly in acute bronchitis, antibiotic treatment is necessary; oral penicillin is often ordered. If the patient's rest is disturbed by persistent cough, which is usually a feature of bronchitis, a sedative linctus is prescribed at night.

Acute Bronchitis

This is usually due to a descending infection and follows such conditions as coryza, measles or whooping cough. It most frequently occurs in the very young or the elderly.

In babies it is characterized by dyspnoea with gasping respirations, cyanosis, restlessness, cough, pyrexia and anorexia. In the elderly there is a dry unproductive cough, tracheitis, wheezing respirations, dyspnoea, cyanosis and pyrexia.

Treatment is bedrest, copious fluids, steam inhalations (often in a tent) mouth toilet, oxygen if cyanosis is severe, and antibiotics.

Chronic Bronchitis and Emphysema

Chronic infection of the bronchial tree is a common condition, especially in middle-aged and elderly men and causes much disability often leading to many serious complications. The condition may begin insidiously with winter cough and sputum at first, followed later by symptoms throughout the year, or it may date from an episode of severe bronchitis or pneumonia. The patient tends to have a slowly increasing disability with cough, sputum and shortness of breath and may suffer from exacerbations of more acute chest infection. The cause of chronic bronchitis is uncertain, but the main factors seem to be: (1) chronic or recurrent bacterial infection of the bronchi, and (2) irritation of the bronchi by atmospheric pollution and by excessive smoking. The combination of infection and irritation causes an over-secretion of mucus from the bronchial tree which is shown by the production of sputum. This excess of mucus may render the bronchi more liable to further infection.

Chronic bronchitis leads inevitably to the condition of emphysema. In this there is thinning and breakdown of the alveolar septa; the lungs become overdistended and lose their normal elasticity. These changes impair the ability of the lungs to take up oxygen and get rid of carbon dioxide due to the decreased surface area of the alveoli which instead of resembling a blackberry (many little sacs) tend to look more like a cherry (Fig. 4). The patient with emphysema suffers from pro-

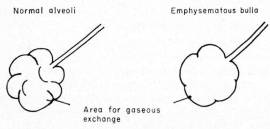

Normal alveoli   Emphysematous bulla

Area for gaseous exchange

FIG. 4. Effect of emphysema on alveoli.

gressive dyspnoea, his breathing is observed to be laboured and the chest appears rigid and moves very poorly with respiration.

Patients with chronic bronchitis and emphysema are very liable to develop pneumonia, which in them is a serious complication. In addition, emphysema imposes a strain on the right ventricle and heart failure of the type known as cor pulmonale often develops in the later stages.

There is no specific treatment for chronic bronchitis and the general aim is to regulate the patient's life as far as possible in order to avoid known irritants, such as fog or a dusty atmosphere and to improve his general state of health. Few sufferers from this condition are able to take the advice so often given that they should live in a dry, mild climate, but the patient should, however, be encouraged to be out of doors whenever the weather is suitable, but to avoid exposure to fog. Breathing exercises, improvement in posture and the encouragement of nose breathing rather than mouth breathing, may help to improve the vital capacity of the lungs. Tobacco is an irritant and should therefore be restricted or forbidden. A sedative linctus to be taken at night and ephedrine tablets for the relief of bronchial spasm may be ordered. Steam inhalations may help the patient to get rid of tenacious sputum. Prophylactic antibiotics may be prescribed in the winter.

The bronchitic subject needs help and encouragement in learning to live with a disability of a chronic nature, but one which can to some extent at least be alleviated by simple measures directed towards maintaining his general health.

The nurse is often in a position to help the patient by making sure that he understands the medical advice he is given and by finding out any difficulties in the home circumstances, particularly if the patient is elderly and living alone. Where some assistance is needed suitable arrangements can usually be made if the circumstances are known.

Bronchiectasis

Bronchiectasis is a dilation of the bronchi and bronchioles in a section of the lung; the dilation may be either saccular or fusiform in type.

The condition is produced by bronchial obstruction from any cause, with infection of the bronchi beyond the block. The weakened and infected walls of the bronchi dilate and this increases the liability to infection.

The patient has a chronic and troublesome cough with copious sputum which is muco-purulent, and often offensive. The amount of sputum produced is usually greatest in the early morning after it has accumulated during the night. Haemoptysis is not uncommon.

Recurrent infections cause fever, loss of weight, loss of appetite and the cough becomes still more troublesome. The patient's life becomes more and more restricted by the debility caused by frequent exacerbations of his chest condition. Clubbing of the finger tips is seen in long-standing cases of bronchiectasis. X-ray examination of the chest assist in diagnosis, and a bronchogram, i.e. an X-ray taken after the injection of an opaque medium into the bronchial tree, is the usual procedure (Fig. 5). The opaque medium used for this is an organic iodine compound, Dionosil. The opaque fluid may be introduced into the bronchi through a special syringe with a

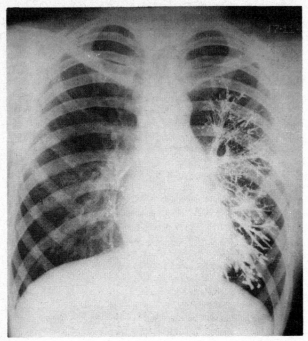

FIG. 5. Bronchogram showing bronchiectasis of left lower lobe.

curved dropper, passed over the tongue into the pharynx and dropping the fluid into the trachea. A local anaesthetic, cocaine, and a spray are required to anaesthetize the pharynx and larynx. Alternatively a short curved trocar and cannula is introduced through the cricothyroid membranes into the trachea and the opaque medium is injected directly into the trachea. Premedication with a sedative such as codeine and an injection of atropine may be ordered. Usually food is withheld for 6 hr prior to the examination as the patient may vomit during the procedure and inhale the vomit into the air passages. When the injection is completed and the X-rays have been taken he should not be allowed to eat or drink until the effects of the local anaesthetic have passed off and the cough reflex is reestablished. Failure to observe this precaution can result in any material which the patient tries to swallow passing down the trachea into the lungs.

Treatment

Postural drainage assisted by physiotherapy is a useful measure in relieving the symptoms of bronchiectasis (Fig. 6). Most bronchiectatic lesions are in the lower lobes of the lung

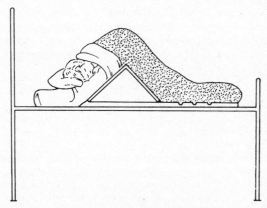

FIG. 6. Postural drainage for bronchiectasis.

and the patient should lie in such a position that his chest, neck and head are lower than the pelvis. This position will vary according to the site of the bronchiectasis and may be determined by X-ray. The patient will often discover for himself the portion which gives maximum drainage. A special bed can be used or the patient can lie in the prone position across the bed with his head and folded arms resting on a pillow on the floor. Drainage will usually be carried out at intervals during the day, beginning when he first wakes in the morning. Direct drainage through a bronchoscope may be carried out, particularly in preparation for resection of the lung.

Physiotherapy includes slapping the chest wall over the affected area, encouraging effective coughing and breathing exercises.

Any associated infection, such as infected nasal sinuses, requires treatment with antibiotics and these drugs will also be used at the first sign of any worsening of the chest infection.

Patients who are suitable for surgical treatment usually make a complete recovery from bronchiectasis following lobectomy or segmental resection of the lung. Elderly patients with extensive bilateral disease are not usually good surgical risks.

Rest is a necessary part of the treatment. Temperature, pulse and respiration rates should be regularly recorded, any rise is an indication of worsening of the infection. The amount of sputum should be recorded daily and a specimen kept for observation. Fresh air, cheerful surroundings and good nutrition all help to improve the patient's general condition and to assist in overcoming the toxic effects of chronic sepsis.

Pneumonia

Pneumonia is an inflammation of the lung which can be caused by a variety of micro-organisms. Exudate produces consolidation of the inflamed area with diminished breathing capacity. There are two main groups of pneumonia:

(1) **Lobar pneumonia,** most commonly due to infection with *Streptococcus pneumoniae* (pneumococcus), can also be caused by other specific organisms such as *Staphylococcus aureus*, *Streptococcus pyogenes*, Friedländer's bacillus, *Haemophilus influenzae*, and also viruses, as for example influenza virus and the virus of psittacosis which can be acquired by human beings from infected birds. In this type of pneumonia the whole of one or more lobes of the lung are affected.

(2) **Bronchopneumonia,** or aspiration pneumonia, in which an important factor is the aspiration of infected material from the upper respiratory tract. The resulting inflammation has a patchy distribution often affecting areas in both lungs. The organisms responsible are likely to be those found in the mouth, nose and throat, such as staphylococci, streptococci and *Haemophilis influenzae*. A lung abscess may result from aspiration of highly infected material.

The onset of lobar pneumonia is sudden, with rapid rise in temperature to 39·4° to 40°C (103° to 104°F), often accompanied by a rigor, rapid respiration and quickened pulse rate, pain in the chest on the affected side due to pleurisy and a tight cough.

The patient feels ill, nausea and vomiting are not unusual and he may complain of severe frontal headache. The onset of bronchopneumonia is less acute, with a slight rise in temperature, increase in the pulse and respiratory rates and cough. This type of pneumonia often complicates bronchitis or infectious fevers such as measles. It is also a possibility to be constantly borne in mind in the nursing of patients who are unconscious, or who have had major chest or abdominal operations. Such patients need to be turned if possible every 2 hr to prevent the collections of fluid in the alveoli.

Treatment

Whatever the cause or type of pneumonia, treatment follows the same general lines. The causal organism is identified if possible from a smear of sputum and a sample of blood for culture is often required. Chemotherapy is started as soon as the diagnosis is made and the drug used will depend on the causal organism. Penicillin is the most frequently used antibiotic in pneumococcal infection, and treatment with the drug may be begun without waiting for laboratory reports. Other antibiotics used are tetracycline, streptomycin and, less frequently, chloramphenicol.

In the majority of instances the infection is arrested and the temperature becomes normal in 2 to 3 days. The dosage of the antibiotic used and the duration of its use depend on the severity of the illness and the response to treatment. Although the symptoms usually abate rapidly the consolidation in the lungs due to inflammation will take some time to resolve. Patients who are cyanosed or severely dyspnoeic require oxygen and this is usually given by means of a face mask. The plastic mask is light, and comfortable to wear, it is cheap and can be destroyed when the patient no longer requires it; this prevents possible cross-infection from this source. The 'Venturi' mask is designed to give more accurate control of the concentration of oxygen reaching the patient and so ensure that while relieving anoxia, it is not sufficient to produce respiratory depression. An oxygen tent may be used and the newer types are made of light plastic materials. Patients suffering from pneumonia complicating chronic bronchitis and emphysema are not generally nursed continuously in the tent; an example of the routine that may be used is 10 min in the tent and 20 min with the tent open.

One danger of oxygen therapy is an accumulation of carbon dioxide in the blood which can lead to carbon dioxide narcosis. (see p. 59). Where oxygen therapy is used the patient must be kept under continuous observation.

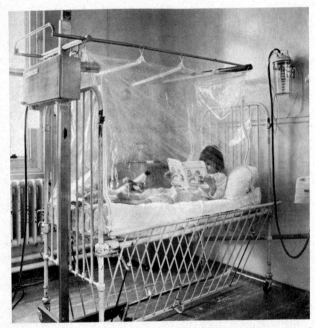

FIG. 7. Oximist tent. For purposes of illustrating the tent, an active child has been photographed and the cot sides let down. Usually, of course, the cot sides should not be left down.

Hypnotic drugs, such as phenobarbitone, may be ordered to be given at night to ensure adequate sleep. Pleuritic pain may be relieved by hot applications such as a kaolin poultice, an electrically heated pad, or if severe, by a local injection of procaine. If heat is applied care must be taken not to burn the patient and a poultice must not be too heavy or secured by tight bandaging both of which will hinder respiration.

The patient is nursed in the sitting position, comfortably supported by sufficient pillows. During the febrile stage rest is important and all nursing attention is given with as little disturbance of the patient and as little activity on his part as possible. As soon as the cough becomes productive, coughing is encouraged. In the early stages of the illness the sputum is tenacious and may be brownish red in colour due to blood (rusty sputum); later it becomes mucopurulent. The expectoration of tenacious sticky sputum may be helped by sips of Compound Mixture of Sodium Chloride, B.P.C., 40 ml in a tumbler full of hot water. This mixture contains sodium bicarbonate, sodium chloride and flavouring agents.

The diet need not be restricted if the patient feels able to eat, but more important is a liberal fluid intake, sugar or glucose can be added to drinks if the patient is disinclined to eat. The temperature, pulse and respiration rate should be taken and recorded 4-hourly, unless there is any reason to require any one of these observations to be made more frequently. Physiotherapy has a useful part in the treatment of pneumonia, and the nurse will often be required to help in carrying out breathing and other exercises prescribed for the patient under the supervision of the physiotherapist.

Complications are not now common if adequate chemotherapy is available, but those which may be seen include:

(1) Empyema (see p. 61).
(2) Failure of the pneumonia to resolve.
(3) Lung abscess.

(2) and (3) may occur if the causal organism is especially virulent or because carcinoma of the bronchus is the underlying disease, or because the patient's resistance is lowered by reason of some other disease.

(4) Carbon dioxide narcosis. This complication affects patients with severe chronic bronchitis and emphysema who develop pneumonia. The normal stimulus to increased depth of breathing is increase of carbon dioxide in the blood, but these patients have become habituated to an abnormally high pressure of carbon dioxide in the blood and in them the stimulus to breathing is shortage of oxygen (anoxia). If this stimulus is removed by making the patient breathe a high concentration of

oxygen, as in a test, his breathing may become inadequate, so that further retention of carbon dioxide occurs. It is therefore essential for the nurse to observe a bronchitic patient having oxygen treatment for the signs of carbon dioxide poisoning. These consist of warm extremities, bounding full pulse, muscular twitching and mental confusion going on to stupor and even coma. Because of the risk of carbon dioxide narcosis these patients are often given oxygen intermittently, and may be given respiratory stimulants such as nikethamide or amiphenazole (Daptazole).

(5) Mental confusion and delirium may occur in very virulent infections or in alcoholic subjects. Severe toxic delirium leads to a dangerous degree of exhaustion, and therefore needs immediate treatment. Paraldehyde by intramuscular injection is a valuable sedative; one of the barbiturate drugs, such as phenobarbitone or nitrazepram (Mogadon) may be ordered.

(6) Cardiac failure may be a complicating factor in elderly patients, particularly those with pre-existing heart disease and will be shown by such signs as increasing breathlessness, cyanosis and irregularities of the pulse. The treatment of this condition is the administration of digitalis, often rapid digitalization (see p. 96) is necessary.

Pleurisy

Pleurisy, inflammation of the pleura, may occur with or without effusion, i.e. 'wet' or 'dry' pleurisy. If the fluid becomes purulent the condition is then called empyema.

The commoner causes of pleurisy are pneumonia, tuberculous infection of the lung when the pleurisy occurs soon after the primary infection, carcinoma of the bronchus and infarction of the lung. Pleurisy may also occur as a result of trauma, such as fractured ribs or wounds of the chest. A pleural biopsy may be needed in order to determine whether a pleural effusion is tuberculous or malignant in origin. An Abram's biopsy needle is commonly used for this and is inserted in the posterior chest wall, the exact side being decided after physical and radiological examination.

The inflammation is accompanied by pain in the chest, particularly on inspiration, and this produces rapid shallow breathing in an attempt to limit the movements of the chest wall. For the same reason the patient will lie on the affected side. Pain is increased by coughing, the cough is dry, short and non-productive. There is usually some degree of fever.

When pleural effusion develops the pain on breathing disappears, but if the effusion is large there will be increased dyspnoea, cyanosis and possibly an increase in the febrile symptoms. If the fluid becomes purulent then the patient is more severely ill with a swinging temperature and increased pulse rate; profuse sweating when the temperature is on the downward swing is often noted.

Treatment

The treatment is directed at the underlying cause of the pleurisy and at relieving the symptoms. Suitable chemotherapy is begun or continued. Pain can be alleviated by hot applications applied to the chest wall on the affected side to restrict movements and so reduce pain, or a local injection of procaine is given to relieve pain and allow free movement of the chest wall.

A small pleural effusion is usually reabsorbed without difficulty. Larger effusions require aspiration. This is usually carried out by puncture of the chest wall with a stout needle to reach the pleural space; the fluid is then withdrawn by means of a syringe with a two-way stopcock to prevent introduction of air during the aspiration.

Empyema. The thick purulent fluid of an empyema cannot as a rule be withdrawn through a needle in this way and surgical drainage by inserting a tube into the pleural cavity will be required; the tube is connected to a length of rubber tubing with an under-water seal in a bottle at the patient's bedside (Fig. 8).

Nursing care includes all general measures for the care of an ill patient confined to bed, maintaining the patient's strength by encouraging his appetite with food which he finds attractive and with as high a calorie value as possible. Where necessary the bowels are regulated with a gentle aperient; if as a result of confinement in bed constipation is troublesome, a Dulcolax (bisacodyl) or glycerine suppository may be ordered.

Physiotherapy is usually a part of the treatment and the nurse often assists with the breathing exercises and by the arrangement of pillows and supports to maintain a good posture in bed and free movement of the chest wall.

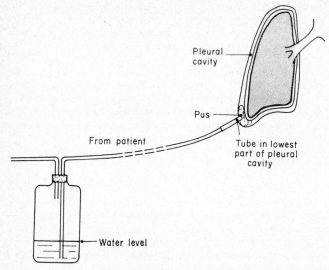

FIG. 8. Closed drainage of an empyema.

Pleural effusion not due to inflammation (hydrothorax) is most commonly seen as part of a generalized oedema in congestive cardiac failure and sometimes in glomerulonephritis. Large pleural effusions commonly occur in connection with malignant growths in the lung, either a primary carcinoma of the bronchus or secondary growths spreading from a carcinoma in another organ; in women the primary growth is often in the breast.

Pulmonary Tuberculosis

Pulmonary tuberculosis is the commonest manifestation of infection with *Mycobacterium tuberculosis*. In this form of tuberculosis the organism usually gains entrance directly through the upper respiratory tract in inhaled dust or droplet infection from a tuberculous person.

The nurse can help in educating the public to regard pulmonary tuberculosis sensibly. Although now uncommon in the indigenous population in the United Kingdom it is often found in the recent immigrant. It can be arrested and, with new methods of treatment it has ceased to be the 'white scourge' of the last century. There is no reason why the majority of those who have to undergo a course of treatment should not be able to live the full, normal life of those in whom the disease has never been manifested.

Primary infection is common and often produces no symptoms; the lesion heals without any ill-effects. The Mantoux test, i.e. an intradermal injection of old tuberculin, is used to detect whether or not infection has taken place. It is generally held that persons who have had a symptomless primary infection, as shown by a positive Mantoux test, and no subsequent tuberculous illness, have developed some degree of resistance to tuberculosis.

Except in miliary tuberculosis the infection is localized, but the toxins are absorbed into the blood. The bacillus produces an inflammatory reaction in the tissue which forms the 'tubercle'; a barrier forms, chiefly composed of lymphocytes, to localize the infection, and within it death of tissue occurs. The dead tissue degenerates firstly into a thick cheesy substance; this process is known as caseation, later it develops into definite pus. If the resistance is good the disease can be arrested before this stage is reached, and fibrosis and, in some cases, calcification occurs. With further progress of the disease, however, the pus escapes, usually by rupture into an air passage, and is coughed up, leaving a cavity which may not heal and remains a seat of infection. Spread is by the lymphatics or by direct ulceration, further areas of the lung become infected, and in advanced cases the other lung also.

Types of the Disease

(1) Primary infection, which is usually symptomless, but can cause enlargement of the hilar glands and pulmonary collapse in young children (Fig. 9). Within a few months of the primary infection serious forms of tuberculosis [e.g. those described under (2) and (3)] are likely to arise unless the individual's resistance to the infection is good.

(2) Miliary or generalized tuberculosis, which may or may not be associated with tuberculous meningitis (see p. 338).

(3) Primary tuberculous pleural effusion.

(4) Erythema nodosum and phlyctenular conjunctivitis are

tuberculous manifestations which may occur early in the course of the infection.

(5) At a later stage the adult type of pulmonary tuberculosis develops either from breakdown of an early focus of infection or by fresh infection; there is a variable amount of disease in one or both lungs, often with cavitation.

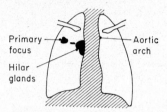

FIG. 9. Primary complex in the right lung.

The earlier the diagnosis and recognition of the disease, the greater are the chances of cure. The main difficulty in diagnosing pulmonary tuberculosis in the early stage is that no symptoms may be present until the disease is advanced. The only certain method of detection is by an X-ray examination of the chest, which will reveal the local focus of infection. The following manifestations only appear when the disease is well established:

(1) Haemoptysis (usually slight) due to rupture of a small vessel during the inflammatory stage.

(2) Spontaneous pneumothorax, caused by ulceration of a small focus of infection, by which an air passage connects with the pleural cavity.

(3) Pleurisy with effusion (Fig. 10).

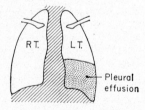

FIG. 10. Pleural effusion.

Signs and symptoms which are more vague than the foregoing and may escape attention until the disease is firmly established are:

(4) Lassitude and general tiredness, with loss of appetite.

(5) Persistent cough (often remaining after a cold or other respiratory infection).

(6) Progressive loss of weight.

(7) Evening rise of temperature, which may be very slight, but in advanced cases the hectic, intermittent type of fever is often seen.

(8) Night sweats, which become very pronounced in the late stages.

These signs and symptoms are produced by the presence of toxins in the blood.

Treatment

Chemotherapy is the most important measure in the treatment of pulmonary tuberculosis. The drugs used are streptomycin, isoniazid (INH) and para-aminosalicylic acid (PAS). At least two and sometimes all three of these are used in combination, as the organisms are very prone to become drug-resistant if the drugs are used individually. Drug resistance is also likely to develop if for any reason the patient does not follow the full course of treatment. Where this resistance is established and the patient has a relapse his chances of eventual cure are much more remote. Chemotherapy is continued for 2 years. Other antibiotics, e.g. viomycin and cycloserine, are available for cases where resistance to streptomycin, PAS and INH has developed.

Rest is also important, but strict confinement to bed is now usually only insisted upon for febrile or seriously ill patients. The patient may be nursed at home if the conditions are suitable or in a sanatorium. Sanatorium treatment offers several advantages, e.g. a better environment for the city dweller, since these hospitals are situated in open country, education of the patient in looking after himself and understanding the nature of his illness, the hygienic precautions used to prevent the spread of infection, and the way of life to be followed when his disease is cured. A planned programme of rehabilitation, and if necessary resettlement, is a part of the work of the chest hospital. Surgical treatment, in the form of thoracoplasty and lung resection, is required in a few patients, especially those whose infection is due to resistant bacilli. Collapse of the affected lung by an artificial pneumothorax or pneumoperitoneum is a form of treatment that is now seldom used.

Haemoptysis may occur during the course of the illness and may be slight if it is caused by capillary oozing or severe if a large blood-vessel is ruptured. This is an alarming occurrence, but haemoptysis is seldom the cause of death. The greatest danger is the spread of infection by the aspiration of blood containing bacilli into other parts of the lungs. The doctor should be informed at once; a sedative such as an injection of phenobarbitone sodium, 60 to 200 mg (1 to 3 gr.) may be ordered. Opinions differ as to the advisability of giving morphine which, although an effective sedative, inhibits coughing. The patient's apprehension should as far as possible be allayed, and he can be encouraged to expectorate the blood and to cough, but without making vigorous efforts. He should be propped up in a comfortable position and kept at rest. Mouthwashes are cleansing and comforting, and sips of water will be acceptable. Blood-stained clothing and sheets should be removed as soon as possible with the minimum of disturbance.

Nursing care of the tuberculous patient consists in carrying out the treatment ordered for the patient, including the administration of drugs, and ensuring that when bed rest is ordered this is adhered to and all nursing attention is given. Building up the patient's resistance to tuberculosis is helped by generous and attractive meals, fresh air and a cheerful atmosphere. Occupational therapy and participation in social activities form part of the treatment as the patient progresses. Resettlement in a suitable occupation may be needed for some patients after recovery.

Measures to prevent spread of infection and to protect the nurses and other persons working in a hospital for tuberculous patients are those described on page 47. Any person handling sputum mugs should be provided with a protective apron and rubber gloves.

If a patient with an active lesion is treated at home, the safety of other members of the family must be considered. Since the patient's sputum is the greatest source of danger, he must use care not to soil his hands or bedclothes but to expectorate into a sputum cup containing disinfectant, such as Roccal 1 : 10. Sputum can then be flushed down the water closet and the container boiled in a pan kept for that purpose. Paper handkerchiefs should be used and promptly burnt. Toilet articles must be kept strictly separate from those of the rest of the family, and the same applies to crockery and cutlery. The patient will need to be warned that close contact with others, and particularly kissing children, should be avoided. All dusting must be carried out with a damp duster, and floors should either be washed or cleaned by vacuum suction. Protective clothing such as an overall, rubber gloves, and a face mask should be worn by those who attend to the patient, handle sputum cups, or clean his room.

ALLERGIC CONDITIONS

Hay Fever

Hay fever is an allergic catarrhal condition affecting the conjunctiva of the eye and the nasal mucous membrane. Attacks commonly occur in the summer when pollen dust from grasses is in the air, hence its name. The sneezing, running eyes and nose are caused by the individual's sensitivity to hay pollens, and the condition may persist for weeks.

Desensitizing the patient by a course of injections of pollen extracts may be successful, and the treatment should be given in the early months of the year so that immunity has time to develop before the summer. Any source of infection, such as nasal polypi or sinus infection, should be looked for and where necessary treated. Antihistamine drugs such as Benadryl will often give relief during an attack, or ephedrine tablets may be prescribed.

Asthma

Asthma is a condition in which spasm of the walls of the bronchial tree produces dyspnoea, inspiration of air is not greatly affected, the difficulty is mainly expiratory. The cause of these attacks is often difficult to determine, in some cases a definite sensitivity (allergy) to a protein which may be animal, such as fur or feathers, or vegetable, such as pollen, is responsible. Emotional factors may play a part in precipitating an attack. In some instances infection of the respiratory tract or nasal sinuses may be responsible; hereditary tendency is a factor in some cases.

Asthmatic attacks not infrequently occur at night; the patient is awakened by extreme breathlessness. He sits up in bed using all his accessory respiratory muscles and gripping the sides of the bed to make this easier by fixing the shoulder girdle. The expiratory effort is extreme, wheezing can often be heard from a distance, the patient's face is congested and sometimes cyanotic. The attack usually passes off with administration of an antispasmodic, but repeated attacks may follow one another in quick succession and exhaust the patient; this condition is known as status asthmaticus.

Immediate Treatment

Patients who repeatedly suffer from asthmatic attacks may have an inhaler which when squeezed produces a fine spray of an antispasmodic drug or drugs which the patient breathes in and thus obtains relief. Drugs commonly used in these inhalers are isoprenaline, salbutamol (Ventolin) and compounds of ephedrine and aminophylline. If no relief is obtained by this method, antispasmodic drugs may be given systemically.

Adrenaline 1 : 1000 solution by hypodermic injection is the most generally effective antispasmodic. The dosage depends on the severity of the attack; 0·2 to 0·5 ml (3 to 8 minims), which can be repeated after an interval of $\frac{1}{2}$ to 1 hr if necessary, may be given. Aminophylline given by mouth or by injection or as a rectal suppository is another useful drug. Corticosteroids may be successful in status asthmaticus which does not respond to adrenaline. In addition, if the patient is found to have any respiratory infection, this must receive prompt treatment with a suitable antibiotic. Oxygen inhalation may alleviate dyspnoea in severe or repeated asthmatic attacks.

Interim Treatment

Any cause that may act as the precipitant of an attack is sought for and where possible treated or corrected, as for example evidence of bronchitis or emphysema, of allergic factors, unsuitable working or living conditions, and psychological difficulties. Physiotherapy is valuable in most cases, breathing exercises and correction of poor posture are directed at making the chest wall more mobile.

A combination of ephedrine and aminophylline is often ordered and these two drugs may be combined with a sedative such as phenobarbitone. Taken in the evening this combination of drugs is often successful in preventing attacks during the night. Isoprenaline, a derivative of adrenaline which is free from the cardiovascular effects of adrenaline, may be given in the form of tablets to be placed under the tongue: the dosage is 5 to 20 mg. The patient is instructed to take the prescribed drugs at the first warning of symptoms in order to prevent the development of a severe attack. Salbutamol (Ventolin) may be used in place of isoprenaline; it is slower in action and has less effect on the heart.

The nursing care of the patient is mainly supportive; because of the chronic nature of the disease the patient may need considerable encouragement to persevere with and co-operate in his treatment, as for example regular attendance at physiotherapy classes. Where the patient is a child the parents are naturally extremely worried and often frightened by the attack. This anxiety may lead to an over-protective attitude and creates an atmosphere in the home which can be a contributory cause of the child's asthmatic attacks. It is therefore essential that the parents should be given all possible help and should be made aware of the nature of the illness, the possible precipitating causes and the treatment to be given when an attack occurs.

INJURY

Pneumothorax

Pneumothorax means that there is air in the pleural space and this may be the result of trauma such as a fractured rib or penetrating wounds of the chest, or may arise spontaneously. Spontaneous pneumothorax may be:

(1) A benign condition occurring in young and otherwise healthy men who show no evidence of tuberculosis, and is probably due to the rupture of a small bullae on the surface of the lung.

(2) A complication of pulmonary tuberculosis.

(3) A complication of other lung diseases, such as advanced emphysema, asthma and some forms of pneumoconiosis.

Symptoms of a pneumothorax are pain in the chest and dyspnoea, of sudden onset.

Treatment

The patient is put to bed and supported comfortably in the sitting position. The pleural pain is treated by hot applications such as kaolin poultices and analgesics. If dyspnoea is marked the air in the pleural space must be removed. This may be carried out by inserting a needle, e.g. Morland's chest needle, into the pleural space and connecting it to an artificial pneumo-thorax machine adapted to take off air, or by introducing a small size catheter into the chest with a trocar and connecting this to an underwater seal in a bottle at the bedside. In some cases the catheter may be connected to a low-pressure suction pump.

NEW GROWTHS

Carcinoma of the Bronchus

Carcinoma of the bronchus has become an increasingly common form of cancer in this country. More men than women are affected although this pattern is changing possibly due to changes in smoking habits. The patient is usually middle-aged and there is often a history of heavy smoking.

The growth may be discovered because the patient becomes ill with a chest infection. The growth blocks the bronchial tube and collapse of the area of lung distal to the obstruction favours the development of infection, which may be manifested as a penumonia which fails to resolve, bronchiectasis, or a lung abscess. Collapse of a part of the lung as a result of obstruction from any cause and absorption of air from the area behind the blockage may occur and is known as atelectasis. Other symptoms of carcinoma of the lung are haemoptysis, cough and pain in the chest.

The diagnostic procedures likely to be required are an X-ray examination of the chest, direct inspection of the bronchus by means of a bronchoscope and removal of a piece of tissue for examination. The preparation of the patient for bronchoscopy is the same as that for bronchography which is given on page 54.

Treatment

In many cases unfortunately the disease has advanced to the stage where spread to the mediastinal and other glands or to the liver, brain or other organs has occurred before the symptoms cause the patient to seek medical advice.

Mass miniature chest radiography, which has assisted in the early diagnosis of pulmonary tuberculosis, is also one of the ways in which a carcinoma of the bronchus may be detected in the older age group at a comparatively early stage. If at all possible surgical treatment, resection of the lung, is advised. In other cases radiotherapy may control the disease for a longer or shorter period. Antibiotic treatment may be required to clear up any infection in the lung. Although surgical treatment has a low immediate mortality, less than 10 per cent, the expectation of life for a patient with carcinoma of bronchus seldom exceeds 5 years and is often less, whatever form of treatment is employed.

Pneumoconiosis

Pneumoconiosis is a term used to describe a group of industrial diseases which affect the lungs, due to inhalation of minute particles of dust during the course of work. A form of fibrosis results which becomes incapacitating, and finally fatal, if not treated at an early stage. Some types of pneumoconiosis are particularly liable to lead to pulmonary tuberculosis.

According to the type of dust inhaled, this condition can be subdivided into:

Aluminosis (aluminium)   Siderosis (iron)

Anthracosis (anthracite coal)   Silicosis (stone)

Asbestosis (asbestos)

Beryllium disease (berryllium is a metal used in the manufacture of fluorescent lamps).

It can also be caused by the inhalation of chalk or zinc in powder form in the manufacture of medicated talcum powder.

Treatment

Many legislative measures are in force to prevent this type of disease, such as compulsory requirements for effective ventilation systems and the damping of dust. If the condition develops removal from contact with the dust is the only way of checking its progress and this is not always effectual.

Other treatment is palliative, to control the cough and to relieve dyspnoea and breathlessness. Ample nutrition, fresh air, adequate rest and freedom from economic anxiety are also essential. In the later stages, congestive heart failure, chronic bronchitis or pulmonary tuberculosis require the usual treatment for these conditions.

4

Disorders of the blood and blood-forming organs

THE main groups of blood disorders are those arising from abnormalities in the number or type of blood cells. More rarely, as in the bleeding diseases such as haemophilia and purpura, the cause is a defect in the clotting mechanism of the blood or in the capillary walls. It will be readily seen therefore that laboratory examination of the blood is an essential part of the understanding and diagnosis of these disorders.

EXAMINATION OF THE BLOOD

Specimens of blood can be obtained by pricking the tip of the finger or lobe of the ear and drawing a few drops of blood into special pipettes. This is usually sufficient for a cell count, but if other tests or a number of tests are required blood is collected from a vein.

Blood tests include:

(1) *A cell count*. This gives the number of red cells, white cells and platelets per cubic millimetre (mm^3); the haemoglobin content is usually estimated at the same time. Normal values are:

Red Cells	4 500 000 to 6 000 000 per mm^3 (men)
	4 300 000 to 5 500 000 per mm^3 (women)
Haemoglobin	in g per 100 ml
	15 to 16, men (100 to 105 per cent)
	13 to 15, women (95 to 100 per cent)
White Cells	5000 to 10 000 per mm^3
	Neutrophils 40 to 60 per cent
	Lymphocytes 20 to 40 per cent
	Monocytes 4 to 8 per cent
	Eosinophils 1 to 3 per cent
	Basophils 0 to 1 per cent

Neutrophils, eosinophils and basophils form the group of white cells known as polymorphonuclear cells, meaning having nuclei of many shapes; furthermore the nuclei are so deeply indented that they appear to be a group rather than one nucleus. The term neutrophil indicates that these cells do not stain with an acid red dye or a basic blue dye, whereas eosinophils readily pick up eosin a red dye and basophils stain with blue dyes.

Platelets   200 000 to 500 000 per mm^3

Red cell counts and haemoglobin estimation are valuable aids in detecting the presence of anaemia from any cause. White cell counts may help in the diagnosis of infections where the number and type of cells will often indicate the type of infection, as for example increase of polymorphonuclear cells in pyogenic infections, increase of lymphocytes in glandular fever. Increase of white cells with abnormal types of cell is found in leukaemia.

Examination of the blood cells in the bone marrow may be required in cases of pernicious anaemia and leukaemia. Specimens of bone marrow are obtained by puncturing the sternum or iliac crest with a sternal puncture needle and withdrawing some of the marrow.

(2) *Estimation of the red cell (erythrocyte) sedimentation rate (ESR)*. The sedimentation rate measures the speed at which the red cells fall in one hour when a column of blood is allowed to stand vertically in a tube of fine, uniform bore which is graduated in millimetres. The height of the column of clear plasma above the sediment of red cells is read at the end of one hour. Several different methods are used; the normal readings in two of these methods are:

Westergren, 3 to 5 mm (men); 4 to 7 mm (women) in 1 hr
Wintrobe, 0 to 9 mm (men); 0 to 20 mm (women) in 1 hr

This test is not diagnostic, as the sedimentation rate is raised in most infections, but it is useful in judging the activity of the disease in some cases, as for example rheumatic fever and tuberculosis. Active infection is accompanied by a high sedimentation rate; as the condition improves the sedimentation rate falls.

(3) *Blood grouping.* The blood group according to the ABO classification and the presence of Rhesus antigens, is a necessary estimation before blood from a donor is given to a patient. The stored blood obtained from the Blood Transfusion Service is labelled with the ABO and Rhesus group, the date on which the blood was collected and the date after which it should not be used for transfusion. It is obviously necessary to know the recipient's group, but even if this is known the precaution of directly cross-matching the donor's and the patient's blood is taken, as it is recognized that there are subtypes as well as the main ABO and Rhesus groups and therefore possible incompatibility even between the blood of members of the same main group (see also p. 86).

HEREDITARY CONDITION

Haemophilia

Haemophilia is a hereditary disease in which the clotting power of the blood is deficient or absent, so that the slightest injury produces a severe, and potentially fatal, haemorrhage. The hereditary defect only appears in males, but is always transmitted by the female line; thus a woman may hand on the defect to a son and to a daughter, the son may be a haemophiliac but not the daughter; however, the daughter can pass on the haemophiliac tendency to her offspring.

The blood coagulation time is increased beyond the normal limits of 5 to 15 min, and when the clot does form it is often soft, friable and easily destroyed. In addition to excessive bleeding from injury, bleeding takes place into tissues (so that the haemophiliac subject bruises very easily) and into joint spaces causing pain and swelling.

Treatment

As far as possible haemophiliacs must be protected against injury of any kind. Bleeding from a slight injury or from a tooth extraction can often be arrested by the local application of fibrin foam or Russell viper venom. Surgical operations are only undertaken if absolutely necessary. Fresh blood transfusions are needed to control prolonged or severe haemorrhage, or in preparation for an operation, stored blood rapidly loses the anti-haemophilic globulin and therefore is not effective.

Haemorrhage into a joint space is treated by resting the limb or by splinting and a firm bandage. Fibrosis is apt to follow the absorption of the blood and may cause limitation of movement. As soon as it is considered safe to do so movements and exercises are started to lessen the subsequent disability as far as may be.

DEFICIENCY DISEASE

Anaemia

By anaemia is meant the group of signs and symptoms which denote deficiency in *quantity* or *quality* of the red blood corpuscles. The symptoms, which will be present no matter what the cause, are:

Cardiovascular system. Pallor, especially noticed in the lips and conjunctiva of the eye.

Breathlessness on exertion, due to deficiency of oxygen-carrying power in the blood.

Palpitations, owing to lack of oxygen to the heart muscle.

Oedema of ankles, caused by increased diffusion of fluids through the capillary walls as the result of anoxia (lack of oxygen) in the cells of the capillary walls.

Alimentary tract. Dyspepsia is a common symptom.

Nervous system. Headaches and dizziness, lack of powers of concentration, irritability, lassitude and tiredness.

Anaemia is due to loss of blood by haemorrhage, or to failure to produce sufficient numbers of normal red blood corpuscles, or as a result of their excessive destruction within the body. Haemorrhage is a common cause, either one severe haemorrhage or continuous smaller losses, as for example from haemorrhoids, excessive menstrual loss, peptic ulcer, or purpuric blood diseases in which there is bleeding from mucous surfaces and into the body tissues. In some parts of the world hook worm infection causes a severe anaemia (see p. 161).

The causes may, therefore, be classified as follows:

(1) Loss of blood.

(2) Failure to produce blood because of: (a) non-absorption of vitamin B_{12} in pernicious anaemia; (b) deficiency of vitamin B_{12} or of folic acid or non-absorption arising from various intestinal diseases, e.g. steatorrhoea, or following intestinal operations; (c) dietary deficiency of iron or of other factors

necessary for blood formation (haemopoiesis), such as protein and vitamin C; (d) depression of the bone marrow by radiation, certain drugs or unknown factors causing aplastic anaemia; and (e) depression and/or replacement of bone marrow in leukaemia, chronic infections, cancer and chronic renal disease.

(3) Excessive destruction of red blood cells, haemolytic anaemia, which can be due to a hereditary factor as in sickle-celled anaemia in Negro races, and acholuric jaundice of the congenital type, also as a result of repeated attacks of malaria or prolonged administration of certain of the sulphonamide drugs.

Examination of the blood helps in diagnosis; cells which are small and poor in haemoglobin but only slightly reduced in numbers are found in iron deficiency anaemia; by contrast in pernicious anaemia large cells, each with a normal complement of haemoglobin, but considerably fewer in number than normal are found.

Macrocytic Anaemia

Normally vitamin B_{12} in the food eaten is altered by a substance present in the gastric juice, called the intrinsic factor, in such a way that it can be absorbed in the small intestine into the blood-stream. In the type of macrocytic anaemia known as pernicious anaemia there is atrophy of the gastric mucosa, the intrinsic factor is not produced, and therefore vitamin B_{12} is not absorbed. The anaemia and the complications that involve the nervous system result from deficiency of vitamin B_{12}.

The patient suffering from pernicious anaemia will show the signs common to any severe anaemia, weakness, palpitations, pallor which has a yellowish tinge, and in addition such manifestations as dyspepsia, gastritis, glossitis (a sore red tongue) and loss of appetite, are usually marked. There is achlorhydria, i.e. absence of hydrochloric acid in the gastric juice, and no acid is secreted in response to an injection of histamine.

Schilling's test for absorption of cyanocobalamin uses radio-active cobalt incorporated with vitamin B_{12}. The patient is given the radioactive test dose by mouth and the amount taken up by the liver can be estimated and compared with normal absorption.

The symptoms due to nervous system complications are numbness and tingling in the hands and feet, loss of motor control with rigidity, unsteady gait and possibly loss of sphincter control.

Treatment

The specific treatment is to supply the essential vitamin B_{12} by parenteral injections of cyanocobalamin. The dosage required for the initial treatment and for maintenance therapy will depend on the severity of the anaemia, the presence of complicating factors, and the response to treatment. Patients must be made fully aware of the need to continue with treatment throughout life and of the risk of relapse and permanent disability if treatment is neglected. If there is also iron deficiency, ferrous sulphate tablets may be ordered. Some patients have become so severely anaemic by the time they first present for treatment, that preliminary blood transfusions may be indicated; if these are necessary they should be given very slowly in the form of packed cells, since patients suffering from chronic anaemia may readily develop heart failure if given too much fluid by intravenous infusion.

A severe degree of anaemia requires rest in bed. An adequate well-balanced diet should be given, but special diets are not now considered of value in these cases.

The neurological symptoms, if present, are improved by large doses of cyanocobalamin, and physiotherapy will help to re-educate the muscles and improve the patient's gait. If loss of sphincter control is evident the skin of the buttocks and thighs need to be protected and a silicone barrier cream may be used after washing and drying the skin.

Deficiency of folic acid can also cause a macrocytic type of anaemia. This is seldom a dietary deficiency, except occasionally in pregnant women whose need for folic acid is increased. It more commonly develops as a result of decreased absorption from the small intestine, for example, in the condition known as idiopathic steatorrhoea (see p. 152).

The treatment is the oral administration of folic acid in doses of from 5 to 30 mg daily. The daily requirement of this vitamin is so small that even where absorption is impaired the dose given is large enough to ensure that this is met. Folic acid is never used in the treatment of pernicious anaemia, as although it may correct the blood abnormalities, it does not prevent the onset of the neurological symptoms referred to above. For this reason it is usual to give cyanocobalamin in all cases of pernicious anaemia.

Iron Deficiency Anaemia

Iron deficiency anaemia may be due to dietary deficiency, severe bleeding or repeated loss of blood, or to toxins from chronic infections or other chronic diseases. Women need considerably more iron than men because of the blood lost at the menstrual periods and in pregnancy iron has also to be supplied to the fetal blood cells. This type of anaemia is therefore more common in women than in men.

Nutritional anaemia is not very often seen in persons taking a normal diet, but may occur if the diet is severely restricted for any reason and iron is not supplied by other means.

The essential feature of iron deficiency anaemia is a low haemoglobin content of the red cells and the treatment will depend on the haemoglobin level. Mild degrees of anaemia, when the haemoglobin is not below 60 per cent, can be treated by giving iron compounds such as ferrous sulphate tablets by mouth. Patients with a more severe anaemia, or those in whom iron by mouth produces dyspeptic symptoms, may be given parenteral iron in the form of intramuscular injections of an iron–Dextran compound, Imferon. Extreme degrees of anaemia, particularly if associated with loss of blood, are likely to require blood transfusion. It is sometimes necessary to give a blood transfusion in cases of severe anaemia without associated blood loss. In these cases the maximum number of blood cells are given in the minimum amount of plasma, i.e. 'packed cells'. This prevents the circulation being overloaded with fluid and the danger of heart failure. Unfortunately because of the high viscosity of the blood, such a transfusion is often difficult to keep running and there is a tendency for clotting to occur within the apparatus. Simple nutritional iron deficiency anaemia responds rapidly to adequate administration of iron. Anaemia due to some underlying cause will usually show some improvement but is not likely to be completely controlled unless the cause can be found and treated. An unsuspected peptic ulcer, a malignant growth, or a chronic septic focus are examples of conditions which may be brought to light in investigating the cause of the anaemic condition.

Unless there is any contra-indication, the diet should be generous and contain adequate amounts of protein, since protein is necessary for blood cell formation. Once the haemoglobin level has been brought up to normal by iron therapy the patient whose anaemia was due to poor nutrition will need advice as to a diet which provides sufficient protein, vitamins and iron to maintain health (see p. 28). It is possible that some patients, for example, an old person living on a small pension may not be able to afford proper food, and in this case some form of social assistance should be arranged.

Agranulocytosis

Agranulocytosis is a condition in which there is a great reduction in, or complete absence of, the granulo-polymorphonuclear cells (neutrophils) in the blood. It results from the toxic action of certain agents, including some drugs such as the sulphonamides, chloramphenicol and thiouracil, particularly if given over long periods. The use of drugs known to be a possible cause of agranulocytosis is avoided if other less toxic substances are available; if it is thought essential to use such a drug its administration is not continued for longer than absolutely necessary.

The symptoms of agranulocytosis are of sudden onset, with fever, inflammation and ulceration of the mouth and throat which rapidly spreads. The patient is seriously ill, and unless treatment is effective he may die. If the suspected cause is a drug which the patient is taking, this is promptly discontinued. Antibiotics are given to combat the infection, either a broad spectrum or the most appropriate antibiotic after identifying the organism. Transfusions of fresh blood are often given.

The patient should be nursed in a single room and all precautions taken to protect him from avoidable infections. Gentle cleansing of the mouth and frequent mouthwashes should be given. Soreness of the mouth and throat make eating difficult and painful; fluids or soft solids are usually all that the patient can swallow. Fluid intake may need to be supplemented by intravenous infusions.

IDIOPATHIC DISEASE

Leukaemia

Leukaemia is a disease whose cause is at present unknown but which is regarded as a malignant condition affecting the tissues which produce leucocytes, i.e. the bone marrow and lymphoid tissue. In the majority of cases there is an increase in the number of white cells in the blood and abnormal types of the cells are also present. In some instances there is no increase in the number of leucocytes in the circulation.

The disease in an acute form attacks children and young adults more commonly than older persons, in whom it tends to run a more chronic course. There is at present no known cure for this disease although treatment may produce remission. Anaemia, which may be severe, is associated with the leucocytosis; this is due to destruction of normal cells and also to the tendency for bleeding to occur spontaneously. Purpuric patches in the skin, and bleeding from the nose, mouth, alimentary tract and genito-urinary tract are not uncommon. Retinal haemorrhage, causing loss of vision, may be the first symptom for which the patient with chronic leukaemia seeks advice.

The spleen is enlarged, in many cases grossly so and often palpable lymph nodes can be found, especially in the lymphocytic type of leukaemia. Resistance to micro-organisms is lowered, and the patient is very prone to intercurrent infections.

In acute leukaemia the course may be a few weeks or possibly months, and death often results from the profound anaemia usually complicated by infection, often in the mouth and throat. Chronic leukaemia, which is described as 'myeloid' or 'granulocytic' when the bone marrow is the seat of the disease and 'lymphocytic' when the lymphoid tissue is mainly responsible for producing abnormal white cells, is more responsive to treatment and although at present there is no known cure, patients may be kept in fairly good health for a considerable time, often for many years.

Treatment

Carefully controlled X-ray treatment to the enlarged spleen and to the leukaemic deposits, which may occur anywhere in the body, will relieve symptoms due to pressure.

Splenectomy may be beneficial in some cases, and occasionally is necessitated by splenic infarcts which produce an acute abdominal emergency, with sudden onset of severe pain and vomiting. Drugs which depress the activity of the bone marrow and blood-forming tissues have been constantly used for a number of years and additions to this group are constantly under trial in the hope that eventually the disease can be totally arrested: at the present time arrest of its progress is all that can be expected. These drugs are described as 'cytotoxic' or 'anti-mitotic'; examples are nitrogen mustard, chlorambucil, mecaptopurine and Myleran. Corticosteroids and ACTH are effective in some cases of acute leukaemia and reduce the tendency to bleeding. Which drugs are to be used, the dosage and the frequency with which the drug is given depends on the type of leukaemia and the effect on the blood as shown by the blood count.

Blood transfusions may be required to combat anaemia and to control bleeding.

General measures to maintain health, avoidance of over-fatigue, an adequate diet, supplemented if necessary by vitamin preparations and protection, as far as possible, against infection will help to prolong life. These patients usually attend a follow-up clinic and should be advised to seek medical help even for what may appear to be a trivial ailment. Any minor surgical procedure such as tooth extraction is best undertaken in hospital.

Many patients suffering from chronic leukaemia may not require admission to hospital as an in-patient until the terminal stage when no form of anti-leukaemic therapy is effective. Once this stage has been reached an overwhelming infection often ends the patient's life without prolonged suffering.

The patient suffering from acute leukaemia is obviously severely ill and the symptoms which first necessitate admission to hospital are often those due to haemorrhages into various parts of the body, accompanied by pain and fever. The diagnosis of leukaemia is established by examination of the blood and of the bone marrow.

As the patient is often a child, or a young adult the situation makes great demands on the skill and personal qualities of the nurse. All necessary nursing care, bed-making, bathing, attention to sanitary needs, must be carried out with the utmost gentleness to avoid unnecessary pain and the bruising which so readily occurs.

Feeding is often difficult owing to the sore condition of the mouth and gums. Fluid and soft diet such as custard and ice cream are usually most acceptable, although any food that the patient happens to fancy should be given. Frequent mouthwashes and gentle cleaning of the mouth and teeth help to make the patient more comfortable, but the use of a toothbrush should usually be avoided, as brushing will cause bleeding and soreness of the gums.

Analgesics such as codeine, to relieve pain and hypnotics, e.g. phenobarbitone, will be ordered in most cases.

Although the patient must be protected as far as possible from the danger of intercurrent infection, strict isolation is only enforced if the patient is having extensive radiotherapy or cytotoxic drug treatment and is therefore at a great risk. The patient, particularly if a child, needs the comfort of seeing other people around him, and his environment should be as cheerful as possible. It need hardly be said that his parents should be allowed to spend as much time as they can with him. The mother will gain some comfort in these sad circumstances if she can help in the care of her child, and will find it a little easier to maintain her normal attitude towards him if she is occupied in this way from the first days of his admission to hospital.

Polycythaemia Vera

Polycythaemia is a condition in which there is an increase in the number of red blood cells, usually also of white cells, and the total volume of the blood is increased. The blood pressure is raised and the patient complains of headache, giddiness, and ringing sounds in the ear (tinnitus). His appearance is flushed and congested, and superficial capillaries are engorged. Haemorrhages and venous thrombosis may occur.

Treatment

The cause of the disease is unknown, and treatment is therefore aimed at controlling the excessive number of blood cells and alleviating the symptoms. Radioactive phosphorus given intravenously, or by mouth, inhibits the excessive production of blood cells and a patient whose disease is controlled by this treatment may remain in reasonably good health for many years. Venesection is a useful measure which by reducing the blood volume relieves the symptoms due to hypertension.

Usually the patient is told of the nature of his illness and the need for regular medical checks including a blood count. As far as possible he should avoid strain and over-fatigue, but otherwise may lead a normal life.

NEW GROWTHS

Lymphadenoma (Hodgkin's Disease)

Lymphadenoma is a malignant condition affecting the lymphoid tissue. The superficial lymph nodes and the spleen are the organs first noticeably enlarged, but the disease can affect lymphoid tissue anywhere in the body and therefore the symptoms may be multiple and varied. Diagnosis is established by biopsy of one of the enlarged lymph glands. Anaemia becomes marked as the disease progresses. Bouts of fever often occur; the temperature remains high for some days after a gradual rise, then slowly declines and remains normal for a period; this is known as Pel-Ebstein fever.

Lymphadenoma is, at present, an eventually fatal disease, but its course may vary in duration from a few months to many years. Deep X-ray treatment and antimitotic drugs, e.g. chlorambucil or nitrogen mustard, bring the condition at least temporarily under control.

General measures include rest in bed during a febrile phase, maintenance of general health by good nutrition, adequate rest and a reasonable amount of exercise. Blood transfusions may be needed if the patient is markedly anaemic.

Purpura

Purpura is a condition in which bleeding takes place into the skin and subcutaneous tissue and also into mucous surfaces and joint spaces. The purpuric rash is seen in the form of purple blotches on the skin; if small these are known as petechae, if resembling large bruises they are called ecchymoses.

Purpura is a symptom of many diseases and can arise from a number of causes, of which the following list gives the main groups:

(1) Infection, especially typhoid fever, meningococcal septicaemia and subacute bacterial endocarditis.

(2) Thrombocytopenic purpura, i.e. due to lack of thrombocytes or platelets. This condition may be secondary to a blood disease such as leukaemia, or to the administration of certain drugs, e.g. gold, chloramphenicol. An idiopathic type occurs which usually affects children and young adults.

(3) Allergic purpura (Henoch-Schönlein disease), in which the precipitating factor may be an allergy to some factor in food or drugs or to infection. The patient is usually a child. A purpuric rash appears on the skin, abdominal pain is often present due to bleeding into the alimentary tract and blood and mucus are passed in the stool. The condition may be mistaken for intussusception and indeed intussusception has been known to start from an area of thickening in the bowel wall due to infiltration of blood.

(4) Scurvy (see p. 182).

(5) Clotting disorders, such as haemophilia, or those resulting from excessive amounts of anticoagulant drugs.

Treatment

The treatment of purpura depends on the underlying cause; when it occurs as part of an infection it will disappear as the infection is overcome. When it is one of the symptoms of a disease such as leukaemia or scurvy it can be expected to disappear if the disease responds to treatment. Splenectomy is sometimes required for the idiopathic type of purpura, which is liable to become a chronic condition. Fresh blood transfusions may be given during an acute attack. Bleeding in Henoch–Schönlein purpura usually ceases in a few days. Corticosteroids may be used both in this type and for idiopathic purpura.

BLOOD TRANSFUSION

Blood transfusion is a very common procedure in the treatment of diseases of the blood and many other conditions; the nurse should be familiar with the possible danger and side effects.

Blood Groups

Transfusion of blood from one person to another is fraught with great risks unless it can be proved that the blood of the donor is compatible with the blood of the recipient. Every individual has substances in his blood which react against 'foreign' proteins, including, in some cases, the proteins in the blood cells of another human being. The effect of these antibody substances is to cause agglutination, or clumping, of the red blood cells. Sometimes, however, the individual will produce no antibodies in response to foreign red cells entering his blood stream and in this case the blood of the donor is said to be compatible with that of the recipient; in other words both these individuals belong to the same blood group. Human blood is therefore classified according to the type of red cell present and the most important classifications of these substances are known as the ABO and Rhesus (Rh) systems. Both donor and recipient must belong to the same ABO and Rh group. As a further check, since subgroups may also be present and because people acquire agglutinating bodies in addition to the 'natural' antibodies, it is also necessary to carry out direct tests matching the recipient's blood against the blood to be donated.

ABO system. Human blood falls into one of four ABO categories, A, B, AB or O. Groups AB and B are comparatively rare amongst European populations, most of whom belong either to the A or the O group.

Group A.   This group has A antigens in the red cells and anti-B antibodies in the plasma.

Group B.   This group has B antigens in the red cells and anti-A antibodies in the plasma.

Group AB.   This group has both A and B antigens but the plasma contains no Anti-A or B antibodies.

Group O.   This group has no A or B antigens in the red cells but has both anti-A and anti-B antibodies in the plasma.

Group A therefore cannot receive blood from Group B as the B group contains Anti-A antibodies.

Group B similarly cannot receive from Group A.

Group AB has no anti-A or B antibodies and therefore, at least theoretically, can receive blood from all other groups.

Group O has both anti-A and anti-B antibodies and can therefore receive only Group O blood, but as Group O contains neither A nor B antigens this group can give to all other ABO groups since the red cells of O group will not be agglutinated by the recipient's plasma. Group O is sometimes referred to as the 'universal donor group' and may in cases of extreme emergency be given to a patient without awaiting the results of full cross-matching tests.

Rhesus group system. The Rhesus, or Rh group, was given this name as it was found that the same system of antibodies was present in the blood of the rhesus monkey. In this system the most important factor is labelled 'D'; the majority of Europeans have this D substance in their blood and are therefore described as Rh positive. About 15 per cent of the population, however, do not have the Rh factor and are said to be Rh negative; transfusion of Rh positive blood to a Rh negative individual can be dangerous, since the Rh negative blood will produce antibodies to destroy the transfused cells. The effect of a first transfusion may be slight but the individual is liable to become sensitive to the D factor and further transfusions with Rh positive blood may produce a serious reaction. A similar reaction can take place in the blood of the fetus in cases where the mother's blood is Rh negative but that of the fetus is Rh positive. The maternal blood then produces antibodies which enter the fetal circulation via the placenta and destroy the fetal red blood cells. The fetus may die or, if it survives to term, the infant may be born with a severe type of haemolytic jaundice. Since sensitivity to the D factor takes some time to develop it is unusual for this reaction to occur in a first pregnancy. If a Rh negative girl or woman of child-bearing age is transfused with Rh positive blood this can also be the cause of a haemolytic reaction should the woman become pregnant with a Rh positive fetus, as her blood will in the meantime have produced Rh antibodies.

Syphilis, malaria and infective hepatitis can be transmitted by blood transfusion. Persons giving a history of malaria or infective hepatitis are not suitable blood donors. Wassermann tests of the blood will ensure that no blood giving a positive reaction to this test for syphilis is used in a transfusion.

The bottles containing whole blood supplied by the Blood Transfusion Services are labelled to show the ABO and Rh groups and also the date of collection and the date after which the blood is unfit for transfusion.

Stored whole blood contains 120 ml of an anticoagulant solution (1·66 per cent disodium hydrogen citrate and 2·5 per cent glucose) in each pint bottle.

Management of Transfusions

In all cases where a blood transfusion is likely to be needed 5 ml of the patient's blood is obtained and sent to the laboratory for grouping and direct cross-matching tests with the sample of the blood to be transfused.

The correct blood for the individual patient is then labelled with his name, number and ward, and the statement that the blood is compatible is signed. The particulars on the label should be checked when the bottle or bottles are moved from the bank to the ward in order to ensure that the right blood is given to the right patient. Almost every case of incompatible transfusion is the result of an administrative error, e.g. incorrect labelling or failure to check the label carefully, particularly when there are two patients in the same ward with the same name.

Stored blood must be kept at a temperature between 4° and 6°C (39° to 43°F) in a thermostatically controlled refrigerator. It should never be cooled below 4°C (39°F) or heated in any way. Bottles containing blood must always be carefully handled to avoid shaking the contents.

Whole blood may be used up to 21 days after withdrawal from the donor, provided that it is properly stored. Red cell suspensions (packed cells), which are prepared by siphoning off the plasma from one or more bottles of whole blood and pooling the red cells, must be used within 24 hr of preparation (Fig. 11).

Rate of flow. Forty drops per minute is the usual rate for a slow transfusion. Rapid transfusion may be needed to replace a severe and sudden loss of blood and in such cases one or more bottles of blood may be given as rapidly as the blood will flow into the vein. In extreme urgency intra-arterial transfusion has been given, but is now little used.

Changing bottles. A full bottle must be obtained from the bank and checked before the bottle in use is empty. The fresh

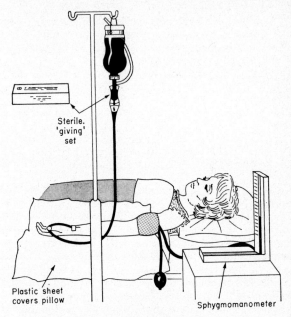

Sterile.
'giving'
set

Plastic sheet
covers pillow

Sphygmomanometer

FIG. 11. Blood transfusion.

bottle is placed at the bedside. When the blood level is just
above the neck of the bottle in use the tubing clip above the
drip chamber is closed; a second clamp may be applied as an
extra safeguard against air entry. The bottle is unhooked and
put alongside the new bottle; the washer of this bottle is removed
and the bung with the delivery and air inlet tubes is transferred
from the old bottle. If a disposable container is used, all that is
needed is to remove the piercing needle from the old bottle and
insert it into the new bottle after removing the adhesive strip
that protects the sterile bung. The needle must not be allowed
to touch the edge or the outside of either bottle during this
procedure. The full bottle is then suspended from the transfusion stand, the tubing clamp opened and the transfusion
continued at the prescribed rate.

Difficulties that May Arise During a Transfusion

(1) Difficulty in maintaining the flow of blood may be due to one of several causes. The vein may go into spasm. This may be overcome by gently warming the limb or by stroking along the vein above the injection site.

The tubing may become kinked or pressed upon and this possibility should always be borne in mind and careful inspection made.

The needle may become dislodged. An attempt may be made to alter the position of needle by gently lifting the mount to depress the point. This may be successful, but if the needle has punctured the wall of the vein the transfusion will have to be stopped and if necessary started again using another vein.

An air-lock may block the flow of blood from the bottle. This should not occur if due care is taken to expel all air from the delivery tubing before connecting it to the needle or cannula. If, however, an air-lock should be present the apparatus must be disconnected from the needle and blood allowed to run freely through the tubing before it is again connected to the intravenous needle.

(2) The introduction of large volumes of blood, or any other fluid, into the blood-stream can give rise to cardiac and respiratory distress as a result of overloading the circulatory system. This danger is greatest when large quantities of fluid are rapidly introduced, but can occur with a slow transfusion particularly in elderly patients with a weakened heart muscle or chronic anaemia. Signs which should be watched for and reported to the medical officer immediately are: rising pulse rate, laboured breathing, cough, pain in the chest and oedema. A fluid intake and output chart should always be kept for a patient who is receiving parenteral fluid.

(3) A severe reaction occurring soon after the transfusion has been started may be due to incompatibility of the blood and haemolysis of the red cells. The symptoms are: shivering and rise of temperature, the patient may complain of severe pain in the lumbar region. The transfusion must be stopped at once. There is great danger of renal failure due to the blocking of the renal tubules by haemolysed blood cells with subsequent suppression of urine and uraemia. The bottle of blood must be

kept so that investigations can be carried out to discover the cause of the reaction.

(4) Pyrexial reaction due to the introduction of foreign protein into the blood can also give rise to rigors, fever and an increased pulse rate. The rate of the transfusion should be slowed, or the transfusion may have to be stopped.

(5) Thrombosis of the vein is not uncommon. It may be limited in extent and cause little trouble, but if extensive there is considerable pain in the limb and there may be a rise in the patient's temperature. The transfusion may have to be discontinued and a hot application may be ordered for the relief of pain.

(6) A haematoma may form at the site of the transfusion. This results from the needle becoming dislodged from the vein and the blood is then extravasated into the surrounding tissues. The transfusion may be stopped and the limb elevated. An injection of Hyalase may be given into the swollen area. There is some danger when the swelling occurs on the anterior aspect of the forearm and elbow that the arteries supplying the forearm may be compressed and careful watch should be kept on the radial pulse and also on the fingers for blueness and coldness.

(7) Sepsis may occur at the site of the infusion. This is more liable to occur when a cannula is tied into the vein than with the use of an intravenous needle.

(8) Air embolism is a rare occurrence but one which must be borne in mind. It is prevented by making sure that air is entirely expelled from the tubing before the transfusion is started, by taking care that the bottle is not allowed to run dry, and by seeing that the arm into which the transfusion is running is never raised above the level of the patient's heart as this can cause air to be sucked into the vein if the bottle is empty. If it is necessary to increase the rate of flow this can be done by raising the level of the bottle; pressure should never be used to make the blood run faster. The patient may complain of a variety of sensory disturbances, e.g. tingling in the fingers, and may collapse. The immediate treatment is to lower the patient's head.

Transfusion of Plasma and Plasma Substitutes

Dried plasma or serum with sterile pyrogen-free fluid for reconstitution is supplied by the United Kingdom Blood Transfusion Service. Plasma transfusions are most useful in the immediate treatment of severe shock and where large amounts of plasma have been lost as is the case in extensive burns. Dried plasma can be stored indefinitely without deterioration, and can be used in an emergency without waiting for agglutination tests. The main disadvantage of plasma transfusion is the possibility of transmitting serum jaundice, a virus infection (see p. 169). Plasma is expensive and various substitutes are used which have the same osmotic pressure and are also free from danger of virus infection. Examples of these substitutes which are widely used are Dextran and Dextraven, substances which have the necessary viscosity and molecular weight to enable them to act as 'plasma expanders'. The aim here is to avoid strain on the heart and kidneys by maintaining the correct circulatory volume and viscosity.

Plasma substitutes have, however, some disadvantages. They tend to produce rouleaux formation of the red blood cells which makes blood grouping tests more difficult to carry out. Blood samples for grouping should therefore be collected before treatment with intravenous plasma substitute is started. Sensitization reactions are not common, but have been known to occur.

5

Disorders of the cardiovascular system

DISORDERS of the cardiovascular system, as the name implies, includes diseases of the heart and blood vessels and in many countries, particularly those with a high level of 'Western' civilization, this group of disorders is one of the chief causes of ill-health in middle age and old age. Some of the common manifestations of heart disease are diminished exercise tolerance and impaired function of other organs, such as the lungs, digestive system and the kidneys, as a result of decreased efficiency of the circulation of the blood. Pain is not a constant feature, but in some types of heart disease severe pain is a prominent symptom. Abnormalities of the pulse are common in cardiovascular disorders but these, as the student nurse has no doubt already discovered, are not confined to these conditions. However, accurate observations and recording of the rate and other features of the pulse form an extremely important part of the nursing care of cardiac patients and will be discussed in some detail before considering the main groups of cardiovascular diseases.

THE PULSE

The pulse is the wave of distension in the elastic arteries produced as the left ventricle of the heart contracts and pushes blood into the aorta. It can be felt most easily at a point where a large artery is near the skin surface and lies over a bone, the most convenient artery for this purpose being the radial artery on the anterior surface of the wrist. The points to be noted when feeling the pulse are the rate, the volume and the rhythm.

Rate

This is usually between 70 and 88 per min in the adult, but some may have a normal pulse rate as slow as 50 and others as fast as 90 per min. In infancy the pulse rate is more rapid; in the new born infant it is between 120 and 140, and gradually slows to reach the normal adult rate about the age of 11 or 12 years.

An increase in the pulse rate is found in shock, haemorrhage, overactivity of the thyroid gland, disorders of cardiac rhythm (fibrillation and paroxysmal tachycardia), and a failing heart muscle. Some drugs increase the pulse rate, for example atropine and amyl nitrite.

In healthy persons the rate increases with exercise but quickly returns to its normal rate with rest. During sleep the pulse rate may be as much as 10 beats per min slower than during the waking hours. Athletes, as a result of training, often have a relatively slow pulse rate even after strenuous exercise; the heart muscle responds to the demands made upon it by increasing the strength of the contractions rather than their frequency. Strong emotion, such as fear or excitement, has the effect of rapidly accelerating the heart beat. In some persons a persistent, unpleasant or alarming situation produces such cardiac symptoms as rapid pulse rate, dyspnoea, palpitations, pain in the chest, which are not related to any disease of the heart but are psychological in origin.

Pathological decrease in the pulse rate, bradycardia, is found in diseases of the conducting tissue of the heart (heart block), in conditions where raised intracranial pressure stimulates the vagus nerve, for example cerebral tumour or head injuries, or as a result of depression of the vital centres in the brain by drugs, notably morphine.

Volume

Volume indicates the propulsive power of the heart and the volume of fluid in circulation. Thus a pulse may be described as having poor volume, or 'thready', when the heart muscle is failing or when the volume of the circulating blood is decreased as a result of shock or bleeding. A pulse of large volume, described as a bounding pulse, is noted in most fevers.

Rhythm

Normally the spacing and force of the beats is even, but in illness and in health irregularities may occur.

Irregularity can be of two main types. These are sometimes called:

'*Regular irregularity*', in which one beat is missed after every two (pulsus bigeminus) or every three contractions (pulsus trigeminus) with otherwise even rhythm.

'*Irregular irregularity*' when the pulse beats are uneven both in time and force. This is the type which is seen in auricular fibrillation.

Abnormalities in the Pulse Rate and Rhythm

Auricular (Atrial) Fibrillation

This is most commonly present in rheumatic heart disease, especially mitral stenosis, in coronary artery disease and in thyrotoxicosis. The heart rate is irregular both in time and

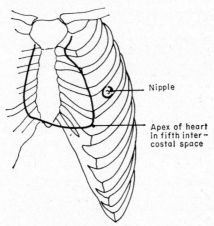

Nipple

Apex of heart in fifth inter-costal space

Fig. 12. Position of apex beat.

force. The auricles (atria) have lost their ordinary rhythmic power of contraction, and a series of small waves pass over them at the rate of about 450 times per min. Only some of these stimulate the ventricles, so that the ventricles may contract at any rate up to about 220 per min. Not all of the contractions are strong enough to give a pulse wave at the wrist, so the radial pulse rate is less than the ventricular rate. This discrepancy which is known as the pulse deficit, is characteristic.

To ensure accuracy in recording the contractions, the heart apex beat (Fig. 12) should be counted and complete reliance is not placed upon the radial pulse rate. All nurses should accustom themselves to counting the heart beats through a stethoscope, so that this can be recorded in cases where it is especially important. The radial pulse rate is also taken and the two marked on the chart in differently coloured inks, or reported as apex rate over pulse rate, e.g. $\dfrac{136\ A}{90\ R}$ The difference between the two numbers is the pulse deficit, i.e. in the example given the figure is 46.

Treatment. Fibrillation due to organic heart-disease is usually treated by the administration of digitalis in doses large enough to keep the heart beat at a more normal rate, and it does so by cutting out the minor ventricular contractions and thus making the rate slower and the individual contractions stronger. The drug will probably have to be continued permanently. Some preparations in use are:

Digitalis Tablets, B.P.
Digoxin Tablets, B.P.
Digoxin Injection, B.P.

The usual procedure is to give a large initial dose by mouth, or by intravenous injection if very rapid digitalization is necessary, followed by a smaller maintenance dosage. For example, an initial dose of 1·5 mg or more of digoxin in tablet form may be given spread over a period of 24 hr, followed by a maintenance dose of 0·25 to 0·5 mg daily.

Signs of overdose must be watched for, as the drug is excreted more slowly than it is absorbed. These are slowing of the pulse rate to below 60 per min from an initially high pulse, e.g. 180 beats per min, in a short period. Before giving a dose of digitalis it is important to check the heart apex rate and compare the last recorded rate with the present one. A rapid decrease in rate is dangerous, and no further dose should be given without reporting and seeking medical advice. Other signs of digitalis overdose are coupling of the pulse, vomiting, diarrhoea and decrease in the output of urine.

In cardiac failure with oedema any improvement in the circulation produces diuresis, and the urinary output must be carefully measured. If a reduction in the amount of urine passed occurs in any patient taking digitalis this fact must be reported, as the drug may be accumulating in the blood-stream with consequent toxic effects.

Quinidine is also used in selected cases, particularly if the fibrillation is of recent onset in a young patient. A test dose is usually given first to exclude idiosyncrasy to quinidine. The patient must be kept lying flat in bed and carefully watched whilst this drug is being taken, so that no unnecessary exertion is made, as sudden collapse may occur. Dizziness, dyspnoea and palpitations are signs which indicate intolerance.

Ventricular Fibrillation

Ventricular fibrillation continuing for any length of time is incompatible with life, since under such circumstances the heart cannot maintain the circulation. Normal rhythm may be restored by the use of the electric defibrillator and while the apparatus is being prepared resuscitation and cardiac massage must be instituted and continued for as long as is necessary.

Auricular (Atrial) Flutter

Auricular flutter is a condition similar to auricular fibrillation, but the contractions are regular as a rule, those of the ventricle being about half those of the auricle (atrium) which may be 250 per min. It may occur in arteriosclerosis, myocarditis and sometimes after acute infection.

Treatment. This is the same as for auricular fibrillation, digitalis being the drug usually prescribed.

Premature Contraction (Extrasystole)

Extrasystole is a common form of irregularity in which an abnormal stimulus in either the auricle or the ventricle causes a contraction, which may be too weak to reach the wrist, before the anticipated time. As the ventricle is not ready to carry out the normal contraction, a longer interval before the next beat then follows and the pulse at the radial artery appears to have missed a beat.

The patient feels the contraction of the heart after the prolonged pause as a 'thump'.

This irregularity occurs in persons with normal hearts but may be a sign of myocardial disease, raised blood pressure, or some toxic agents, e.g. tobacco, or sepsis.

The treatment is that of the condition found in association with it, if there be one.

Sinus Arrhythmia

In sinus arrhythmia the rate of the pulse is increased in inspiration and lessened with expiration, due to respiratory associaton with the nerve control of the sino-auricular (sino-atrial) node. It is common in children, is not pathological and no treatment is necessary.

Paroxysmal Tachycardia

Paroxysmal tachycardia is an attack of tachycardia, which starts suddenly and terminates as abruptly, the pulse rate being 150 or more per min, but unlike the rapid pulse found in auricular fibrillation there is no irregularity of rhythm. The condition is common in young adults and no myocardial disease may be evident. In older persons and those with a history of cardiac disease the condition is more serious. Oedema, congestion of the lungs and other signs of heart failure may occur as a result of repeated and prolonged attacks and the patient may suffer from anginal pain. He complains of shortness of breath and feels the 'flutter' of the heart in the chest.

Treatment. The patient may be able to stop the attack by holding his breath and contracting the abdominal muscles, or by putting his head between his knees. Pressure first on one carotid sinus where the carotid artery is felt in the neck at the side of the trachea, for about 10 sec and then pressure on the carotid artery on the opposite side, is often effective. Sedatives such as barbiturates or a tranquillizing drug, e.g. chlorpromazine, may be prescribed. Improvement of the general health and avoidance of causes which appear to precipitate the symptoms are helpful. Quinidine or procainamide hydrochloride (Pronestyl) may be ordered.

Heart Block

Heart block results from failure of the conducting tissue in the heart to transmit all impulses from the auricles to the ventricles. Every other impulse may be checked (incomplete or two-to-one heart block) or all may be interrupted (complete heart block) when the ventricles take on a rhythm of their own at a rate of about 35 per min.

Toxins of infectious diseases, e.g. rheumatic fever or diphtheria, syphilitic disease of the heart and myocardial infarction are some of the possible causes of heart block. Overdose of digitalis causes partial heart block.

In any of these cases complete standstill may occur, lasting for some seconds and give rise to Stokes–Adams attacks in which there is cessation of the pulse for several seconds, so that if the number of beats are counted for a complete minute the total is about 6 to 8 beats. Convulsions, unconsciousness and sudden death may occur, especially when the condition is due to myocardial failure.

Treatment. Absolute rest is essential and the cause must be treated, for example, if the condition is due to syphilis, antisyphilitic treatment is necessary. Stokes–Adams attacks are treated by injections of adrenaline. Ephedrine or isoprenaline, in the form of sublingual tablets, is given to patients with heart block to prevent these attacks. Pacemakers are frequently used; the internal pacemaker requires the operation of thoracotomy— two electrodes are placed in the heart to stimulate rhythmic contractions at a rate of 35 or more per min. These electrodes are connected to an internal battery and using such a device the patient may return to normal life. The batteries have to be recharged at intervals, varying from 1 to 2 years. Electronic and atomic devices may be used which increase this interval.

BLOOD PRESSURE

Hyperpiesis or hypertension, raised blood pressure, is frequently related to acute or chronic renal disease where there is impairment of renal circulation, and much experimental work is being done on the cause of this rise in pressure. When hypertension occurs with no evidence of renal disorder it is known as essential hypertension, and is often associated with arteriosclerosis. Therefore it is a condition which is most often seen in the later years of life, although it is not entirely unknown in the young. Usually the hypertension increases gradually, but there is a particularly acute and progressive form, with poor prognosis, known as malignant hypertension.

Raised blood pressure may cause no symptoms until or unless cardiac, cerebral or renal complications ensue; sometimes there may be a complaint of frequent headaches. As has already been mentioned, hypertension can be a cause of left ventricular failure. Cerebral haemorrhage due to rupture of a blood-vessel is perhaps the commonest complication, less commonly renal failure may supervene.

Treatment

In progressive order, according to the increasing severity of the hypertension, the following hypotensive (pressure-reducing) drugs are commonly prescribed:

(1) Mild sedatives such as small doses of phenobarbitone.

(2) Chlorothiazide, a diuretic drug with some hypotensive effect.

(3) Drugs which block both sympathetic and parasympathetic nerve ganglia, e.g. mecamylamine (Inversine), pempidine (Perolysen), methyldopa (Aldomet) orally, and hexamethonium by injection.

(4) Drugs which block the sympathetic nerves only, e.g. guanethidine (Ismelin), bethanidine (Estabal) given orally.

Large doses of pressure-reducing drugs can produce symptoms of hypotension, dizziness and faintness when standing, and the patient needs to be warned of this possibility. Constipation may be troublesome following the administration of the drug mentioned under (4) above and a laxative such as Senakot or Dulcolax tablets may be ordered. Guanethidine may cause diarrhoea.

A low-sodium diet is sometimes ordered, and patients who are overweight will benefit from a reducing diet aimed at a gradual reduction in weight; otherwise a special diet is not required unless necessitated by some complicating factor.

High blood pressure, or simply 'blood pressure', has a sinister meaning for the lay person. A simple explanation of the situation usually allays fear and gains the co-operation of the patient and his family. A placid attitude to the minor irritations of life and a tranquil home environment are a great help to the hypertensive patient.

Hypopiesis describes a low blood pressure unrelated to any obvious organic disease. It may be due to loss of muscle tone, especially in the small arteries (hypotension or hypotonia).

Anaemia may be a cause of hypotension, or it may be associated with excessive fatigue. In some cases the blood pressure may fall on change of position, e.g. on standing upright, when it is called orthostatic hypotension.

SOME SPECIAL INVESTIGATIONS USED IN CARDIOVASCULAR DISEASE

The Electrocardiogram

An electrocardiogram is a graphic record of the fluctuation in the electrical current produced by the heart muscle during the cardiac cycle of systole and diastole. This examination is of value in a number of conditions such as cardiac arrhythmia, heart block, congenital heart disease and myocardial infarction.

Interpretation of the electrocardiogram is made by comparing the pattern recorded with normal cardiac pattern. Not all heart diseases produce abnormal electrocardiograms, and it is possible that variation from the normal pattern can be found in persons who have no cardiac disease.

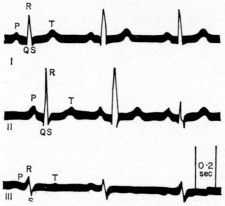

FIG. 13. Normal electrocardiogram.

The normal electrocardiogram. The record obtained is illustrated in Fig. 13. It consists of a series of five main deflections of an electrical wave, namely PQRST. The P wave is due to the auricular contraction. The QRST waves are due to the ventricular contraction. The time interval between the beginning of the P wave and the beginning of the Q (or if absent, R wave) is termed P–R interval and normally is within 0·2 of a second. The time interval from the beginning of the Q (or if absent, R wave) to the end of the S wave (termed the QRS complex when normal) must be within 0·1 of a second.

Monitoring of heart activity. In many cases of acute heart disease a continuous record is made of the heart's activity and the electrocardiograph is shown continuously on a screen similar to a television set. Such apparatus normally has an alarm system fitted so that a bell rings in cases of cardiac arrest.

X-Ray Examinations

(1) An X-ray of the chest will show the outline of the heart and give information as to its size and position, it will also show the presence of pericardial effusion.

(2) **Cardiac catheterization.** This is chiefly used in investigation of the particular type of defect, or combination of defects in congenital malformations of the heart. A long radio-opaque catheter is passed into a vein in the right elbow; its passage through the brachial vein, the innominate vein, the superior vena cava into the right side of the heart is watched under the X-ray screen (Fig. 14). Samples of blood can be obtained from the vena cava, right auricle, right ventricle, and the pulmonary artery. The tip of the catheter may be able to demonstrate an aperture in the septum of the heart.

(3) **Angiocardiography.** This is an investigation of the heart and great blood-vessels after the direct injection of a radio-opaque medium, e.g. diodone, into a vein or artery through a catheter. Serial radiographs are taken immediately after the injection. For examination of the aorta in suspected coarction (narrowing of the vessel) or aneurysm, the catheter may be introduced either into the right brachial or the common carotid artery. In the case of an investigation of the right side of the heart in Fallot's tetralogy or in patent ductus arteriosus (see p. 105) the catheter is introduced into the right cephalic vein at the elbow or the right saphenous vein of the thigh.

As a considerable quantity of the iodine opaque compound has to be used in this examination there is a possibility of iodine poisoning occurring, with dizziness, shock and collapse. Some individuals are particularly sensitive to iodine and a sensitivity test may be carried out before this examination. The patient is given a small dose of the contrast medium; if he has an idiosyncrasy to iodine symptoms of upper respiratory catarrh appear.

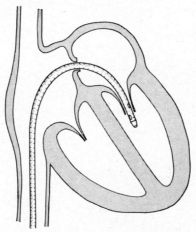

FIG. 14. Cardiac catheterization demonstrating an atrial-septal defect

A local anaesthetic is generally sufficient for adult patients undergoing these examinations, but a general anaesthetic is usually given to a child.

DISEASES OF THE HEART

'Heart disease' suggests to the lay person a condition in which the sufferer can only hope to survive if he leads the life of a complete invalid and which is likely to cause his death at any moment. It is a well-known fact that a large number of the deaths occurring suddenly in middle age, particularly amongst men of the business and professional groups, are due to heart failure resulting from disease of the arteries supplying the heart muscle. Less generally appreciated is the fact that many people with damaged hearts are still able to lead useful, active lives. Advances in medical knowledge continue to discover means of treating some conditions where there was previously little hope of improvement, as for example remedying congenital defects by successful surgery and the use of antibacterial drugs in some infective conditions.

However, in any medical ward a considerable proportion of the patients of all ages occupying the beds at any given time are suffering from some form of cardiac illness, and the nurse should understand the causes which may be responsible for the failure of the heart muscle to work with its normal efficiency.

The following classification gives the main heart diseases:

(1) Congenital defects.
(2) Chronic rheumatic heart disease.
(3) Ischaemic and hypertensive heart disease associated with atheroma of the coronary arteries.
(4) Heart disease secondary to chronic lung disease (cor pulmonale).
(5) Syphilitic heart disease.
(6) Heart disease due to thyrotoxicosis, acute infections and, more rarely, other toxic causes.

Congenital Heart Disease

Various forms of developmental errors in the structure of the heart can occur (Fig. 15); the defect may be so gross that it is incompatible with life, or on the other hand it may have little effect on the efficiency of the heart. Not all children with congenital heart disease are 'blue babies'; there are several types of congenital defect which do not cause cyanosis, for example atrial septal defect and ventricular septal defect, when a hole in the septum between the left and right sides of the heart allows some blood to be forced through from the left side to the right (left to right shunt); patent ductus arteriosis, when this vessel, which is necessary for the fetus but normally closes at birth, remains patent and some of the blood pumped into the aorta from the left ventricle passes through the ductus arteriosus back into the pulmonary artery; coarction or narrowing of the aorta which requires additional effort from the heart muscle to get the blood through the narrowed opening.

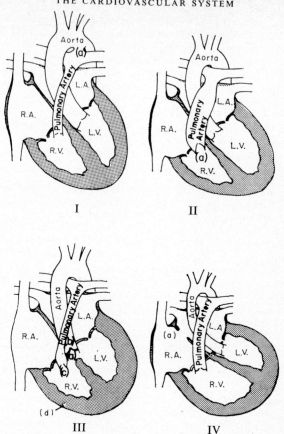

FIG. 15. Congenital malformations of the heart and great vessels. (I) Patent ductus arteriosus (a). (II) Pulmonary valvular stenosis (a). (III) Fallot's tetralogy: (a) ventricular septal defect, (b) dextro position of aorta, (c) pulmonary valvular stenosis, (d) thickened wall of right ventricle. (IV) Atrial septal defect (a).

The cyanotic form of congenital heart disease of which the combination of defects known as Fallot's tetralogy is the commonest type, gives the typical picture of a child with serious circulatory impairment, whose life is likely to be restricted and brief unless the defects can be remedied. Fortunately the outlook in this and in other congenital cardiac conditions has improved considerably with the recent advances in cardiac surgery which have made it possible to repair septal defects, 'holes in the heart', and deal with other mechanical faults by valvotomy and operations on the blood-vessels.

Chronic Rheumatic Heart Disease

Chronic rheumatic disease of the heart often follows an attack of acute rheumatic fever or chorea, but sometimes arises without any previous history of such an illness.

The rheumatic condition is generally ascribed to the allergic effect of a streptococcal infection which damages serous membranes, particularly those of the joints, and the tissues of the heart. In some patients the infection affects the tissues of the brain and in this case the obvious manifestation is chorea, a condition characterized by jerky restless movements; in these cases the heart is also often damaged.

When the acute stage of the illness subsides the cardiac condition may also clear up completely, but in a proportion of cases the valves of the heart are permanently damaged, so that they do not close completely, thus allowing blood to regurgitate through the valve and at the same time when the valve is open the orifice which it guards is narrowed, making it more difficult for the blood to be pumped through. The valve most commonly affected is the mitral valve, between the left auricle and ventricle; less frequently the aortic valve in the left ventricle at the opening of the aorta is damaged. In suitable cases, where the chief defect is narrowing or stenosis of the valve, the operation of valvotomy is performed, but, particularly if the heart is further damaged by repeated rheumatic infection, there is always the possibility of congestive cardiac failure supervening. Other complications include auricular fibrillation as a result of the dilation of the left auricle, embolism and infection of the damaged valves with the development of subacute bacterial endocarditis.

Subacute bacterial endocarditis is an inflammation of the endocardium occurring in patients who have an existing valvular disease or congenital defect. The organism responsible is usually the *Streptococcus viridans*, and it reaches the heart via the blood-stream. Irregular masses of fibrinous clot containing the organisms are deposited on the valves and are known as vegetations. Small emboli from these vegetations may be carried to any part of the body. In the skin small purpuric spots appear and in the deeper tissues, particularly in the extremities, painful hard lumps. Clubbing of the fingers is often noted. Emboli cause local pain and symptoms wherever they occur, for example in the brain, spleen, kidneys and joints.

The constitutional symptoms are fever, malaise, lassitude, loss of appetite and loss of weight. The onset is often insidious and the temperature may be only intermittently raised and then only $0.5°$ to $1°C$ ($1°$ to $2°F$). Anaemia is progressive, and the patient looks ill and pale, sometimes with a distinctive tinge in the skin described as a 'cafe-au-lait' colour. The treatment of acute bacterial endocarditis is the administration of large doses of penicillin, 4 mega-units or more daily. Streptomycin may be combined with penicillin. The disease if untreated is fatal, and before the antibiotic era there was no cure. It is still a very serious condition, death may occur from emboli in the brain, kidney or mesenteric blood-vessels, or the added cardiac damage may result in congestive cardiac failure.

Ischaemic and Hypertensive Heart Disease

Ischaemic and hypertensive heart disease is caused by a diminution in the blood supply to the heart and is usually due to atheroma of the coronary arteries and their branches. Hypertension throws a strain on the left ventricle and these two causes of heart disease often co-exist. Atheroma narrows the lumen on the blood-vessels by the deposition of plaques of fatty material in their walls. A clot of blood, or thrombus, may form on the plaques so that a blood-vessel may be blocked either by the atheromatous deposit or by a blood clot or by a combination of these factors. Because thrombus formation was thought to be the cause of blockage in these cases, the condition has been called coronary thrombosis until recent years but, as the actual cause of the obstruction can be determined only by post-mortem examination, the term myocardial infarct is now commonly used because death of tissue, or infarction, will always occur in that area of the myocardium which loses its blood supply from whatever cause. Atheroma is often, but not always, associated with a raised blood pressure.

The severity of the symptoms of ischaemic heart disease will depend on the degree of interference with the blood supply to the heart muscle. If the heart is still able to meet most of the demands made upon it, signs of diminished blood supply will only be shown when some extra effort is required. This effort produces pain which is known as angina, or angina pectoris; its characteristic feature is that it is always associated with effort and ceases with rest. It varies in severity and is felt behind the sternum, radiating to the left shoulder and down the left arm, and sometimes also the right arm. Exposure to cold, emotion and exertion after a heavy meal are factors which may precipitate an attack.

The attacks may increase in severity and frequency, and death may occur from coronary occlusion. Coronary occlusion, i.e. complete blocking of a branch or branches of a coronary artery, causes a myocardial infarction; an area of the heart muscle is deprived of its blood supply and this area therefore degenerates.

The cutting off of the blood supply causes acute pain, lasting longer than that of anginal attacks which is relieved as soon as the spasm responsible for it ceases. Infarction is more serious, as on its extent depends whether the area of heart muscle not affected is sufficient in amount and in strength to maintain the circulation and therefore the life of the patient following acute myocardial infarction. This disaster may be immediately fatal and is the commonest cause of sudden death (see p. 110 on 'Cardiac Arrest'). In many cases, however, the damage is not so extensive and the patient survives; the symptoms are severe pain in the chest similar in distribution to anginal pain, but it is not associated with exertion and does not cease with rest. Nausea and vomiting sometimes accompany the attack. The patient shows signs of shock, the skin is cold and sweaty, the pulse is rapid and the blood pressure falls. The patient may die within a few hours or days of the onset and further attacks are liable to occur; however, a considerable proportion of patients survive and may lead a reasonably active life for many years.

Some 24 hr after the onset the patient may have a moderate degree of fever, which is associated with necrosis of the myocardial infarct. There is always the danger of congestive cardiac failure following an infarct, and the damaged heart muscle may show various types of arrhythmia, such as ventricular tachycardia, auricular fibrillation and heart block. Other possible complications are pulmonary oedema, venous thrombosis, usually in the legs, pulmonary embolism and arterial embolism.

Treatment

The treatment of anginal attacks is to give nitrites in some form; these drugs have a rapid but transient effect on the coronary arteries, causing them to dilate. The usual preparation is Glyceryl Trinitrate Tablets, B.P., which must be chewed slowly and not swallowed whole. The patient must learn to regulate his life within the limits imposed by his anginal pain. If it is imperative that he should make some effort which usually brings on an attack he can take one or two of the tablets before undertaking this exertion. In general he must learn to avoid circumstances that may precipitate an attack, such as hurrying to catch a train, sudden exposure to cold and heavy meals. If he can cultivate a placid attitude of mind and not be readily roused to anger or excitement this is all to the good. Overweight patients benefit by a reduction in weight, which must, however, be gradual and under medical supervision.

The immediate treatment of coronary occlusion and myocardial infarct is the treatment of shock and the administration of morphine to relieve pain; 15 mg of this drug is given and repeated in one hour if this is necessary. Complete rest in bed in the most comfortable position is essential, and every effort should be made to allay the patient's anxiety. Severe degrees of shock may require the use of vasopressor drugs, e.g. noradrenaline (Levophed), and oxygen may be necessary for the relief of dyspnoea accompanied by cyanosis. Anticoagulant drugs are often used to reduce the risk of the blood clot in the coronary artery spreading, the development of further clotting and the possibility of pulmonary embolism. Heparin is a rapidly acting anti-coagulant, and is usually given intravenously for immediate effect. Oral anticoagulants can be given to maintain the action, and one such drug in general use is phenindione

(Dindevan). The individual dosage required is checked in every case by examination of the blood in order to determine the prothrombin level; at first this is done daily and the dose withheld until the result of the examination is known. Overdosage may cause bleeding into the tissue or from the nose, the urinary tract or the rectum, and careful watch must be kept for signs of such bleeding. Phytomenadione (Konakion) Vit. K is a specific antidote should bleeding occur. Recently the value of anticoagulants in the treatment of coronary thrombosis has been questioned and in some cases their use has been abandoned.

The period of rest in bed depends on the severity of the attack and medical opinion is divided as to its value, but in all but mild cases the patient is encouraged to rest in bed for most of the day for about 7 days, although usually he is allowed up to use a commode, and then resumption of any further activities must be gradual. For a further 2 weeks he slowly resumes a more active life, first sitting out of bed for increasing periods, later walking around the bedroom, and then being allowed to go to the bathroom and toilet. A month of convalescence follows, and if all goes well at the end of 3 months from the date of his attack, the patient may be allowed to work provided this does not involve mental or physical strain.

Throughout the illness the nurse must be constantly on the alert for signs of complications. Such symptoms as dyspnoea, and haemoptysis, suggests the presence of pulmonary embolism, pain in the calf of the leg is a symptom of venous thrombosis. Substernal pain with dyspnoea, irregularities of the cardiac rhythm and oedema are indications of further damage to the heart or the onset of cardiac failure. Having said this, it is necessary to add that encouragement and a cheerful atmosphere will help the patient to accept his present condition and to look forward to the time when he can again lead a normal, though possibly somewhat restricted life.

Cardiac Arrest

This may occur due to the diminished supply of oxygenated blood to the heart muscle. Unless the heart is restarted within 3 minutes the lack of oxygen to the brain cells will cause irreparable damage.

With the patient lying flat the heart should be massaged by

placing the heel of both hands on top of one another over the lower part of the sternum, depressing it firmly and then releasing at a rate of 12 times per min. At the same time oxygen should be got to the lungs by mouth-to-mouth respiration. Medical help must be obtained immediately.

Both these techniques should be learnt and practised on a dummy so that proficiency is gained. The length of time such a technique is continued is decided by the doctor. It will not be successful in all cases and the nurse must realize that final control over life and death is not in her hands. The decision when to resuscitate or not is a difficult medical one but generally the method is only successful in cases of acute arrest and not useful in chronic disease.

Heart Disease Secondary to Chronic Lung Disease (Cor Pulmonale)

Cardiac failure is a not uncommon complication of long-standing chronic diseases of the lung, such as bronchitis and silicosis, with fibrotic changes, and emphysema. The patient will give a history of chronic chest disease and is likely to have a productive cough and considerable dyspnoea.

Treatment is aimed at clearing any respiratory infection that may be underlying the condition, together with rest in bed and appropriate measures according to the degree of congestive cardiac failure present (see p. 113).

Syphilitic Heart Disease

Syphilitic infection may attack the aorta or the aortic valve. Syphilitic aortitis produces weakening of the wall of the artery and the development of an aortic aneurysm. Disease of the aortic valve causes the cusps to become thickened and shrunken resulting in aortic regurgitation. When the left ventricle contracts to pump the blood into the aorta the valve should open completely and then close after the contraction to prevent blood regurgitating back into the ventricle. If the aortic valve is incompetent the ventricular muscle has to work harder in order to empty the ventricle. So long as the muscle is able to do this it can compensate for the defective valve, but in so doing the ventricle becomes dilated and hypertrophied. When compensation fails symptoms of congestive cardiac failure appear.

Syphilitic disease may also involve the coronary arteries, producing anginal pain and possibly coronary occlusion.

Treatment

If syphilis is proved to be the underlying cause, appropriate antibiotic therapy, usually penicillin, is indicated. The heart symptoms require the same treatment as those arising from any cause.

Heart Disease Caused by Thyrotoxicosis or Other Toxic Factors

Thyrotoxicosis and other toxic conditions, such as acute infections, are liable to lead to auricular fibrillation and congestive cardiac failure. If the toxic state can be controlled, for example by drugs, radioactive iodine, or surgical operation in the case of thyrotoxicosis, the cardiac condition will usually disappear or improve, but if persistent will require the appropriate treatment for auricular fibrillation or cardiac failure from any cause.

Pericarditis

Inflammation of the pericardium may be due to a variety of causes, such as rheumatic heart disease, myocardial infarct from coronary occlusion, uraemia, some infectious diseases, including tuberculosis, and from secondary new growths invading the pericardium.

Pericarditis without effusion usually causes few symptoms apart from pain, which in some cases is very severe and similar to the pain of myocardial infarction.

Pericarditis with effusion may interfere with the action of the heart, reducing the cardiac output and blocking the venous return; this condition is known as 'cardiac tamponade'.

Chronic constrictive pericarditis produces a hard fibrotic pericardium, sometimes with calcium deposits, and is almost always due to tuberculous infection. The constriction obstructs the venous return to the heart and produces symptoms very similar to congestive cardiac failure with oedema and ascites.

Treatment

The cause of the pericarditis is treated, for example salicylates in the treatment of acute rheumatic fever and antibiotics for tuberculous and other types of bacterial infection. Pain may be so severe as to require the administration of analgesics such as codeine or, in some cases, morphine. Oxygen is useful if dyspnoea and cyanosis are present.

Pericardial effusion which is hampering the heart's action may be drained by aspiration with a 20-ml syringe and a suitable needle. Constrictive pericarditis is treated surgically by removal of as much as possible of the thickened pericardium.

Patients suffering from pericarditis need careful nursing. Rest in bed in the most comfortable position, usually semi-recumbent, is essential. The patient with a pericardial effusion should be carefully lifted for such nursing attention as making his bed and care of pressure areas; turning the patient from side to side is not allowed as this may further embarrass the action of the heart. He should not be allowed to undertake any exertion, such as feeding himself or washing his own face and hands and cleaning his teeth, until the physician gives permission. At least 4 weeks' rest in bed is usually required.

Congestive Cardiac Failure

All the cardiac diseases previously mentioned may lead to the condition of congestive heart failure, when the cardiac muscle is no longer able to maintain an efficient circulation. There is pulmonary congestion and a raised venous pressure. Retention of sodium and water in the tissues leads to oedema.

The first symptoms that the patient complains of are usually breathlessness, which he first notices on mild exertion and later when he is at rest, swelling of the feet and ankles, and 'indigestion', possibly nausea and vomiting. He may also say that he has poor nights and feels irritable and depressed.

Examination reveals venous congestion in the veins of the neck, a rapid pulse which is often irregular in rhythm due to auricular fibrillation and decreased output of urine, which often contains protein. Oedema is due to salt retention, and as the condition progresses the dependent parts of the body, the legs when the patient is up, the thighs, abdomen, and back when he is in bed, become grossly swollen with fluid. Oedematous fluid also tends to collect in the serous cavities of the peritoneum and pleura; these collections are known as ascites and hydrothorax respectively.

The symptoms relating to the alimentary tract, nausea and vomiting, tenderness over the liver and the decreased efficiency of the kidneys, are due to venous engorgement.

Increasing dyspnoea adds to the patient's discomfort, and often he can only breathe with any degree of ease if he is sitting upright and leaning forward; this condition is known as orthopnoea.

Pulmonary congestion is also shown by cough and sputum which may be blood-stained; more marked haemoptysis is due to an infarct in the lung, and the patient may complain of pain in the chest due to pleurisy. Patients with marked pulmonary congestion and oedema may suffer from paroxymal attacks of acute dyspnoea which usually occur at night when the patient wakes up struggling to breathe. The condition is known as 'cardiac asthma'. Distressing cough with the expectoration of large quantities of water sputum indicates pulmonary oedema, a serious complication of cardiac failure.

Treatment

General nursing care. The first principle of treatment is rest; the heart muscle has a chance to recover some of its power if the demands made upon it can be reduced to a minimum. The position in which the greatest degree of rest can be ensured is almost always sitting upright, well supported with pillows. A bed table and pillow on which the patient can lean forward and rest his arms often help to give him a slight change of position and to assist his breathing difficulties. He can be supported in the sitting position with his legs hanging down, so that oedema will tend to collect in the legs rather than in the abdomen; this will also help to make him comfortable. A 'cardiac bedstead' which can be adjusted to a chair position is very useful, but if this is not available the patient may spend part of the day in a comfortable armchair. Sleep is important, and a careful note should be made of the number of hours' sleep that the patient gets in a 24 hr period; if necessary a hypnotic will be ordered, such as phenobarbitone 30 to 120 mg, or paraldehyde, 5 to 10 ml by intramuscular injection. In some cases morphine, 10 to 15 mg, may be necessary. Measures that can be taken to promote the patient's comfort at bedtime include a light and easily digestible evening meal, remaking the bed and providing warmth if necessary by an extra light blanket or wrap round his shoulders, ensuring adequate ventilation without draughts, and seeing that the patient has an opportunity of emptying his bladder before settling to sleep.

Care of the areas of the body subjected to pressure often presents difficulty. Since the patient must remain in the sitting position day and night it is essential to relieve the pressure on the buttocks by the use of an air-ring, sponge rubber ring or sheep skin pad. The skin over oedematous tissue is particularly liable to break down and form a sore and constant care is necessary. Three nurses may be needed to give adequate attention to the washing and massage of the back of a heavy, oedematous and dyspnoeic patient.

While the patient requires complete rest and is not allowed to exert himself bed-bathing must be skilfully carried out, and again adequate help is necessary to move the patient and to ensure that all areas of the skin are properly washed and also inspected for any sign of redness.

Measurement of the daily urinary output must be kept. Constipation will require a mild aperient or a rectal glycerin or Dulcolax suppository. If the patient is spending part of the day in a chair, or if permission is given for him to sit out of bed, he will often use a bedside commode more comfortably than a bedpan.

Discretion with regard to visiting and visitors may be needed; the patient should not be over-tired or worried by domestic or business matters, but a short daily visit from members of his family or close friends who can talk to him cheerfully and interestingly helps to prevent boredom.

Diet at first must be light, and small dry meals are less likely to cause gastric discomfort than a fluid diet. Sodium is usually restricted, and no additional salt is allowed, although a small amount may be used in cooking. Carbohydrates, such as toast, biscuits and sugar; proteins, in the form of fish, chicken and eggs, prepared in various ways, are the main constituents of the diet. Adequate nutrition is important and vitamin supplements may be ordered.

Medical treatment. Digitalis increases the efficiency of the heart muscle, and is one of the main drugs used in the treatment of congestive cardiac failure. It is particularly useful if auricular fibrillation is a feature (see p. 95).

Oedema is treated mainly by the administration of diuretics, although in ascites and hydrothorax fluid may need to be removed by paracentesis. The mercurial diuretics have been successfully used for many years, and mersalyl by intramuscular injection and mercaptomerin by subcutaneous injection are examples of this group of diuretics. Ammonium chloride is often ordered to increase the action of these mercurial diuretics. Oral diuretics such as chlorothiazide such as Frusemide (Lasix) is one of the diuretics which is often used. It is convenient as its action is immediate, and also it can be given either by intravenous injection or orally: dose, 40 to 120 mg. Following the administration of any of these diuretics very large amounts of urine are passed and the measurement must be carefully recorded.

Mechanical methods of reducing oedema include:

(1) Paracentesis of the abdomen, using a large trocar and cannula, or a small Southey's tube, inserted into the left or right iliac fossa. It is essential that the bladder should be empty before the trocar is introduced.

(2) Paracentesis of the pleural cavity, using an aspirating needle and a syringe with a two-way stopcock.

(3) Acupuncture of the legs, i.e. small incisions made into the superficial tissues to allow the fluid to drain, or the insertion of Southey's tubes into the oedematous tissues.

All these procedures must be carried out with strict aseptic precautions; infection readily occurs in oedematous tissue. With the effective use of diuretic drugs these mechanical methods of treating oedema of cardiac origin are now seldom used.

Pulmonary oedema may require the administration of oxygen and venesection. Morphine is given, possibly with atropine, and an intravenous injection of aminophylline. In acute pulmonary oedema with hypertensive heart failure, one of the hypotensive drugs, e.g. hexamethonium, may be given intravenously.

Improvement in the heart's action is shown by decreasing dyspnoea and oedema, and increased appetite. The patient is able to lie back on his pillows, and with better nights and less discomfort his mental outlook improves. While complete rest is essential in severe degrees of cardiac failure, gradual return to activity marks the recovery stage. The patient is first encouraged to move about more freely in bed and to help himself. The physiotherapist may be asked to teach and supervise leg exercises and breathing exercises.

As the patient will have to live within the limits imposed by the state of his heart muscle, he and his relatives need help in planning the type of diet that will suit him, the amount of activity he can undertake, the understanding of his condition and the importance of keeping his regular appointments for medical examination. Some rearrangement of living conditions may be advisable, and the social worker will help here, for example a cardiac patient living in an upper storey flat without a lift may be found other more suitable accommodation.

Although the patient must lead a quiet existence, he should be encouraged to live his necessarily restricted life to the full: too great an insistence on inactivity is not good for the patient's morale or that of his family and, furthermore, too much rest favours venous thrombosis. How far the patient himself should be told of the seriousness of his cardiac condition and the prognosis is a matter for the decision of his doctor in view of all the circumstances in the individual case.

DISEASES OF THE ARTERIES

Aortitis and Aneurysm

Aortitis is a chronic inflammatory condition in which the elastic wall of the artery undergoes a fibrotic degeneration, and local stretching of the weakened wall may produce a swelling which is known as an aneurysm. Syphilis is one of the commoner causes of aortitis; this usually affects the arch of the aorta, and is often associated with inflammation of the aortic valves of the heart.

There are three types of aneurysm (Fig. 16), described as: (a) fusiform, (b) saccular (according to their shape), and (c) dissecting. A dissecting aneurysm is caused by separation of the coats of the arterial wall and bleeding into the separated layers. It is usually a complication of arteriosclerosis.

Symptoms of aortitis are pain in the chest and, probably, heart failure due to aortic valve incompetence. An aneurysm will cause signs and symptoms of local pressure. An aneurysm of the aortic arch can be seen and felt as a pulsating tumour. There may be difficulty in swallowing as a result of pressure on the oesophagus, and dyspnoea due to pressure on the air passages. As the swelling increases in size it erodes bone, and may destroy areas of the vertebral column or the sternum.

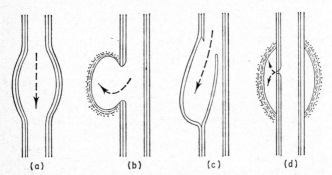

FIG. 16. Types of aneurysms: (a) fusiform, (b) saccular, (c) dissecting (showing blood leaking *between* the layers of the vessel), and (d) false (showing blood leaking *out* of the vessel to form a swelling enclosed in fibrous tissue).

Dissecting aneurysms are liable to produce symptoms similar to coronary occlusions and myocardial infarct. The patient experiences a sudden agonizing pain, and collapses with severe shock; death commonly occurs shortly after the initial attack.

Treatment

If aortitis is due to syphilis then antisyphilitic treatment is indicated (see p. 351). Aortic aneurysm may be treated surgically; the weakened area is replaced by arterial graft or by a synthetic Dacron or Teflon graft. As a palliative measure attempts may be made, for example by the insertion of silver wire, to produce clotting along the walls of the aneurysm. Rupture of an aortic aneurysm is a constant risk, and should it occur blood will escape into the trachea, bronchi and oeso-phagus with inevitable death.

Arteriosclerosis

'Arteriosclerosis' means hardening of the arteries and, is a degenerative change in which the walls of the vessels become less elastic, thickened, or sometimes calcified. Atheromatous plaques, already referred to under coronary occlusion, may obstruct the vessels. There is an hereditary tendency to the development of arteriosclerosis, but in most individuals advancing age takes its toll and the blood-vessels share in the degenerative changes of senility.

There is no effective treatment for the condition, but it is not incompatible with a reasonably active life. Moderation in alcohol and tobacco are usually advised. The complications of arteriosclerosis are coronary occlusion, renal failure and cerebral haemorrhage.

Intermittent Claudication

Intermittent claudication is a symptom of arterial disease in which there is reduced circulation to the lower limbs (or limb), thereby causing severe muscular pain on walking which ceases with rest. The condition may occur as a manifestation of thrombo-angiitis obliterans, an inflammatory condition of the arteries and veins in the legs, or of arteriosclerosis. Gangrene may result if efficient circulation is not maintained.

Treatment

Adequate rest is essential, and fatigue must be avoided by instructing the patient to walk slowly and to rest as soon as he feels pain. Physiotherapy in the form of special exercises for the feet and legs may be ordered. As there is danger of gangrene great care should be taken to prevent even the slightest injury of the feet. Cutting the toe-nails and treating corns and callosities should be done by a chiropodist. Very hot or very cold water is to be avoided, and after bathing in warm water, the feet should be well dried and dusted with a good powder. Socks should be of wool, and shoes well fitting but not tight. Bed socks should be worn at night. All clothing should be warm and loose. Moderation in diet is advisable and tobacco is usually forbidden.

Improvement in the condition is slow, and it is likely that the attacks may continue for a long time.

Surgical treatment in the form of endarterectomy or vascular grafts is successful in selected cases.

6
Disorders of the alimentary tract

DISORDERS of the digestive system include conditions affecting the alimentary tract from the mouth to the rectum and the associated glands, the liver with the bilary tract and the pancreas, whose secretions are essential for the digestion of food. Common manifestations of these disorders are dyspepsia or 'indigestion', nausea, vomiting, abdominal pain, diarrhoea and constipation, although it should be noted some of these symptoms, such as vomiting and constipation, are not necessarily confined to diseases of the digestive system.

THE MOUTH AND PHARYNX

The care of the mouth and teeth is one of the duties of the nurse in the care of any sick person. It is referred to in many places in the text and is obviously not confined to the nursing of patients suffering from disorders of the digestive system.

Descriptive Terms in use in Describing Diseases of the Mouth and Pharynx:

Stomatitis: inflammation of the mouth.
Tonsillitis: inflammation of the tonsils.
Pharyngitis: inflammation of the pharynx.
Glossitis: inflammation of the tongue.
Gingivitis: inflammation of the gums.
Parotitis: inflammation of the parotid glands.
Pyorrhoea: sepsis of the gums.
Vincent's angina: a mixed infection of the tonsil and fauces by a species of spirillum and a fusiform bacillus.
Ludwig's angina: cellulitis of the floor of the mouth.

Hygiene of the Mouth

In health the mucous membrane of the mouth is well able to withstand the various forms of minor damage to which it may be subjected, such as the effect of ice cold or very hot food or drink and the mastication of hard substances, such as crisp toast. The flow of saliva in the mouth helps to keep the surface in good condition as well as moistening the food and beginning the process of digestion. Halitosis, 'bad breath', in apparently healthy individuals is often associated with dental, sinus or tonsillar sepsis, but may be due to poor oral hygiene. Neglect of the teeth, with resulting bacterial decomposition of particles of food in the crevices between the teeth, causes halitosis and often leads to dental decay.

In illness the normal cleansing action of the saliva may be missing because the patient is not eating, and drying of the mouth lowers the resistance of the mucuous membrane to bacterial infection. All patients who are able to do so should be supplied with a suitable toothbrush, dentifrice and mouthwash for cleaning the teeth and mouth at least twice a day, and it is the duty of the nurse to see that this part of the patient's toilet is satisfactorily carried out. Dentures should be removed and cleaned twice daily. Where a patient is too ill to attend to his own toilet the nurse is directly responsible for the care of the mouth (see p. 13). Particular attention is needed in the case of patients who are either not taking a normal diet or the normal amount of fluid by mouth, as for example the nephritic or cardiac patient whose fluid intake is restricted, the patient with a peptic ulcer who is fed by a continuous intragastric 'milk drip'. The mouth is also apt to become excessively dry in febrile patients, in unconscious patients and in those cases where drugs such as belladonna and atropine which check the mucous and salivary secretions, are used.

Stomatitis

Stomatitis may take various forms. It may be a simple inflammation or vesicles may form and ulcers may develop. Predisposing causes are malnutrition and lack of care and cleanliness of the mouth; children are most commonly affected. The actual cause is not always known.

Types of Stomatitis

Thrush. This is due to a fungus (*Candida albicans*), and may spread into the pharynx or oesophagus.

Ulcerative stomatitis. A form which is most commonly seen in children who are ill-nourished and neglected.

Stomatitis due to avitaminosis. This condition is associated with scurvy, pellagra, pernicious anaemia and sprue.

Aphthous stomatitis. This form is caused by the virus of herpes simplex and appears first as vesicles, which rupture and form ulcers.

The symptoms of stomatitis are soreness of the mouth to a degree governed by the amount of ulceration present, reluctance to take food because of the pain caused by chewing and often only food which needs no mastication can be tolerated at all, bland fluids are more acceptable than acid fruit drinks. The mucous membrane of the tongue and cheeks is red and swollen and the indent of the teeth may be seen on the tongue. The breath is usually foul, especially in the ulcerative type and the submaxillary glands are sometimes enlarged. Salivation is usually marked and bleeding may occur, especially from ulcerated gums. Some cases, but not all, show constitutional disturbances such as slight fever, headache and malaise.

Treatment

Cleanliness of the mouth is of major importance, and treatment must be carried out before and after feeding. Mild and soothing lotions are best, e.g. bicarbonate of soda or normal saline solution. Chlorate of potash or permanganate of potash in weak solution can be used. Painting the patches with 1 per cent gentian violet is useful in the treatment of thrush. Nystatin tablets or dequalinium lozenges are antifungal agents that may be ordered and in severe cases penicillin will be given systemically.

Great care must be taken to be very gentle when attending to the mouth in order to avoid giving pain, damaging the mucous membrane and causing bleeding. For young children the nurse should use old linen, cotton wool or a gauze swab wrapped around an orange stick. Metal forceps should be very carefully handled and should clip the swab firmly, so that it cannot be dislodged and inhaled, possibly causing asphyxia.

The lips tend to become easily cracked and sore and should be kept clean and moist with a suitable emollient such as glycerin and borax, liquid paraffin or petroleum jelly.

Since most of these cases are infective great care should be taken to prevent spread to others and to the nurse herself. All necessities for cleansing the mouth and the feeding utensils should be kept for the patient's individual use and the nurse should be careful to wash her hands thoroughly after contact with the patient. Efficient ventilation and fresh air help to prevent spread of infection and will assist in the patient's recovery. Contact with other persons should be reduced to a minimum to prevent possible droplet infection. Children in particular should be kept away from the patient.

Considerable persuasion is often needed to get the patient to take sufficient nourishment, which should be provided in concentrated and non-irritating forms until the soreness of the mouth is less. Thickened demulcent fluids or semi-solids, such as egg and milk drinks, custards, milk jelly and junket, are likely to be taken better than others. In severe cases a piece of soft rubber tubing on the spout of a feeding cap may be the least painful method of drinking. For infants spoon feeding will be more satisfactory than a bottle, as sucking is painful and the bottle feed is then refused. In extreme cases, where there is dehydration, fluid may have to be given parenterally. The bowels must be regulated as necessary.

In the septic ulcerative form of stomatitis there is special danger of bronchopneumonia, therefore the patient should be propped up in bed, to lessen the danger of the infected material passing down the trachea. A child should be turned well over on to his side so that drainage from the mouth can take place, and the foot of the bed may be raised on blocks to drain the discharge away from the air passages.

Tonsillitis

Tonsillitis is an acute infection of the tonsils, which involves the peritonsillar and pharyngeal tissues to a greater or lesser extent. The cause is often *Streptococcus haemolyticus*, but a number of other micro-organisms can be responsible and not infrequently tonsillitis complicates a catarrhal upper respiratory tract infection.

The patient is usually a child or young adult; he complains of a very sore throat and pain on swallowing, the temperature is raised and may be as high as 39·4° to 40°C (103° to 104°F), and there are general symptoms of fever; headache, malaise and loss of appetite are commonly present. On examination the tonsils and adjacent area of the pharynx are red and swollen, yellow patches of purulent exudate may be seen on the tonsils and the submaxillary lymph glands may be swollen and painful. Occasionally the infection spreads to the deeper tissues and a peritonsillar abscess or 'quinsy' develops.

Treatment

Streptococcal infections are treated by the systemic use of antibiotics, usually penicillin. Prompt treatment is usually effective, and the occurrence of a peritonsillar abscess is now much rarer than it was in the era before chemotherapy was available.

Domiphen bromide (Bradosol) antiseptic lozenges are often useful. Painting the throat with Mandl's paint (iodine, potassium iodide and glycerin), although less common, may be ordered. Aspirin gargles given before meals are particularly useful in relieving pain and so allowing the patient to swallow with less discomfort. The patient should remain in bed until the temperature is normal and the local inflammation has subsided. Food should be soft and in the acute stage, semi-fluids and fluids are usually most acceptable. Two-hourly warm saline mouthwashes help to keep the mouth clean and are comforting, and some patients may appreciate hot external applications such as a kaolin poultice. If needed an aperient should be given.

Recurrent attacks of tonsillitis lead to enlargement of the tonsils and of other areas of lymphoid tissue in the nasopharynx forming adenoids, which partially block the nasopharynx preventing adequate nose-breathing, and also block the pharyngotympanic (Eustachian) tubes leading to the middle ear, causing partial deafness. The child who has recurrent attacks of tonsillitis with enlarged adenoids is likely to be at a great disadvantage as a result of frequent absence from school and moreover when he does attend, he may appear slow and dull due to deficient hearing. Streptococcal infection may lead also to nephritis and acute rheumatic fever; tonsillectomy and removal of the adenoidal tissue is therefore usually advised when the patient has recovered from the acute infection.

Ulceration of the Pharynx

Pharyngeal ulcers may arise from a number of causes, for example tuberculous or syphilitic infection, new growths, carcinoma of the tonsillar area, or a type of sore throat known as Vincent's angina.

The treatment is the treatment of the cause of the ulceration. Vincent's angina produces a yellowish membrane somewhat similar to diphtheritic membrane. The actual micro-organism responsible is doubtful, but examination of a throat swab will distinguish this condition from pharyngeal diphtheria. The infection may be accompanied by some degree of fever and malaise, and also by enlargement of the local lymph glands. Penicillin usually produces a rapid cure, but as the condition is often associated with septic infection in the mouth, examination and treatment by a dental surgeon may be necessary.

DISEASES OF THE OESOPHAGUS

The most prominent symptom of disease of the oesophagus is difficulty in swallowing which is known as dysphagia. Dysphagia of acute onset is usually caused by a foreign body obstructing the passage. Stricture of the oesophagus, caused by ulceration with the formation of fibrous tissue which gradually contracts, or the presence of a new growth, results in a gradually progressive dysphagia. Where narrowing of the oesophagus is associated with inflammation, as may happen in hiatus hernia and some cases of malignant obstruction, swallowing is painful as well as difficult.

Cancer of the Oesophagus

The oesophagus is a fairly common site for carcinoma, particularly in middle-aged or elderly men. In its early stages it is often symptomless and even when some difficulty in the passage of a solid, bulky bolus of food is experienced the patient may not seek medical advice. As the obstruction increases there is more and more difficulty, and the patient begins to lose weight rapidly. Such food as the patient takes may be regurgitated, and in the later stages of the disease the patient suffers constant pain.

Treatment

An opening into the stomach, gastrostomy, through which the patient can be fed with a high joule fluid diet, is often the first step. In some cases excision of the growth is possible; in others where this is not considered feasible deep X-ray treatment may be given. The patient is likely to require considerable doses of morphine or other powerful analgesic drugs to relieve his pain.

Achalasia of the Cardia

Achalasia is a term used to describe a condition in which the cardiac sphincter at the gastric end of the oesophagus does not relax normally during swallowing. Food is held up in the oesophagus above the sphincter until the weight of the accumulation in the oesophagus forces the sphincter to open. In course of time considerable dilatation of the lower end of the oesophagus results and this can be demonstrated by X-ray examination while the patient swallows an opaque meal containing barium. The appearance as shown on the X-ray film distinguishes this condition from other causes of dysphagia, particularly malignant disease of the oesophagus. Another differential point is that although the patient is often underweight and may have pain and regurgitate food, the condition remains stationary and his general health does not show the deterioration associated with cancer.

Treatment

Antispasmodic drugs may be ordered, such as belladonna or propantheline bromide (Pro-Banthine). In some cases dilatation of the cardiac sphincter by graduated weighted bougies may be carried out. The patient will usually find that foods which are soft or semi-fluid are more easily passed than solid, dry foods. Heller's operation of splitting the muscle of the cardiac sphincter may be necessary in severe achalasia.

Oesophageal Varices

Oesophageal varices are large varicose veins which develop at the lower end of the oesophagus as a result of obstruction in the portal circulation such as may occur in cirrhosis of the liver. In this situation communicating veins between the portal and systemic circulation take a considerable proportion of the venous blood back to the heart, but there is always a possibility that these oesophageal veins, as a result of the increasing volume of blood which they carry, may rupture, and when that happens large quantities of blood are vomited.

Treatment

The immediate treatment of bleeding from oesophageal varices is absolute rest and blood transfusion. An inflatable tube, Sengstaken tube, may be used to control further bleeding. This apparatus has three component tubes; it is passed through the oesophagus into the stomach and a thin rubber balloon near the end of one tube is distended with water. The tube is then withdrawn until resistance shows that the balloon is pressing against the cardiac sphincter. A second sausage-shaped balloon which lies in the oesophagus is now blown up with air to a pressure of 20 mmHg and the tube through which the balloon is inflated is clamped. The third tube allows a check to be kept on the amount of bleeding taking place, by aspiration at regular intervals, or continuous gastric suction may be used. An alternative treatment is intravenous administration of pituitrin by the drip method, which sometimes stops the bleeding. In some suitable patients, particularly if no extensive liver damage is present, surgical treatment such as making an anastomosis between the portal vein and the inferior vena cava may successfully reduce the venous pressure which causes the oesophageal varices.

Hiatus Hernia

Hiatus hernia, or diaphragmatic hernia, is the condition in which part of the cardiac end of the stomach is able to slide up through the normal diaphragmatic opening which allows the lower end of the oesophagus to pass through from the chest to the abdomen. A small hiatus hernia may give rise to no symptoms at all, but where it does give rise to trouble the usual symptoms are dysphagia, 'heart-burn', sometimes with regurgitation of food, and epigastric discomfort. These symptoms are always worse if the patient lies down after a meal. Ulcers sometimes occur as a result of acid gastric juice leaking into the oesophagus.

Treatment

The patient is advised to take small easily digested meals and to avoid strenuous exercise or lying down flat after a meal. He will find that he suffers less from heart-burn and discomfort if he sleeps in a semi-sitting position, supported by an 'armchair' arrangement of pillows. Antacid preparations, magnesium trisilicate or aluminium hydroxide (Aludrox), are usually effective in relieving the symptoms. If medical treatment does not effect an improvement and the patient's symptoms are progressively more severe, surgical repair of the hernia may be considered.

DISEASES AND DISORDERS OF THE STOMACH AND DUODENUM

Descriptive Terms Used

Dyspepsia, or indigestion, is a somewhat vague term used to describe discomfort, often associated with flatulence, which is experienced after eating. It can be caused by eating too much at one time, by eating hurriedly or when under emotional stress. Chronic dyspepsia may be due to a number of causes and is quite commonly a symptom of diseases of the biliary system and gall-bladder.

Gastritis is inflammation or irritation of the mucous lining of the stomach from any cause.

Hyperchlorhydria is the name given to excess hydrochloric acid in the gastric juice, which is a feature in patients with a duodenal ulcer.

Hypochlorhydria is diminished secretion of hydrochloric acid, a condition which may be found in atrophy of the gastric mucosa in chronic gastritis and in carcinoma of the stomach.

Achlorhydria, the absence of hydrochloric acid, is found in pernicious anaemia. If no secretion occurs in response to an injection of histamine, the achlorhydria is said to be 'histamine-fast'.

Nausea describes the unpleasant sensation of internal discomfort, 'feeling sick', sometimes accompanied by giddiness and faintness.

Vomiting (or emesis) is the forcible ejection of the contents of the stomach via the mouth, and is frequently, but not always, preceded by nausea.

Haematemesis is the term used to describe the vomiting of blood.

Vomiting

Vomiting is a common symptom in gastric disorders, but is also a symptom of many conditions, for example toxic states such as uraemia, the onset of acute infections, accompanying the severe pain of renal or biliary colic, intestinal obstruction, appendicitis, cerebral conditions, disturbances of the semicircular canals causing sea-sickness and other forms of motion sickness. Infants and young children vomit very readily, often for no apparent cause; sometimes it may be the result of over-feeding.

When vomiting is a symptom, the nurse should note the amount vomited, the frequency of vomiting, and the character of the material vomited. Observations should also be made as to whether nausea precedes vomiting, whether it occurs in relation to taking food, for example immediately or shortly after a meal, whether effort is involved or if vomiting is an effortless regurgitation of the stomach contents and whether pain is present and if it is relieved by vomiting.

The material vomited is usually food which is partially digested and will often by very acid. Vomit which contains bile and is yellow or green in colour is seen in any condition in which vomiting continues after the stomach has emptied its immediate contents; if intestinal obstruction is the cause, this will be followed by vomiting of brown fluid which may be foul-smelling and is often referred to as 'faecal vomiting'.

Vomiting of clear watery fluid occurs in the 'early morning sickness' of the early months of pregnancy. Vomiting of large quantities of food or fluid often indicates that there is obstruction to the passage of food through the pylorus into the duodenum and consequent dilatation of the stomach. This condition may be due to congenital pyloric obstruction, to the formation of scar tissue from healing ulcers, or to a new growth, or acute dilatation of the stomach, a complication that occasionally follows the administration of a general anaesthetic.

Haematemesis, or vomiting of blood, most commonly occurs in cases of peptic ulcer. Oozing of blood from an ulcerated surface probably occurs in all these cases, and small amounts of blood will be passed in the stools which can usually only be detected by chemical examination. If, however, the ulcer erodes large vessels in the gastric or duodenal mucosa, not only will large quantities of blood be vomited but will also be passed in the stools. The blood vomited may be altered in colour by the action of the gastric juice and will then have a 'coffee grounds' appearance. Other causes of haematemesis are carcinoma of the stomach, oesophageal varices and bleeding in purpuric and leukaemic states. Following operations or injury to the mouth, nose or throat, blood may be swallowed and later vomited.

There may be some difficulty in certain cases in deciding whether blood has been vomited or if it has been coughed up, i.e. whether the patient has had a haematemesis or a haemoptysis. The previous medical history of the patient will be of value here, and also information from any relative or other person present as to whether the patient coughed while bringing up blood or if it appeared to be vomited, and the appearance of the vomited material. In haematemesis the blood is likely to be dark in colour and at first may be mixed with food; in haemoptysis the blood will be bright in colour and may be frothy from mixing with air. In very profuse bleeding, however, in either case bright blood may gush out in a continuous flow and these points cannot be distinguished. The patient who bleeds freely from an eroded artery in the stomach will usually feel faint before vomiting occurs, also he will pass tarry, melaena stools sooner or later. If the bleeding is from the lung the patient will continue to cough up some blood or blood-stained sputum for a period of 24 hr or longer.

Investigations and Tests used in the Diagnosis of Gastric Disorders

Tests of Gastric Function

Gastric function tests estimate the hydrochloric acid content of the gastric juice, and also the amount of the residual contents, 'resting juice', in the stomach after 12 hr fasting. The most commonly used tests are:

(1) *Aspiration of gastric residuum.* The patient must be given nothing by mouth for 12 hr prior to the test; as this test is usually carried out in the early morning the usual instructions state that the patient must have nothing to eat or drink after early supper on the previous evening until the test has been completed.

A Ryle's or Refuss's tube is passed via the nose into the stomach and the gastric contents are aspirated with a syringe. The entire amount aspirated is measured, placed in a container, labelled and sent to the laboratory.

A further elaboration of this test is to leave the intragastric tube in position and to give a hypodermic injection of histamine (0·3 to 0·8 mg). After this injection the stomach is aspirated at intervals of 10 or 15 min over a period of 1 hr or, in some cases, longer. Histamine is a powerful stimulant to the gastric mucosa and if no acid is secreted in response to the injection, the condition of achlorhydria is established.

Histamine may produce unpleasant symptoms, such as generalized flushing, throbbing in the head and neck, and headache, as a result of its vasodilator action. These symptoms can be prevented by giving one of the antihistamine drugs, e.g. promethazine hydrochloride (Phenergan). Synthetic gastrin is now often used in place of histamine and it is a more potent stimulator of acid secretion.

(2) *Diagnex test* also known as the 'tubeless' test. No preparations containing aluminium, calcium, iron or magnesium must be given during the 24 hr prior to the test. The patient should fast for 12 hr before the commencement of the test and should have nothing but the test substances and water by mouth until the test is complete.

(a) At the specified time, e.g. 06.00 hours, the patient is asked to empty his bladder and this urine is discarded.

(b) He is given two capsules containing caffeine sodium benzoate 250 mg with a glass of water. This preparation is a gastric simulant.

(c) If an injection of histamine or gastrin has been ordered it is given at 06.45 hours.

(d) At 07.00 hours the patient again empties his bladder, the entire amount passed is saved and sent to the laboratory in a container labelled 'control urine'.

(e) Immediately after emptying his bladder the patient is given the Diagnex (Azure A Resin) blue granules suspended in about 60 ml (2 fluid ounces) of water. The granules do not dissolve and the patient must be instructed not to chew them but to swallow them whole. A further 60 ml of water is given to ensure that no granules are left in the glass.

(f) Two hours later, 09.00 hours, the patient empties his bladder and all the urine passed is saved and sent to the laboratory in a container labelled 'test urine'.

If the gastric juice contains hydrochloric acid an exchange of hydrogen irons can be effected with the azure A resin in the test substance. Azure A resin is then absorbed and excreted in the urine.

The test cannot be repeated until at least a week has elapsed and therefore the nurse should be sure that she understands the instructions and carries them out accurately.

The patient may continue to pass blue or greenish-blue urine for some days after the test.

(3) *Fractional test meal.* This type of test is now less commonly used than the two tests described above.

The test is usually carried out in the early morning and the patient should be given nothing by mouth after supper on the previous evening.

A series of specimen bottles, or test tubes, is needed. One is labelled 'resting juice' and the remainder are numbered 1 to 12.

(a) An intragastric tube is passed, the 'resting juice' is aspirated as in the gastric residuum test, and a sample is placed in the labelled test tube.

(b) If alcohol is to be used for the test meal, 200 ml of 5 per cent alcohol is injected down the intragastric tube. Gruel (made by boiling 55 g of fine oatmeal with 1 litre of water until the volume is reduced to 0·5 litre), is sometimes used, in which case this is left to the patient to drink with the intragastric tube left in position.

(c) A sample (about 5 ml) of the gastric content is aspirated every 15 min and put in the appropriate test tube beginning with no. 1.

(d) When no further material can be aspirated the series of the test tubes in a labelled rack is sent to the laboratory. The procedure usually takes 2 to 3 hr. The results of the test will include an analysis of the 'resting juice' and the amount of free hydrochloric acid in the successive specimens aspirated.

X-Ray Examination of the Stomach

In order to demonstrate the shape, size and contour of the stomach it is necessary to fill it with a substance which is opaque to X-rays. The medium used is barium sulphate, which is prepared as a suspension with starch mucilage or tragacanth powder, sweetened and usually flavoured to form a 'barium meal'. Should the patient be taking any preparation containing bismuth this must be discontinued for at least 2 days before the examination, and no aperient should be given within 24 hr of the barium meal. It is essential that the stomach should be empty and no food or drink is allowed for at least 6 hr, some radiologists may say 12 hr, before the examination. During the examination the patient will be required to stand, and if he has been confined to bed a few days must be allowed in order that he may be up and able to stand before the visit to the X-ray department.

After the initial examination further films are taken and instruction will be given as to when the patient may have food. Usually an aperient is ordered when the examination is completed.

Gastroscopy and Biopsy

Gastroscopy is carried out by passing a flexible tube with telescopic lenses and mirrors via the mouth and oesophagus into the stomach and, so mirroring those areas of the gastric mucosa which can be seen by this method. Useful information in respect of the presence of inflammation or ulceration may be obtained, but there are some areas of the stomach which cannot be visualized through the gastroscope. Biopsy of a section of the gastric mucosa may be carried out at the same time as the gastroscopy examination, which will be undertaken in the operating theatre. No food or fluid should be given by mouth for 12 hr beforehand; premedication in the form of morphine to 10 mg and atropine 0·6 mg may be ordered.

Gastrophotography

This is similar to gastroscopy except that the end of the tube contains a small camera with which photographs of the stomach mucosa can be obtained.

Tests for Occult Blood

Very small amounts of blood mixed with the intestinal contents may be passed in the faeces and not be recognizable as such. Its presence can, however, be detected by chemical tests, and a specimen of the stool may be required for laboratory examination for the presence of haemoglobin. A simple test which is now in general use is the Haematest. A thin smear of faeces is placed on the test paper provided, a Haematest tablet put in the centre of the smear and 2 drops of water added to the tablet. A positive result is shown by a diffuse area of blue colour appearing on the paper around the tablet within 2 min.

Gastritis

Acute gastritis may be the result of too much rich or indigestible food or too much alcohol which acts as an irritant to the gastric mucosa, to bacterial food-poisoning, viral infections or chemical irritants.

The main symptoms are epigastric discomfort or pain, particularly severe if a chemical poison such as a strong acid or alkali is the cause, nausea, vomiting and headache. The temperature may be raised to a moderate degree.

Treatment

Rest in bed is necessary, food should be restricted to fluids, and alkalis such as aluminium hydroxide may be given. If the condition is due to irritant poisons the appropriate antidote and usually a stomach wash-out will be urgently needed and also treatment for shock, which may be profound.

Chronic gastritis calls for investigation and treatment of the cause, which may be chronic alcoholism, infection of the gums (pyorrhoea), gastric ulcer or carcinoma, or congestion of the gastric mucosa as a result of congestive cardiac failure or portal vein congestion.

Peptic Ulcer (Gastric and Duodenal Ulcer)

A peptic ulcer occurs either in the stomach, or in the first part of the duodenum, that is in areas which are exposed to the acid gastric juice. Why the mucous membrane should be damaged by this contact is not at all clear, but once an ulcer has occurred the action of pepsin and hydrochloric acid in the gastric juice makes healing difficult. There is some evidence that persons who live under high pressure, who have constant worry and anxiety, whose meal and relaxation times are often irregular, are particularly prone to develop peptic ulcers. However ulcers also occur in persons who show no evidence of nervous strain and whose lives appear to be run along orderly and regular lines. The majority of peptic ulcers are chronic, but occasionally an acute ulcer develops and causes haematemesis, often without any warning symptoms of gastric disorder.

The chronic ulcer is usually deep, penetrating the mucosa down to the muscle layer and producing fibrous scar tissue. In this type of ulceration there is almost always a history of 'indigestion', pain after meals which is relieved by taking an alkaline powder or by food. If the ulcer is in the stomach the pain is often described as 'burning', and the onset is usually 1 to 2 hr after a meal. Vomiting may occur, and when it does the pain is relieved. If the ulcer is in the duodenum the onset of the pain is usually 2 or 3 hr after a meal and is accompanied by a feeling of hunger. The patient usually gets complete relief by taking some such food as a glass of milk and biscuits. In many cases for no clear reason, since the ulcer usually remains active, the patient may have periods when he is completely free from symptoms. Investigations will include those described on page 131, and of these the barium meal X-ray examination usually gives most information (Fig. 17).

Treatment

Rest in bed for a period which will vary according to the severity of the symptoms but is usually 2 to 3 weeks, together with a bland diet, of which milk is the basis, and the administration of alkalis in the form of magnesium trisilicate or aluminium hydroxide (Aludrox) form the basis of treatment in un-complicated cases.

Drugs which reduce the secretion of gastric juice and diminish the motor activity of stomach muscle may be ordered. Examples of such antispasmodic drugs are tincture of belladonna, atropine sulphate and propantheline bromide (Pro-Banthine).

Frequent feeding prevents the stomach from being left completely empty, a state in which the gastric juice, which is secreted

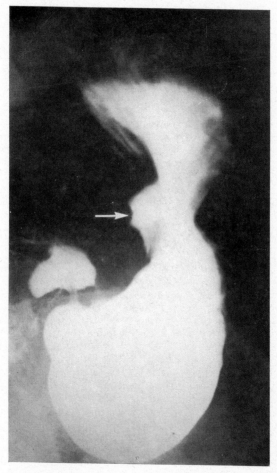

FIG. 17. X-ray photograph of stomach filled with a barium meal showing a large ulcer on the lesser curvature.

continuously, can irritate the ulcerated area. In the early stages of treatment continuous feeding may be given by passing an intragastric tube via the nose into the stomach and connecting it to a drop counter attached by a length of tubing to a blood transfusion bottle containing the feed. The amount to be given in 24 hr is usually 3 litres (6 pints) of milk, to which Complan may be added. This continuous 'milk drip' may be kept going for about 4 days, and is particularly useful for patients who have severe pain at night which interferes with their rest and is only temporarily relieved by food.

The main principles on which the diet for peptic ulcer is based are: (1) regular frequent meals; (2) bland foods which will not damage the mucous membrane and are also non-stimulating to the gastric juice, and (3) adequate calorie, protein and vitamin content to ensure good nutrition and promote healing of the ulcer. Examples of suitable diets which fulfil these requirements, increasing the amount and variety of the food as the patient's symptoms respond to treatment, are given on page 140.

The patient's co-operation is an essential part of his treatment. The reasons for the 'ulcer regimen' and the need to continue to follow the medical instructions should be fully explained. On a regimen of rest and careful feeding the symptoms often clear within a few weeks, and further X-ray examination shows that the ulcer is healing. Nevertheless there is always the possibility of a relapse, and the majority of patients who have had treatment for a peptic ulcer will need to order their lives on the general lines of diet, rest, avoidance of gastric irritants, such as alcohol and tobacco which the physician considers advisable in the particular circumstances. If the patient is going to keep the rules they must not be so strict that he is strongly tempted to disobey them. The directions for diet should cover as wide a variety of foods as possible to avoid monotony and also to help ensure that the meals have adequate nutritive value including vitamins. While milk forms the basis of the feeding in the acute stage and remains an important item in the diet of the patient with a peptic ulcer, it cannot in itself supply all the necessary factors for good nutrition. There is a possible danger that a patient who leaves hospital without proper instructions, or who does not follow the advice given, may when he gets a return of his ulcer pain and finds that a strictly milk diet and dose of alkali will relieve his symptoms, cease to take any other food.

If this practice is continued for some time the patient's nutritional state will suffer; furthermore he may develop a state of alkalosis with such symptoms as vomiting, mental confusion and possibly tetany.

Complications of Peptic Ulcers

Bleeding. Repeated small blood losses from the ulcerated surface may cause a considerable degree of anaemia. Severe haemorrhage occurs if the ulcer erodes a large blood vessel and is shown by haematemesis, usually preceded by feelings of faintness and dizziness, and melaena, the passage of dark tarry stools containing blood. The blood vomited is at first dark brown in colour, due to the action of the gastric juice, but if the bleeding continues, bright blood, which may contain clots, is vomited, and the patient rapidly shows the signs of pallor, weak, rapid pulse and cold skin surface associated with severe haemorrhage.

Complete rest, allaying the patient's fear as far as possible with reassurances that the bleeding will be arrested are the first steps. He should lie flat with the foot of the bed raised and the bed should be comfortably warm but not overheated. Sedation is usually ordered immediately, e.g. morphine 15 mg, or if it is thought that morphine may increase the vomiting, pethidine 50 or 100 mg.

The patient's blood should be typed and cross-matched; blood and plasma should be readily available, as transfusion is needed in all cases of severe haemorrhage. The pulse rate should be recorded hourly and the blood pressure every 2 hr. All vomit and stools are saved for inspection.

If the bleeding is not diminishing surgical treatment may be urgently needed and this must be made clear to the relatives, who will be asked to give their consent for operation if the patient is not able to do this himself. If, however, there is no immediate indication for this the patient may be given chips of ice to suck and frequent mouthwashes will help to keep his mouth clean and to remove the taste of vomited blood. If his condition is improving feeding by mouth is usually begun within 12 to 24 hr, and the Stage I ulcer diet is suitable.

Perforation. A peptic ulcer may perforate the muscular coat of the stomach, and the stomach contents then escape into the peritoneal cavity, with resulting peritonitis. The onset of this complication is sudden, with severe epigastric pain and collapse.

In the majority of cases the treatment is immediate operation. In a few instances, where the symptoms are less acute, continuous gastric suction, with careful observation of the patient's condition, his temperature and pulse rate, may be used.

Pyloric stenosis. Scarring resulting from duodenal ulceration causes a narrowing of the pylorus, obstruction to the passage of the contents of the stomach into the duodenum, hypertrophy and eventually gross dilation of the stomach. This condition can be demonstrated by X-ray examination, and is also strongly suspected if a patient vomits very large amounts at intervals of 24 hr or more. The obstruction may be partly due to spasm or to swelling of the mucous membrane and therefore the condition may be relieved by rest, diet and antispasmodic drugs. If these measures meet with no success then surgical treatment is probably necessary; the most usual operation is partial gastrectomy and duodenectomy.

Malignant changes. These are rare, but it is thought that in a few instances cancer of the stomach may originate in a chronic gastric ulcer. Duodenal ulcers have not been known to undergo malignant changes.

Diet for Patients with Gastric or Duodenal Ulcers
Stage I. 6300 kJ (1500 kcal)

Hour
06.00 Milk 150 ml (5 fl oz), sweetened and flavoured with suitable flavourings, if desired.
08.00 Milk 150 ml (5 fl oz), with 1 beaten egg; *or*
A small portion (approximately 150 ml) sieved porridge.
10.00 Milk 150 ml (5 fl oz), 1 rusk.
12.00 30 g (1 tablespoonful) of flaked fish or minced chicken, rabbit, tripe or sweetbreads, served with white sauce, coloured with tomato juice or finely chopped parsley.
60 g (2 tablespoonsful) of creamed potato.
Milk pudding, custard or milk jelly (150-ml portion).
14.00 Diluted fruit juice, e.g. orange juice, blackcurrant purée, rose hip syrup.
16.00 Milk 150 ml (5 fl oz) sweetened and flavoured, if desired.
2 slices thin, crustless bread and butter, or rusks and butter.
Fruit jelly or sieved fruit, a small portion.
18.00 Cream of vegetable soup 150 ml (5 fl oz).
1 rusk, or thin bread and butter.
Milk pudding, custard or jelly (150-ml portion).

20.00 150 ml (5 fl oz) milk, sweetened and flavoured, if desired.
If awake during night—150 ml (5 fl oz) milk, sweetened and flavoured, if desired.

	Carbohydrate	Protein	Fat
Approximate value (g)	170	58	65

Stage II. 7140 kJ (1700 kcal)

Hour

06.00 150 ml (5 fl oz) milk, sweetened and flavoured with suitable flavourings, if desired.

08.00 Weak, freshly made, milky tea, sweetened, if desired.
1 egg, lightly boiled, poached *or* scrambled.
or fine oatmeal porridge.
2 slices of thin crisp toast (allow to become cold before spreading with butter or margarine) *or*
2 slices of thin bread and butter.

10.00 150 ml (5 fl oz) milk, 1 rusk.

12.00 45 g (1½ tablespoonful) of flaked fish, minced chicken, rabbit, tripe or sweetbreads, served with white sauce, coloured with tomato juice or finely chopped parsley.
60 to 90 g (2 to 3 tablespoonful) of creamed potato.
30 to 60 g (1 to 2 tablespoonful) of sieved vegetables.
A medium helping of cereal pudding, custard or jelly.

14.00 Diluted fruit juice, e.g. orange juice, blackcurrant purée or rose hip syrup.

16.00 Weak, freshly made, milky tea.
2 slices of thin crisp toast, buttered when cold; *or*
3 slices of thin bread and butter.
Jam (without pips or skin), honey or syrup.

18.00 Cream of vegetable soup.   A savoury dish.
Crisp toast.   *or* Thin bread and butter.
Cereal pudding or custard.   Cereal pudding.

20.00 150 ml (5 fl oz) milk, sweetened and flavoured, if desired.
If awake during night—150 ml (5 fl oz) milk, sweetened and flavoured, if desired.

	Carbohydrate	Protein	Fat
Approximate value (g)	200	68	70

Stage III. 8400 kJ (2000 kcal)

Hour

06.00 150 ml (5 fl oz) milk, sweetened and flavoured with suitable flavourings, if desired.

08.00 Weak, freshly made, milky tea, sweetened, if desired.
Porridge or cornflakes, with hot milk and syrup or sugar.
or 1 egg, lightly boiled, poached or scrambled.
3 slices crisp toast, buttered cold, *or* 3 slices of thin bread and butter.
Jelly marmalade or honey.

10.00 Milk 150 ml (5 fl oz), 2 rusks.

12.00 A medium helping of chicken, rabbit, fish, tripe, sweetbread, tender mutton or minced beef.
A medium helping of potato, mashed or creamed.
A medium helping of sieved vegetable.
An average helping of suitable pudding.
Fruit purée whenever possible.

14.00 Diluted fruit juice, e.g. orange juice, blackcurrant purée or rose hip syrup.

16.00 Weak, freshly made, milky tea.
2 slices of thin, crisp toast, buttered when cold, *or*
2 slices of thin bread and butter.
Jam (without pips or skin), honey or syrup, if desired.
Sponge or madeira cake.

18.00 A savoury dish.   Cream of vegetable soup.
Cereal pudding.   *or* A savoury dish.
Fruit purée, whenever possible.

20.00 Milk 150 ml (5 fl oz) sweetened and flavoured, if desired.

	Carbohydrates	Protein	Fat
Approximate value (g)	250	75	78

Convalescent Stage

Breakfast: Choice of: Porridge, puffed rice, cornflakes, with milk and sugar or syrup. One egg, lightly boiled, poached or scrambled, flaked haddock or grilled bacon.
Crisp toast, buttered when cold, or bread and butter (bread should not be new).
Jelly marmalade, honey or syrup.
Weak, freshly made, milky tea, sweetened if desired.

Mid-morning: Milk drink, flavoured if desired. Plain biscuits, sponge or madeira cake.

Lunch: Choice of: A moderate helping of fish, steamed, baked, grilled or boiled; or tripe, sweetbread, chicken, rabbit, lamb or minced beef or mutton.
Potato, mashed or creamed, a good helping.
Vegetable purée, a good helping.

Lunch, *cont*:	Cereal pudding, custard, jelly or a light steamed sponge.
	Fruit juice or purée.
Tea:	Weak, freshly made, milky tea, sweetened if desired.
	Crisp toast or bread (not new), as required.
	Butter or margarine, honey, syrup or jam without skin or pips.
	Sponge cake, swiss roll or madeira cake.
Supper:	Cream of vegetable soup.
	Fish or egg dish, or grated cheese.
	Toast or bread, as required. Butter or margarine as required.
	Choice of pudding.
	Fruit juice *or* purée.
Before retiring:	Milk drink, cake, biscuits or bread and butter.
	During night if awake, milk 150 ml (5 fl oz), flavoured, if desired.

General Instructions for Patients with Peptic Ulcers

Foods to be Avoided

Soups	Meat soups and extracts and rich gravies.
Meat	Tough meat, twice cooked meat, made-up dishes, sausages, pork, veal, salt beef.
Fish	Shell fish, kippers, mackerels, herrings, smoked fish, tinned salmon and sardines.
Vegetables	Peas, beans, celery, onions, leeks, cucumber, roast and fried potatoes. Vegetables must not be cooked in fat but butter or margarine may be added. Coarse salads.
Fruit	Dried fruit such as raisins, figs, currants, sultanas, lemon peel.
	Jam and marmalade should be taken only in jelly form.
Condiments	Mustard, pepper, curry, pickles, chutney, spice, relishes and vinegar.
Various	Avoid all fried foods, pastry, suet puddings, new bread, hot buttered toast, fruit or spiced cake, coarse biscuits such as digestive, rye or wheat crisps, coarse cereals, cooked cheese, strong tea and black coffee.

Foods Allowed

Soups	Cream of vegetable and milk soups.
Fish	Plaice, sole, cod, hake, halibut; steamed, boiled, baked or grilled.

Meat and Poultry	Lamb, mutton, beef (minced if at all tough), rabbit, chicken, tripe, sweetbreads. Meat should be steamed or roasted, not boiled or stewed.
Vegetables	Potatoes, boiled or steamed or baked in jackets, then mashed or creamed. Carrot, turnip, swede, spinach, cabbage, well cooked and sieved, head of cauliflower, lettuce and parsley finely chopped. Tomato purée.
Fruit	Cooked and sieved. Concentrated fruit juices, rose hip syrup, orange juice, blackcurrant purée or syrup.
Puddings	Cereal puddings, custard, junket, fruit fool, ice cream, milk jelly. Light sponge puddings served with fruit purée, trifle, queen of puddings, apple snow.
Sweets	Plain or milk chocolate, with no added fruit or nuts. Boiled sweets.
Beverages	Tea or coffee, weak and freshly made, with plenty of milk, water and fruit juices; drink between meals rather than with meals.
Savoury dishes	Spaghetti in tomato sauce. Soft roes in parsley sauce. Fish custard. Savoury omelette. Creamed rabbit, chicken or fish. Cauliflower in white sauce with grated cheese. Minced ham custard.

Important

(1) Take small meals regularly and at frequent intervals.
(2) Avoid going longer than 2 to 3 hr without food during the daytime.
(3) Do not take a meal whilst tired or cold; rest and get thoroughly warm before eating.
(4) Do not hurry over your meals. Chew your food thoroughly.
(5) Try to rest for a while after eating your food.
(6) Avoid smoking, especially before meals.
(7) Take beer and spirits only on the advice of your doctor.

Congenital Hypertrophic Pyloric Stenosis

Congenital hypertrophic pyloric obstruction is most common in first-born infants, more often boys than girls. The signs appear during the first 3 weeks of life as a rule, and are ejection of food as soon as the stomach is full with projectile vomiting, loss of weight, dehydration and constipation. The infant is always hungry and takes a feed eagerly. If the abdomen is watched during feeding, visible peristaltic waves crossing the stomach from left to right can be seen, and the passage of food is blocked at the pylorus where a tumour-like swelling can be seen and felt.

Treatment

Treatment is usually surgical; Rammstedt's operation of splitting the muscle of the thickened pyloric sphincter can be carried out under a local anaesthetic and usually gives excellent results. Medical methods may be tried if the symptoms are not very pronounced, an atropine preparation known as Eumydrin is given to relieve the muscle spasm at the pylorus and this, with very careful feeding, has been successful, but a complete cure takes some time and needs much patience.

Carcinoma of the Stomach

Carcinoma of the stomach may not cause any marked symptoms until the disease is well established, or there may be a long history of 'indigestion' with loss of weight. Surgical treatment offers the only hope of arrest of the disease, but the survival rate is low, owing to the difficulty in diagnosing this condition in its early stages before secondary growths have developed on the liver and other organs.

DISORDERS AND DISEASES OF THE INTESTINES

Observation of Faeces

Normal stools are light-brown in colour and formed. The colour is due to the presence of bile pigments and the bulk of the faeces is composed of food residue, i.e. undigested or indigestible food, mixed with mucus and water.

Observation of the stools includes noting the colour, consistency, presence of any abnormal substance and the frequency of defaecation.

Blood in the stools, if bright in colour, comes from the large intestine, the rectum or anal canal, and may be due to haemorrhoids, new growths, or ulceration of the bowel as in ulcerative colitis, dysentery, typhoid fever, or acute enteritis from any cause. In infective conditions the stools often contain considerable amounts of mucus as well as blood. Bleeding from the stomach or duodenum as in peptic ulcer produces dark tarry stools, melaena, as the blood is altered by the action of digestive enzymes in the intestine.

Absence of bile pigment in jaundice and the presence of abnormal amounts of fat in the faeces produce light clay-coloured stools which are often bulky, glistening with fat and offensive.

In infancy the stools may sometimes contain milk curds, indicating over-feeding, unsuitable feeding, or digestive disturbance. Frequent green stools are seen in bacterial enteritis of infants. These stools are acid and cause soreness and excoriation of the buttocks.

Foreign bodies which may be looked for in the stools include intestinal parasites, gall-stones, and such articles as safety pins, beads and buttons, which are often swallowed by children.

Laboratory Investigations

Bacteriological Examination

For bacteriological examination the laboratory may require the entire stool, in which case it is sent labelled in the bed-pan in which it has been passed. In infective intestinal conditions where blood, pus, or mucus are present, a small sample of the stool containing this material is sent to the laboratory in a stoppered glass container.

Fat Absorption Tests

Analysis of faeces for fat. No aperient, and particularly no oily drugs such as liquid paraffin, must be given for at least 3 days prior to or during this test or the fat balance test.

If possible the whole stool is sent to the laboratory. If this is not convenient then the material is mixed to a uniform consistency and a sample sent in a suitable container.

On a normal diet the total daily output of fat should be less than 7 g.

Fat balance test. A fat balance test may be necessary if it is considered that the analysis of the faeces on a normal diet does not give a sufficiently accurate result.

The patient is given a standard diet containing 50 g of fat per day for 48 hr prior to the test and during the test. The diet is supplied from the diet kitchen and it is essential that any food not eaten by the patient should be returned to the dietitian.

First day. The patient is given two capsules containing carmine dye before breakfast. The stools are examined as they are passed and when coloured by carmine the whole stool is saved and sent to the laboratory. All subsequent stools are sent to the laboratory.

Sixth day. The patient is given 60 g (2 oz) of powdered charcoal mixed with water. All stools passed are saved until charcoal appears in the faeces. A convenient method of collecting the stools is into a sheet of Cellophane large enough to cover the interior of the bed-pan and hang down over the rim. The edges of the sheet are brought together and the whole stool in the Cellophane wrapping is deposited in a labelled water-proof container.

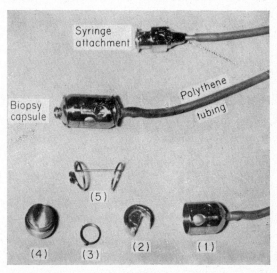

FIG. 18. The Crosby intestinal biopsy capsule. The capsule is attached to a length of polythene tubing long enough to reach the jejunum; at the other end is attached a 20-ml syringe. The cylinder (1) has a side port which receives the mucosal specimen. The knife (2) is a cylindrical block which pivots within the capsule and is activated by the spring (3). The dome (4) normally covers the end of the cylinder. The wrench (5) is a stiff wire key used to cock the instrument.

Intestinal Biopsy

A small sample of the jejunal mucosa can be obtained by means of Crosby's capsule (Fig. 18). The fine flexible tube with the capsule attached is swallowed and passed through the stomach into the small intestine.

Direct Examination of the Rectum and Pelvic Colon

Digital examination is usually the first procedure for rectal examination. The patient lies in the left lateral position with the knees well flexed and the buttocks brought to the edge of the bed or couch. The doctor carrying out the examination requires a right-hand rubber or disposable polythene glove or caped finger stall and a suitable lubricant such as petroleum jelly or a water soluble lubricant. The examination only extends to that part of the rectum which can be reached by the examining finger.

Sigmoidoscopy and proctoscopy are examinations that will permit direct visual examination of the rectum and pelvic (sigmoid) colon, through an illuminated metal tube. The proctoscope is a short tube designed for examination of the rectum and anal canal only. The sigmoidoscope tube will allow inspection of the rectum and colon for a length of about 23 to 25 cm (9 to 10 in). A pair of bellows is attached to the instrument which permits inflation of the bowel, thus straightening out the folds of the mucosa.

Sigmoidoscopy is usually carried out in the theatre and a general anaesthetic may be required. Preparation of the patient varies; sometimes an aperient is given 48 to 36 hr before the examination and no further preparation is required, or a Dulcolax suppository may be given 1 or 2 hr before the patient is examined. Should rectal wash-outs be ordered, the nurse should ensure that the fluid given and the fluid returned are both measured; should fluid remain in the pelvic colon the surgeon will be unable to get a clear view through the sigmoidoscope.

X-Ray Examinations

The opaque meal examination as described on p. 134 is used to investigate some intestinal conditions, as for example suspected appendicitis. The first film is taken 6 hr after the barium meal has been taken.

Examination of the large intestine is, however, more frequently carried out by means of an opaque enema (barium). Before the examination the colon should be cleared of faeces; an aperient is given 36 hr before and a colonic wash-out or a Dulcolax suppository is given about 4 hr before the X-ray examination. The patient is usually allowed a light diet on the preceding day and a cup of tea on the morning of the examination.

One or two litres of barium suspension are introduced slowly through a rectal tube and the filling of the colon is watched under the X-ray screen. After the film has been taken the patient evacuates the enema and a further film may be taken. Films may be required after 24 and 48 hr and no aperient should be given until the radiologist says that the examination has been completed.

Constipation

Constipation is the condition in which the excretion of faeces is infrequent and difficult. The causes of constipation may be:

(1) *Defects in diet:* (a) insufficient roughage, so that there is lack of stimulus to peristalsis, and (b) insufficient fluid intake so that the waste is too solid, or there may be too great an absorption of water.

(2) *Sedentary habits*, whereby lack of exercise causes loss of tone in all muscles, including those of the bowel. Patients confined to bed may be constipated as a result of unaccustomed inactivity.

(3) *Interference with the controlling nervous mechanism*, as may occur from repression of the desire to defaecate, or to avoid the pain incurred when haemorrhoids or fissures are present. Megacolon (Hirschsprung's disease) causes constipation due to abnormality of the sympathetic nerves resulting in absence of peristalsis and a grossly dilated colon.

(4) *The effect of drastic purgation*, which causes a lack of muscle tone and thus defeats its own end.

(5) *Mechanical obstruction* by adhesions or growths in the intestinal tract or from pressure outside the gut.

Treatment

Where there is a specific cause this should be treated. In other cases correction of the condition can be brought about by attention to faulty habits:

(1) Response to the call for defaecation and training in regularity so that this reflex occurs at the same time each day. The process should be unhurried to be really effective.

(2) Correction of diet: (a) adequate roughage supplied by bran, wholemeal bread, vegetables and fruit, and (b) at least 2 litres of fluid daily.

(3) Exercise should be taken regularly and outdoor games may be beneficial.

Aperients or Laxatives

These drugs are used to secure evacuation of the bowel and may be classified as:

(1) Those whose action is mechanical, such as liquid paraffin, agar, methyl cellulose.

(2) Saline aperients, such as magnesium sulphate.

(3) Contact laxatives, bisacodyl (Dulcolax).

(4) Irritant purgatives such as the anthracene group, senna, often given as Senakot, cascara, phenolphthalein and castor oil.

Aperients should always be used with discretion, as their indiscriminate use causes loss of natural function which it may be impossible to regain, due to an atonic muscle wall from over-stimulation, or to failure of the normal nerve stimuli. In the treatment of constipation without obvious cause, all other methods should be tried first, and perseverance and encouragement can do much to correct the condition.

There is no evidence to support the theory that in illness aperients, by promoting free action of the bowels, help in the elimination of any toxins. Patients confined to bed, however, should not be allowed to become uncomfortably constipated. In elderly patients in particular, obstinate constipation may result in the impaction of hard dry faeces in the rectum and colon with symptoms of intestinal obstruction.

Diarrhoea

Diarrhoea is the condition in which frequent loose or fluid stools are passed. It may be due to excessive peristalsis or to over-secretion from the intestinal mucosa. It is commonly caused by:

(1) *Dietary* indiscretions, which may also give rise to colic.

(2) *Infection*, such as occurs in food poisoning, gastro-enteritis, typhoid fever, colitis.

(3) *Irritation* from drugs, e.g. arsenic, mercury, colchicum, excessive use of aperients.

(4) *Emotional* stress.

Diarrhoea may be a serious and troublesome manifestation in some conditions such as septicaemia, extensive burns, or hyper-activity of the thyroid gland.

Alternating diarrhoea and constipation may be a symptom of partial chronic intestinal obstruction due to malignant growth.

Intestinal Colic

Intestinal colic is severe griping pain due to violent peristaltic contractions. The causes are:

(1) Eating unsuitable or irritating foods.

(2) Mechanical obstruction, as in strangulation, intussusception, or malignant growth.

(3) Acute inflammation, e.g. appendicitis.

(4) Poisons, e.g. chronic lead poisoning.

(5) Disturbances of nervous origin, as in the abdominal crises of tabes dorsalis (see p. 271).

The pain may be so severe that collapse occurs with a small, feeble pulse and cold clammy skin. It may be accompanied by vomiting, diarrhoea or constipation.

The immediate treatment of this condition is the relief of pain by the application of heat, a protected hot water bottle or kaolin poultice, to the abdomen; if the pain is very severe morphine or pethidine may be ordered. Further treatment will depend on the cause of the colic.

DISEASES OF THE SMALL INTESTINE

Apart from duodenal ulcer diseases of the small intestine are comparatively rare. The main functions of the small intestine are to complete the digestion of food and to absorb the digested food. One group of diseases is associated with malabsorption of digested food from the small intestine and fat is excreted in the faeces in large amounts; the term malabsorption syndrome is used for this group, which includes coeliac disease, sprue and idiopathic steatorrhoea.

Coeliac Disease

Coeliac disease usually appears in children between 1 and 5 years of age. There is deficient absorption of fat from the small intestine, and this is due to sensitivity to gluten in wheat flour and other foods containing wheat grain. The stools are bulky, offensive and pale in colour, and the child usually has his bowels open several times in 24 hr. Growth is stunted, the abdomen protuberant, while loss of flesh is obvious in the thin stick-like limbs and the wasted buttocks. Anaemia is usually present to some degree. The child is prone to intercurrent infections, and occasionally serious loss of electrolytes and fluid in the copious stools which necessitates intravenous therapy as a life-saving measure.

Treatment

A gluten-free diet is given which excludes all foods made with whole wheat flour or containing wheat grain in any form. Rice flour, cornflour, soya flour and oatmeal are substituted. Additional protein is given in the form of Complan added to milk dishes; iron and vitamins may be prescribed. Physiotherapy helps to develop muscles and to correct poor posture.

Appropriate diet generally leads to considerable improvement and the child is not kept in hospital longer than necessary, since it is most important that he should be encouraged to grow out of invalid habits and should be ready for school at the appropriate age. However, before the child leaves hospital his mother must have plenty of opportunities of learning about the management of her child and his diet.

Steatorrhoea and Tropical Sprue

In both these conditions the main features are copious stools containing fat, and macrocytic anaemia. Loss of weight and a sore tongue are common symptoms. Tetany may occur from loss of calcium.

Treatment is mainly dietary. A high protein, low-fat diet, with added vitamin preparation, is usually prescribed. Vitamin B_{12}, cyanocobalamin, and corticosteroids may form part of the treatment.

Regional Ileitis

Regional ileitis is an acute or chronic inflammation of the terminal part of the ileum. In the acute form the symptoms may be similar to those of appendicitis with abdominal pain and tenderness on the right side. In chronic ileitis extensive inflammation, ulceration and thickening of the bowel wall may give rise to haemorrhage and obstruction. Abscesses and fistulae are possible complications.

Medical treatment includes rest and a bland diet. Antispasmodic drugs, such as belladonna or Pro-Banthine, may be prescribed to relieve colicky pain and corticosteroids may be successful in relieving the symptoms. Relapses are not uncommon; surgical treatment may be advisable, and will be essential if such complications as abscesses, fistulae, persistent haemorrhage or intestinal obstruction develop.

DISORDERS OF THE LARGE INTESTINE

Ulcerative Colitis

Ulcerative colitis is a condition in which there is inflammation and ulceration of any part of the colon, although the area most frequently affected is the pelvic colon and rectum.

The cause is uncertain; there is little evidence that infection plays any important part in producing the disease, although the ulcerated areas become infected. Young adults are most often affected, and the disease is commoner in women than in men. There may be a background of emotional stress, such as prolonged anxiety and possibly inadequate nutrition.

The onset is usually insidious, with increasing diarrhoea, abdominal discomfort and loss of appetite. The stools are fluid offensive and contain mucus and blood. Acute exacerbations with very frequent stools and some degree of fever alternate with remissions during which the patient is comparatively well but is usually anaemic and underweight. Often, however, the general trend is towards deterioration in the patient's condition, with increasingly severe relapses, emaciation and debility.

The diffuse shallow ulceration of the colon, as seen by sigmoidoscopy, and its narrowed pipe-like outline, as shown in the X-ray film after a barium enema, are characteristic of this disease, but further investigations may be undertaken in order to exclude specific infections such as dysentery.

Treatment

In all but mild cases complete rest in bed and warmth are necessary. Antispasmodic drugs such as belladonna or Pro-Banthine, and sedatives such as Compound Tablets of Codeine, B.P., may be ordered for the relief of colicky pain and diarrhoea. If the patient is markedly anaemic, blood transfusion may be necessary; in less severe anaemia iron in the form of ferrous sulphate tablets may be given.

Systemic administration of steroids, e.g. corticotropin (ACTH) intramuscularly, or prednisone by mouth, is often successful in controlling the acute phase of the disease. Retention enemas, such as either hydrocortisone or prednisolone hemisuccinate given in a small quantity, 120 ml (4 oz) of warm normal saline solution, may be ordered. The retention enema should be given at body heat, using a rubber catheter and a small funnel. Tilting the foot of the bed or raising the buttocks above the level of the rest of the trunk and giving the fluid very slowly 20 to 30 min for 120 ml of fluid, will help the patient to retain the enema.

If the patient is mentally restless and anxious, phenobarbitone may be given, or one of the tranquillizing drugs such as chlorpromazine. If any particular cause of emotional stress can be discovered and dealt with this may be of considerable assistance in procuring the mental and physical rest of which the patient stands in such great need.

Diet is of importance in the treatment of ulcerative colitis, as the patient is usually considerably below normal weight and his nutritional balance is disturbed, in particular he needs to build up his protein and vitamin intake. The diet therefore should be of high kilojoule value and should also tempt the patient's appetite, which is apt to be capricious, and at the same time exclude indigestible roughage which will irritate the inflamed and ulcerated bowel. Predigested protein in the form of Complan is often added to milk and other foods, and vitamin preparations are given to supplement those contained in the diet.

If the depletion of water and electrolytes is serious, and the patient is unable to make up the loss by an adequate intake of fluids by mouth, intravenous therapy will be necessary.

Example of a Low Residue High Kilojoule (kcal) Diet

Breakfast:
Tea or coffee with milk and sugar to taste.
Puffed rice, cornflakes or patent barley, with milk and sugar.
Boiled, poached or scrambled eggs, or boiled or steamed white fish, or smoked haddock, or lean ham.
White bread, toast or rusks, sparingly buttered.
Honey, golden syrup, black treacle, jelly marmalade, or jelly such as bramble jelly.

Mid-morning:
Coffee, cocoa, milk or any other form of milk food with added cornflour and sugar to taste.
Plain biscuits, e.g. cream crackers, rusks, petit beurre, or Marie.

Lunch:
Boiled or steamed fish, or rabbit, chicken, sweetbreads, brains, tripe, or minced tender meat.
Gravy or white sauce.
Mashed potatoes, sieved vegetables.
Milk pudding, custard, blancmange, junket, plain jelly or steamed sponge pudding.
Chocolate may be eaten after meals, or used as flavouring.

Tea:
Tea with milk and sugar to taste.
White bread and a small amount of butter.
Honey, golden syrup, black treacle, jelly, cream cheese or Marmite.
Sponge or plain madeira cake, or plain biscuits.

Supper:
Tea, coffee or cocoa made with milk, or any other form of milk food with sugar to taste.
White bread or plain biscuits and butter.
Eggs, white fish, smoked haddock, soft cheese or pudding.

Bedtime:
Cocoa, milk, with added Complan and sugar.
Plain biscuits if desired.

Milk may be reinforced with Complan and flavoured with chocolate or coffee.

Well-strained and sweetened orange, lemon, or grapefruit juice should be taken two or three times a day.

The foods may be arranged according to taste.

Meals should never be eaten in a hurry, and at least 10 min rest should be taken after finishing them.

Foods not allowed include:

Wholemeal bread, rye, and other crispbreads, whole grain cereals, tough meat, whole coarse vegetables, whole fresh or canned fruit (sieved fruit and fruit puree are usually allowed), dried fruits such as figs, currants and sultanas.

Surgical Treatment

In severe cases of fulminating ulcerative colitis, or in those cases where medical treatment produces only very temporary remissions, surgical treatment may become necessary, and an ileostomy is usually performed. Although this operation leaves the patient with a permanent opening into the bowel, the use of disposable ileostomy bags made of plastic or of newer types of latex, makes this condition much more manageable for the patient than it was at one time. Providing the patient is given full instructions and will co-operate in carrying them out over the first few difficult months, he should be able to lead a normal life and in much greater comfort than was possible before the operation.

Total or partial colectomy may be carried out with ileostomy. In a few fortunate patients where the disease is limited, it is possible for colectomy to be combined with anastomosis to the lower end of the rectum, thus doing away with the necessity for an ileostomy.

The nursing care of the patient is on general lines with very special care to prevent pressure sores. If the patient is passing very frequent stools a rubber bedpan helps to relieve pressure, and is more comfortable than metal or plastic types. Careful attention must be paid to the toilet of the anal region which may become excoriated. Application of a barrier cream after cleansing may be beneficial. Frequent cleaning of the mouth is necessary in the acute stage of the disease; when the patient is able to take food and fluid in sufficient amounts the mouth as a rule regains its normal moist, clean state.

Ulcerative colitis tends to become chronic, relapses are common and treatment may be disappointing. Skilful and sympathetic nursing can do much to help the patient over difficult periods of depression and anxiety which are so often a feature of this illness.

Diverticulitis

Diverticulitis is the name given to a condition in which multiple small pouches, or diverticula, along the course of the colon become inflamed and produce symptoms such as colicky abdominal pain, tenderness and constipation, and sometimes localized peritonitis with fever. Abscesses may form, or thickening of the bowel wall may cause intestinal obstruction.

Treatment

A bland low-residue diet and suitable lubricating aperients such as liquid paraffin or Mil-Par (magnesium and paraffin emulsion) to ensure a soft consistency of the bowel contents are usually ordered. Local peritonitis and other complications require appropriate treatment, rest in bed, fluid diet and the administration of sulphonamides or antibiotics such as chloramphenicol or chlortetracycline. Surgical treatment may be necessary to drain an abscess or relieve obstruction.

Diverticulosis, i.e. the presence of diverticula, may be congenital, this condition does not usually cause symptoms and is often only revealed in the course of an opaque enema X-ray examination. Recently it has been considered that a diet deficient in roughage may predispose a person to chronic constipation and to the development of diverticula; this, despite the fact that the individual may have a daily bowel movement. Tests have shown that residue may remain in the colon for many days producing toxic substances which damage the colonic wall. A daily intake of fibre such as bran is advocated to avoid the situation.

Megacolon (Hirschsprung's Disease)

Megacolon is a congenital condition in which the sympathetic ganglion cells in a part of the pelvic colon and rectum are absent, and the colon becomes enormously dilated and fills with faeces.

The child has a distended 'doughy' abdomen which increases in size. He is constipated, but from time to time passes a very large stool. The greatly distended colon can be demonstrated by an X-ray examination with a barium enema. Growth and nutrition are poor, and unless surgical treatment can be successfully undertaken the outlook is not very hopeful. The operation consists of resection of the abnormal area and anastomosis with the anal canal.

New Growths of the Large Intestine

The commonest form of neoplasm, or new growth, is carcinoma of the colon or rectum. The patient is usually middle-aged, and may seek advice because he is passing blood and has become constipated or has alternating diarrhoea and constipation. He may complain of colicky pain, otherwise pain is not a prominent feature, and unfortunately a number of such patients do not consult their doctor until the disease is well advanced. If the condition is diagnosed early surgical treatment is often successful. In the later states only palliative treatment, in the form of colostomy to relieve obstruction, is usually possible.

Helminthic Infections (Intestinal Worms)

Helminthic infections are commonest in countries where standards of personal and community hygiene are low, and are also more prevalent in tropical and subtropical than in temperate climates. Some of these parasites, for example threadworms, are, however, found in every country and in all classes of society. It has been estimated that over 80 per cent of the total world population harbour one or other type of intestinal worms.

Mild infections usually cause little inconvenience to the human host. Heavy and repeated infections produce local symptoms, such as digestive disturbances and abdominal pain, and also general manifestations of ill health and poor nutrition, including anaemia, lowered physical and mental vitality and in children, retarded growth.

Tapeworms (Cestodes)

Tapeworms are long, flat, segmented worms which use animals and man as their hosts both in the embryonic and the adult stages of their life cycle. The three types of these parasites for which man is the host of the adult worm are, *Taenia solium*, whose intermediate host is the pig, *Taenia saginata*, or beef tapeworm, with domestic cattle acting as the intermediate host and *Diphyllobothrium latum*, the fish tapeworm, which is found in fresh-water fish. The embryos develop in the tissues of the intermediate host and become encysted; if the flesh of the infected animal is eaten by man he can become the host for the adult worm. Efficient inspection of animal carcases intended for human consumption and thorough cooking, which kills the embryos, are the main methods of preventing infection with tapeworms.

Taenia saginata is the commonest cause of tapeworm infection. When the encysted form is swallowed in infected beef or veal, the cyst wall dissolves in the stomach, the parasite passes into the duodenum and fastens by the hooklets on its head to the mucous membrane, from which it sucks the blood of the host. A fully developed worm may be as much as 10 m (30 ft) in length. It grows in segments from its head and the largest of these contain mature ova, which are passed out in the faeces, where the segments are easily recognized. There may be other rather indecisive signs, such as colic or vague abdominal discomfort, vomiting, abnormally large appetite, itching at nose or anus, or salivation. Anaemia develops in long-standing cases. Diagnosis can be made only by actual observation of the excreted segments and no curative treatment is adopted until this is proved beyond doubt.

Treatment

Treatment aims at the expulsion of the tapeworm by the administration of an anthelmintic drug. For many years extract of male fern was used in the treatment of tapeworm infection. This drug has been replaced by dichlorphen (Antiphen) and niclosamide (Yamesan) which have a direct effect on all types of tapeworm. There is no need for the patient to fast but the drugs are best given before breakfast. They may cause some nausea and colic. Neither is there need to examine the stools for segments as they are partially digested in the gut after being killed by the drug.

Hydatid Cysts

Hydatid cysts are the cystic form of a tapeworm (*Taenia echinococcus*) whose intermediate hosts are usually cattle or sheep but which may infect man. Dogs are the host for the adult worm; man can become infected through close contact with dogs and contamination from their excreta. When the embryo worms reach the human intestine they penetrate the intestinal wall, and can be carried by the blood-stream to the liver, lung, or other tissues, and there form a cyst which is capable of producing others ('daughter cysts'), sometimes to an enormous extent.

Symptoms vary according to the position of the cysts, the treatment most likely to be satisfactory is surgical removal.

Roundworms (*Ascaris lumbricoides*)

Roundworms are similar in shape and size to the garden worm, but paler in colour. The eggs are excreted in the faeces and may contaminate water or vegetables and so enter the alimentary tract, where the larvae are set free, penetrate the mucous membrane, and thus pass into the blood-stream. Reaching the liver they travel thence to the lungs to penetrate an air sac, ascend the bronchial tree and thus reach the pharynx, when they are again swallowed and once more entering the intestine, develop into adult worms. Roundworm infection (ascariasis) is common in many countries; it has been estimated that in some areas of the tropics almost 100 per cent of the population harbour this parasite. Ascariasis can be a serious condition, particularly in children between the age of 1 and 5 years, causing digestive disturbances, intestinal colic, loss of appetite, debility and retarded growth. If present in large numbers, roundworms can cause intestinal obstruction. The presence of migrating larvae in the lungs may produce symptoms similar to those of pneumonia with fever and persistent cough.

Treatment

The anthelmintic in general use is piperazine (Antepar); no preliminary aperient or fasting are necessary. The usual dosage of Antepar elixir is 24 ml (6 fluid drachms) for infants and children under the age of 5 years, 30 ml (8 fluid drachms) for older children and adults. Antepar is also available in tablet form, the adult dose is 4·5 g and the dose for children is 120 mg per kg of body weight up to a maximum of 4 g. Bephenium granules (Alcopar) may also be used in single dose of 5 g or half that dose for children under 2 years of age. Ascariasis is particularly likely to be endemic in areas where the standards of both personal and environmental hygiene are low. If the faeces of infected persons are deposited on the ground the roundworm ova then develop to the infective stage in the soil. Food and fingers are easily contaminated with these ova which are then swallowed. Every adult worm in the human intestine must develop from an ingested ovum; roundworms do not multiply within the intestine.

While improved hygiene combined with health teaching are obvious steps which should be taken to control this widespread infection, these measures take time to become effective. In the meantime children who are at risk may be given treatment with Antepar at about 3 monthly intervals in order to prevent heavy reinfection.

Threadworms (*Oxyuris vermicularis*)

Threadworms are small worms about 1 cm ($\frac{1}{2}$ in) long which appear like threads in the faeces. The adult parasites develop in the small intestine but pass to the large intestine where they may be present in large numbers. The ova are excreted in the faeces and thus may contaminate water, but commonly the method of spread is from infected clothing and towels, or by the fingers as the result of scratching the skin near the anus. The female deposits eggs on the skin around the anus, causing itching, which is worse at night, producing restlessness and loss of sleep.

The usual anthelmintic is piperazine (Antepar), which may be given as an elixir or in tablet form. The adult dose is 1 to 2 g daily given for 7 days; for children the dose is according to body weight.

To prevent reinfection and allay irritation, the area around the anus can be smeared regularly with a weak mercurial ointment. Children should wear a one-piece sleeping suit fastened at the back to prevent the hands from coming in contact with the anal region during the night. Towels, flannels, and other toilet articles, used by those known to be infected should be kept separate for their particular use and measures taken to disinfect the bed and other clothing which might be a source of spread of the parasite. Hands and nails should be well washed after each visit to the lavatory and before meals, and the nails should be kept short.

Hookworms

Hookworms are small parasites about 1 cm ($\frac{1}{2}$ in) in length which inhabit the human small intestine. Hookworm infection (ancylostomiasis) by the type known as *Ancylostoma duodenale* is prevalent throughout the Mediterranean area, the Middle East, Pakistan and northern India. In Africa south of the Sahara, Central and South America, the West Indies and southern India infection is due to another type of hookworm, *Necator americanus*. Mixed infections with both types occur over wide areas of the Far East.

Infection is commonest in rural areas which lack proper sanitation and where, therefore, the soil is often heavily polluted with human excreta. Any person walking barefoot on such ground may become infected with hookworm larvae which enter the body through the skin. The larvae travel via the lymphatic and the blood circulation, eventually reaching the small intestine where they mature into the adult worms, which live on blood from the tissues of the host.

The most typical manifestation of hookworm infection is anaemia, which is likely to be accompanied by impairment of mental and physical activity. Retarded growth and development may be noted in children and in pregnant women the haemoglobin may be reduced to danger level.

Treatment

One anthelmintic drug used in the treatment of hookworm is tetrachlorethylene, but it is apt to produce unpleasant side-effects such as giddiness. More recently bephenium in the form of Alcopar Dispersible Granules has been successfully used in the treatment of both children and adults. It is dispensed in single-dose sachets containing 5 g of the granules to be given in water when the stomach is empty and at least 1 hour before food is taken. Children under 2 years of age, or under 10 kg in weight, are given half the adult dose. The accompanying anaemia often requires treatment, which in most cases is the administration of iron.

Trichinosis

Trichinosis is caused by infection with the larvae of the worm *Trichinella spiralis*. Pigs can be the host for this worm and the disease is contracted by eating infected pork which has not been thoroughly cooked. When the larvae are swallowed they hatch out in the small intestine and then invade the muscles where they become encysted.

Mild infections may produce no symptoms, severe infections cause vomiting, diarrhoea and fever, followed by oedema, which is particularly noticeable around the eyes, pain and tenderness in the muscles. The majority of patients recover, but in heavy infections death can occur from myocardial failure, or from involvement of the brain causing encephalitis with paralysis and coma.

The treatment of trichinosis is mainly directed towards relieving the symptoms and providing general nursing care. In severe cases cortisone drugs have proved to be of value.

Schistosoma (Bilharzia)

Schistosoma, or bilharzia, are blood flukes which are not, strictly speaking, intestinal parasites since they inhabit the blood vessels of the human host. However, two varieties of this parasite, *S. mansoni* and *S. japonicum*, cause dysenteric symptoms with blood and mucus in the stool. The third type, *S. haematobium*, infects the urinary tract.

The intermediate host is a freshwater snail and infection is acquired through washing, bathing or fishing in water in which these snails have shed the parasites at the infective stage. Schistosoma infection (schistosomiasis) is widespread in Africa, the Middle East, the Far East, Central and South America, and it also occurs in some areas of southern Europe bordering the Mediterranean.

The parasites enter the body through the skin or mucous membrane and then develop into adult worms in the blood vessels of the rectum and the large intestine, or the bladder. The ova deposited by the female worm escape through the walls of these organs causing irritation and bleeding. The same individual may be infected with both the vesical and the intestinal type of schistosomiasis at the same time.

Treatment

Two anthelmintics used for the treatment of all types of schistosomiasis are sodium antimonygluconate (Triostam) and lucanthone hydrochloride (Nilodin). Triostam is dispensed as a sterile powder which must be dissolved in cold sterile water immediately before use. It is given by slow intravenous injection; 3·5 ml of the solution contains 190 mg of Triostam. The total dosage required is based on the patient's body weight and is divided into six equal doses given on six consecutive days. Nilodin is given by mouth; the total dose, calculated on body weight, is given in divided doses, twice daily for 3 days.

7

Disorders of the liver, biliary tract and pancreas

Tests of Liver Function

TESTS of liver function are less satisfactory than function tests of some other organs because the liver has numerous functions any single one of which may be deficient, whilst the others remain relatively intact. Also the liver has a large reserve and has to be very extensively damaged before any of the tests show an abnormal result. No test has yet been devised which tests the liver as a whole, but there are innumerable tests which depend on the different individual functions of the organ. The commonest of these tests are given below.

Bile Pigments

Failure of the liver to excrete bile pigments leads to the accumulation of these in the blood and their excretion in the urine:

(1) *Bilirubin*. The normal level of bilirubin in the blood serum varies from 0·2 to 0·75 mg per 100 ml. Increased serum bilirubin is found in liver damage, obstructive jaundice and haemolytic jaundice. Bilirubin will be present in the urine in all cases of jaundice except haemolytic jaundice.

(2) *Urobilinogen*. This pigment will be present in the urine in cases of incomplete obstructive jaundice, in diffuse liver damage, for example infective hepatitis, and in haemolytic jaundice. In cases of complete obstructive jaundice urobilinogen is absent from the urine.

Serum Protein Tests

These tests are designed to show variations from the normal ability of the liver to synthesize serum proteins. They are not specific tests for liver damage since alterations in the serum proteins may be found in many other diseases.

In liver diseases the serum albumin level is low and the serum globulin is raised. The abnormal composition of the serum proteins is also reflected in the so-called 'empirical liver function tests', for example the thymol turbidity and cephalin–cholesterol tests. These become positive when liver function is impaired— e.g. in cirrhosis of the liver and infective hepatitis.

Not less than 5 ml of whole blood is required for each of these tests.

Serum Enzyme Estimations

Normally only very small amounts of the great number of enzymes involved in cellular process are found in the blood, but when cells are damaged the concentration of certain enzymes rises and estimation of these helps to establish the existence or the amount of cellular damage. The enzymes most commonly estimated are the aspartate transaminase (glutamic oxaloacetic transaminase, or GOT), which is increased in hepatitis and following myocardial infarction, and the aline transaminase (glutamic pyruvic transaminase, or GPT), which is increased in various forms of liver cell damage.

Bromsulphthalein Test

This test measures the ability of the liver to excrete a dye, bromsulphthalein.

The patient should have a fat-free breakfast and no food thereafter until the test is completed.

Procedure

10.00 hours   5 mg per kg of body weight of 5 per cent brom-sulphthalein is injected intravenously very slowly over a period of 3 min. The ampoule must be warmed if any crystals are visible.

10.45 hours   10 ml of clotted blood is collected from another vein, special care being taken to avoid haemolysis.

Interpretation of the test. After 45 min the serum should show that less than 7 per cent of the injected dose is still retained.

Prothrombin Concentration Test

Prothrombin is formed in the liver from vitamin K absorbed from the intestine. A low prothrombin level may be due to liver damage, or to the non-absorption of vitamin K resulting from biliary obstruction. If the prothrombin concentration is low, the test may be repeated after an injection of vitamin K, and if it then returns to normal it is suggestive of biliary obstruction.

Liver Biopsy

Liver biopsy is performed in cases where it is necessary to obtain a sample of the liver substance for examination. A small amount of liver tissue is removed by a puncture made with a special trocar and cannula (Silverman's liver biopsy needle), or with a Menghini's liver biopsy needle. Prior to carrying out this investigation the patient's blood group is ascertained, his blood is cross-matched, the haemoglobin and prothrombin content, the bleeding time and the clotting time are estimated. The biopsy is not usually proceeded with if the prothrombin content is found to be below 70 per cent of the normal.

Bleeding into the peritoneal cavity may occur following liver biopsy and therefore the patient must be under close observation; an hourly pulse chart should be kept for at least 12 hr following this procedure.

Jaundice

Jaundice describes the yellow colour of the skin and conjunctiva of the eyes due to the absorption from the blood of pigments which are normally excreted in the bile. The intensity of the colour can vary from a pale daffodil yellow to a deep greenish yellow. Jaundice may be due to a number of widely different causes, and is classified in accordance with the cause:

(1) *Obstructive jaundice.* Bile cannot pass down the common bile duct into the intestine and the pigment is absorbed into the blood-stream. The commonest causes of obstructive jaundice are impaction of a gall-stone in the common bile duct and a growth in the head of the pancreas which compresses the bile duct.

Since no bile can colour the faeces in this type of jaundice, the patient will pass light, clay-coloured stools. The urine is dark and contains bile pigments.

(2) *Infections.* These cause hepato-cellular jaundice. Examples are infective hepatitis of viral origin, protozoal infection

as in malaria, Weil's disease (leptospiral jaundice) and amoebic infection, bacterial infection which may be secondary to severe septic infection. Some toxic substances such as chloroform, chlorpromazine and TNT, a chemical used in the manufacture of explosives, have a similar effect. In infective jaundice, owing to damage to the liver cells, the pigments brought in the blood are not removed and excreted in the bile in the normal way; thus they are retained in the blood-stream and eventually colour the skin and conjunctiva. Since the amount of bile pigment reaching the intestine is diminished, the stools will be paler than normal, and bile pigments will be excreted in the urine.

(3) *Haemolytic jaundice*. This is due to excessive amounts of bilirubin in the blood from the breaking up of large numbers of red blood cells. The liver is unable to eliminate all this pigment and jaundice develops. Slight jaundice of this type is seen in many new-born infants, it develops a day or so after birth and usually clears up by the end of the first week of life. Severe jaundice which may be present at birth is a symptom of haemolytic disease of the new born, due to anti-Rhesus agglutinins. The same factor can produce haemolytic jaundice if a patient who is Rh negative receives a transfusion of Rh positive blood, when he develops anti-Rh agglutinins and is later given a further transfusion with Rh positive blood (see also p. 87). The stools in haemolytic jaundice are the normal brown colour, the urine contains an excess of urobilinogen, but no bile, and is therefore also normal in colour.

DISEASES AND DISORDERS OF THE LIVER

Infective Hepatitis

Infective hepatitis is an acute disease due to a virus, and may appear as an epidemic. The patient has vague symptoms of loss of appetite, malaise, slight fever, nausea, vomiting and some abdominal pain before jaundice appears. It is then noted that urine passed is darker in colour than normal, and that the stools are pale in colour. Often the general symptoms are subsiding when the jaundice appears. At the end of about 2 to 3 weeks in most cases the jaundice is clearing and the patient feels much better. However, convalescence is often slow, the patient is easily tired and may feel generally depressed and lethargic for 6 to 8 weeks after the acute stage of his illness.

Relapses sometimes occur, and in a small percentage of cases acute liver failure may cause death.

Treatment

Rest in bed is necessary in the febrile stage of the disease, and return to activity must be gradual. While the patient feels nauseated and has no appetite glucose fruit drinks are likely to be all that he can take. As soon as possible the diet should be increased, as a high kilojoule (kcal), high-protein diet helps the liver cells to combat the infection. Fat is not easily digested, and the patient usually feels very averse to taking fatty food. Skimmed milk powder and Complan may be added to milk feeds and other foods to increase the protein intake.

It is probable that the disease is spread by contamination from faeces and urine, therefore the necessary precautions against its spread must be taken (see p. 309). The nurse must be particularly careful to wash her hands thoroughly after attending to the patient.

A variety of hepatitis known as serum hepatitis may result from infection introduced by an intravenous injection given with a syringe which has been used for withdrawing blood and not effectively sterilized, or by a blood or plasma transfusion. The danger of such infection is probably greatest when pooled plasma is used. The infection may also occur when patients are receiving renal dialysis which involves the circulation of blood through a machine. Staff in such units are particularly at risk if the patient's blood contains an antigen known as the 'Australian' antigen. The signs, symptoms and treatment of serum hepatitis are in the main the same as those of infective hepatitis.

Weil's Disease (Leptospiral Jaundice)

This disease is due to infection with a spirochaete, *Leptospira icterohaemorrhagiae*, which is excreted in the urine of rats and can infect soil, water or food. It more commonly occurs in those whose work may bring them into contact with soil or other material contaminated by rats, e.g. sewer workers, miners and farmers.

The onset is sudden, with a high temperature, 40° to 41°C (104° to 105°F), headache, muscle pains, vomiting, sometimes a purpuric rash and nose-bleeding. Jaundice appears about the fourth day of the illness. The kidneys are also involved, proteins and blood appear in the urine, and occasionally, there is complete renal failure with anuria.

Treatment

The treatment is the administration of large doses of tetracycline or penicillin as early as possible. Careful recording of the amount of urine passed and testing for the presence of protein and blood are necessary in order to detect signs of renal failure at their onset.

Acute Liver Necrosis (Acute Yellow Atrophy)

Acute liver necrosis failure may occur as a result of viral hepatitis or from the toxic effects of such drugs as chloroform, gold, arsenic or from phosphorus or TNT poisoning. It is also an occasional complication in the later months of pregnancy.

The initial symptoms are similar to those of infective hepatitis, but are progressively severe, with deepening jaundice, vomiting, headache, confusion and delirium, which may end in coma and death.

Treatment

The treatment is to give intravenous glucose solution, often with tetracycline added. The patient is encouraged to take carbohydrate by mouth in the form of glucose fruit drinks, no proteins in any form are given in the acute stage as it has been found that they tend to increase the mental confusion and delirium.

Cirrhosis of the Liver

Cirrhosis of the liver is a condition in which fibrous tissue forms around and within the lobules of the liver. It may follow acute hepatitis. In some cases it is thought to be due to a nutritional deficiency; liver damage is commonly found in children suffering from deficiency of protein and vitamins in the condition known in Africa as kwashiorkor. In certain cases alcoholism is a causal factor. Considerable enlargement of the liver may be noted, although in the late stages of the condition it usually shrinks.

The symptoms are due to obstruction in the portal circulation or to failure of the liver cells to carry out their function, or to a combination of both factors. A considerable volume of blood is shunted through the collateral circulation and is not therefore subjected to the normal detoxicating action of the liver, inability of the liver cells to perform their function adds to this failure, and neurological symptoms such as mental confusion, result. Jaundice may be present, but not usually to a marked extent. Gastric disturbances occur, e.g. vomiting, especially in the early morning, loss of appetite and furred tongue. Haematemesis may result from the portal congestion which produces enlargement and varicosity of the anastomosing veins at the lower end of the oesophagus (Fig. 19). These veins are very liable to rupture and cause very severe bleeding. The bleeding may be excessive in amount (see p. 127). Haemorrhoids may be a troublesome symptom, and they also result from the enlargement of anastomosing veins in this case in the anal canal. Ascites develops, partly as a result of portal hypertension and partly as a result of poor liver function and reduced protein in the blood. Generalized oedema is also a sequel to lowered blood plasma proteins.

In late stages the patient becomes thin and weak, his eyes are sunken and he is obviously very ill. Death may result from liver failure or from bleeding, but improvement may follow treatment and be maintained for some years.

Treatment

A high-protein diet is given if the patient is oedematous with ascites but has no mental symptoms. If neurological or mental symptoms are present, then a low-protein diet must be given and neomycin may be given by mouth in order to prevent protein break-down by bacteria in the intestinal tract. In certain selected cases surgical treatment may be advised to relieve portal congestion and an anastomosis between the portal vein and the inferior vena cava is carried out.

Diuretics are ordered to lessen the ascites. In some cases with gross ascites, where pressure of this fluid is reducing the urinary output, puncture of the peritoneum, paracentesis abdominis, may be carried out. A many-tailed bandage applied from above downwards and readjusted to maintain

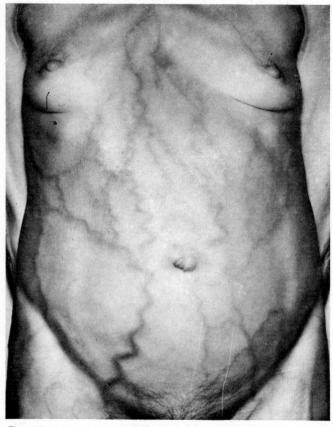

FIG. 19. Infrared photograph showing enlarged collateral vessels in a patient with cirrhosis of the liver and portal hypertension.

pressure as required is helpful during the drainage of the fluid from the peritoneal cavity.

The nursing treatment is on general lines and is directed towards maintaining as far as possible the comfort and well-being of the patient.

DISEASES OF THE GALL-BLADDER AND BILIARY SYSTEM

Cholecystitis

Acute inflammation of the gall-bladder or cholecystitis may be due to infection by *Escherichia coli*, streptococcal or staphylococcal organisms, or rarely by typhoid bacilli. The presence of gall-stones which may obstruct the outlet of the gall-bladder and cause biliary stasis which leads to infection is often associated with repeated attacks of cholecystitis.

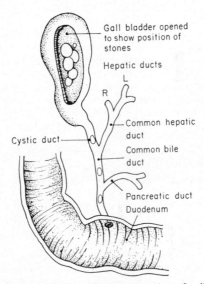

FIG. 20. Diagram to show possible situation of gall-stones.

The symptoms may be indefinite and comparatively mild, dyspepsia, flatulence, with some pain and tenderness on the right side of the upper abdomen. More acute attacks with severe pain and fever may be accompanied by jaundice due to swelling of the bile ducts or obstruction by a gall-stone in the common bile duct (Fig. 20). Suppuration and perforation are complications requiring immediate surgical drainage. In-flammation of the gall-bladder often involves the bile ducts, giving rise to cholangitis. Following an acute attack the patient is likely to develop chronic cholecystitis with the formation of gall-stones, which may at any time block the common bile duct and produce attacks of biliary colic.

Biliary colic is characterized by severe and excruciating pain in the epigastric area or in the right upper quadrant of the abdomen radiating through to the back and upwards to the shoulder. It may be so severe that the patient shows signs of collapse, with sweating and pallor; the pulse rate quickens and vomiting is usual. Later the pain becomes a dull ache, perhaps followed by a fresh acute onslaught.

The stone may be passed out into the duodenum, and so expelled in the faeces. To discover if this is so, the faeces must be examined by washing them through a sieve, when the stone if present will remain behind. The pain ceases when the stone enters the intestine, but may recur if another is forced into the duct. If it becomes impacted in the bile duct, jaundice will occur 24 hr later. If it lodges in the ampulla of Vater, at the point where the pancreatic duct and the common bile duct enter the duodenum, there may be interference with the flow of pancreatic secretion as well as of bile. Infection is likely to spread along the duct and cause acute pancreatitis.

Diagnosis of gall-bladder disease and the presence of gall-stones is assisted by X-ray examination. A straight X-ray of the abdomen seldom shows the presence of gall-stones, as the majority of such stones are not radio-opaque; therefore the examination known as cholecystography, is carried out after the administration of a contrast medium.

Preparation of the patient for cholecystography will be in accordance with the directions issued by the radiologist. Usually an aperient is ordered 2 days before the examination and a low-residue diet is given for these 2 days. After supper on the second day an iodine-containing compound, iodopanoic acid (Telepaque), is given. After this no food or fluid is given by mouth until the first X-rays have been taken on the following morning; then the patient is given a meal with a high fat content, e.g. scrambled eggs, buttered toast and tea or coffee with cream. An hour later the final films are taken.

An intravenous injection of sodium iodipamide (Biligrafin)

may be given and films are taken at 5-min intervals up to 30 or 45 min after the injection, when the dye should be visible in the bile ducts and gall-bladder. A fatty meal is then given as in the oral method.

Serial X-ray films of the biliary tract following an intravenous injection of Biligrafin may be required after the gall-bladder has been opened and drained or removed, in order to demonstrate the presence of stones in the bile ducts or the patency of the common bile duct. This examination is known as cholangiography.

Treatment

During an attack of cholecystitis rest in bed is necessary. Any signs of increasing infection, with raised temperature and pulse rate, persistent vomiting and pain, should be looked for and immediately reported if they occur, as suppuration, gangrene and perforation of the gall-bladder are possible developments which call for immediate operation.

Morphine 10 to 15 mg, atropine 0·4 to 0·6 mg, or pethidine 50 to 100 mg may be ordered for the relief of pain.

If vomiting and distension are prominent features an intragastric or duodenal tube is passed via the nose and suction is carried out. No food or fluids are given by mouth, and intravenous therapy will be required to meet the fluid and electrolyte requirements. In less severe attacks fluids such as sweetened fruit drinks, water, weak tea, can be given at first, followed by light diet, mainly carbohydrate and containing very little fat. Toast, rusks, biscuits, with jam or marmalade, cereals with sugar and fruit juice, fruit jellies, steamed white fish, chicken, small amounts of milk, e.g. half a pint daily, are examples of foods which may be allowed.

When the attack has subsided, cholecystography and possibly liver function tests are carried out and surgical treatment is considered.

Biliary colic necessitates immediate treatment for the relief of pain and spasm. Rest in bed with warmth applied to the abdomen by a well protected hot water bottle or electric pad will help, but injections of morphine or pethidine with atropine are necessary in most cases. Large quantities of fluid by mouth are usually ordered, and sometimes magnesium sulphate by mouth to promote the flow of bile. Since biliary colic is evidence of gall-stones and attacks are likely to be recurrent, surgical removal of the gall-bladder, cholecystectomy, is usually advised.

Pancreatitis

Acute pancreatitis may be associated with diseases of the gall-bladder and biliary tract, or there may be a history of peptic ulcer. The actual cause of the inflammation is uncertain, although it is an occasional complication of mumps.

The attack is characterized by sudden agonizing pain in the upper abdomen radiating to the back and up to the shoulder area, accompanied by vomiting and a considerable degree of shock. The condition may be difficult to distinguish from perforated peptic ulcer or biliary colic and if the diagnosis is in doubt an emergency laparotomy may be undertaken without delay. Otherwise the immediate treatment is that of the shock with intravenous plasma, morphine or pethidine for the relief of pain. No food or fluid is given by mouth, and usually gastric suction is carried out either intermittently or continuously. Fluids are given intravenously, and a careful fluid balance chart must be kept.

As the condition improves small quantities of fluids are given by mouth and followed, if all goes well, by a bland low-fat diet.

If the symptoms suggest an acute abdominal emergency, but the diagnosis of pancreatitis is in doubt, estimation of the amylase content of the blood and urine should be carried out. If time permits, the urine sample should be obtained from urine collected over a period of several hours, but in an emergency a specimen should be obtained immediately and sent to the laboratory. Duodenal drainage may be required in order to obtain a sample of the pancreatic secretion. An injection of secretin or of Mecholyl may be given to stimulate the flow of pancreatic juice.

Chronic Pancreatitis

Chronic inflammation of the pancreas with progressive fibrotic changes, necrosis and the development of diabetes, may follow an acute attack and may be associated with disease of the gall-bladder and biliary tract or with peptic ulceration. The patient may have recurring bouts of pain and digestive disturbance, the stools are bulky and contain excessive amounts of fat.

Treatment

Any associated condition, such as cholecystitis or peptic ulcer, should be treated. A high-calorie high-carbohydrate diet, with reduced fat and protein, is usually ordered. If diabetes develops this will necessitate the administration of insulin.

Carcinoma of the Pancreas

Carcinoma of the pancreas is a disease of middle age, and is commoner in men than in women. Unless the head of the pancreas is involved and causes obstruction by pressure on the common bile duct, symptoms are likely to be few and indefinite in the early stages of the disease. Often secondary deposits have developed in the liver before the diagnosis can be made.

The treatment is surgical resection of the growth if at all feasible; in advanced cases palliative treatment for the relief of biliary obstruction, by making an opening from the gall-bladder to the duodenum (cholecystenterostomy), may be carried out. Sedatives and tranquillizing drugs, such as chlorpromazine, will be needed for the relief of nausea and pain.

8

Nutritional disorders

Under-Feeding and Malnutrition

UNDER-FEEDING, or subnutrition, means that there is an insufficiency of the total food intake to meet the body's needs for growth, repair, maintenance and energy. The term malnutrition is used to describe a serious lack of one or more of the essential constituents of the diet, as for example vitamin or protein deficiency.

An extreme degree of under-feeding, or starvation, is uncommon in any of the economically developed countries with the exception of some instances of old people living alone, where a combination of lack of money, disability and loss of interest may eventually cause starvation, and in circumstances where lack of food is due to a pathological state. One example of such a condition is a disease with a psychological background known as anorexia nervosa, in which the patient loses all desire for food and which can lead to extreme emaciation and even death. Other possible causes are 'slimming diets', which in women may lead to the development of anorexia nervosa, persistent vomiting from any cause, and chronic alcoholism which is frequently associated with a grossly inadequate intake of food.

The most obvious result of under-feeding is marked loss of weight. In children this will be accompanied by retardation of growth, the skin hangs loosely over the wasted muscles, both skin and hair are thin and dry and the eyes are sunken. In extreme degrees of starvation oedema develops as the tissue cells cannot hold their normal amount of water and the lack of plasma proteins leads to exudation of fluid from the blood vessels; this type of oedema is known as 'famine oedema'. The ability to maintain life for considerable periods in such circumstances is an example of the extraordinary ability of the human body to adapt itself to adverse conditions; the basal metabolic rate is lowered, the heart beats more slowly, the individual becomes apathetic, seldom changing his position or making any unnecessary movements, thus reducing his energy needs to a minimum.

The treatment of this condition is equally obvious; food must be given in sufficient quantities to restore the lost weight and vitality. However, caution is needed in feeding a starved patient; small quantities of easily digested foods are necessary at first, since the digestive powers, as all other bodily functions, are impaired and injudicious feeding is very likely to cause vomiting with further deterioration of the patient's condition. Complan containing predigested protein and all essential food requirements is often of value in such cases. Psychological factors, as in anorexia nervosa, will need the help of a psychiatrist.

Deficiency Diseases

Protein Deficiency

Protein deficiency has already been mentioned as one of the factors responsible for famine oedema, where it is a part of a general state of under-nutrition. The condition now known as 'protein malnutrition' in young children is common throughout many parts of the world where the diet of the child after weaning consists mainly of carbohydrates such as plantains, maize and other cereals and where first-class proteins are seriously lacking. Protein malnutrition may be manifested in two forms. The first is marasmus or wasting (Fig. 21), and the other is the condition which has been given the West African name of 'kwashiorkor'. The marasmic child is usually under 1 year old, is obviously wasted with a wizened appearance. The child showing evidence of kwashiorkor is usually in the 1 to 3 year age group and at first sight may not appear to be as malnourished as the marasmic infant, although obviously ill, miserable and apathetic. However, the apparent lack of wasting is due to the presence of oedema which is most marked in the feet, hands and face. The skin loses its dark pigment and develops a scaly rash. The hair also loses its dark colour, changing to a rusty brown, sometimes almost flaxen; it is sparse and straight. Many of these children die from liver damage due to prolonged protein deprivation or to intercurrent infection against which they have little resistance.

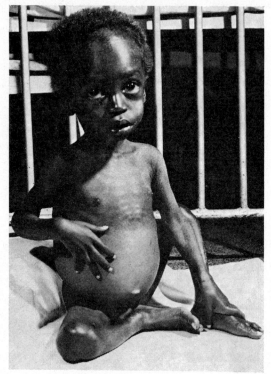

FIG. 21. Marasmus, one form of protein calorie malnutrition.

A child severely ill as a result of protein malnutrition needs hospital treatment, the basis of which is adequate feeding. Frequently the child has no appetite and will not take sufficient food, and in these cases feeding by intragastric tube is necessary. An important aspect of treatment is the admission of both mother and child to hospital.

Dried skimmed milk is a suitable form of protein for these children, and large quantities of this food have been given by international agencies to countries where protein malnutrition occurs as a common condition. At the same time health educational programmes are directed towards improving local eating habits and gaining the co-operation of the parents in planning better feeding for their children, using all available sources and also improved methods of agriculture in order to provide increased supplies of food.

One cause of protein deficiency in babies in developing countries has been the use of dried milks for baby food in place of breast feeding. Because of the cost of the dried milks, many mothers made them up with excess water and so deprived the baby of adequate protein. Health educationalists, both in the countries affected and in the United States, stress the value of breast milk in maintaining adequate nutrition in babies.

Vitamin Deficiency Disorders

Vitamin deficiency as the sole cause of disease is now very seldom seen in this country, but symptoms resulting from lack of vitamins may be seen in association with other conditions or as a result of a restricted diet, if measures are not taken to ensure that these substances are taken in sufficient amounts. In some countries where the daily diet of numbers of the population is deficient in many respects diseases due to lack of these essential factors are not uncommon.

Vitamin A deficiency is chiefly manifested by impairment of vision. This vitamin is necessary for the visual purple in the retina which enables the eye to distinguish objects in a dim light: lack of vitamin A also causes drying of the conjunctiva, softening and degeneration of the cornea; this condition is known as keratomalacia and is one of the causes of blindness among children in some countries. Lack of vitamin A is also associated with a dry, rough skin, and may be responsible for liability to respiratory infection. Synthetic vitamin A preparations are available for the treatment of these conditions.

Vitamin B deficiencies are responsible for two well-defined diseases, pellagra and beri-beri.

Pellagra is caused by lack of nicotinic acid and occurs in areas of the world where maize forms the main part of the diet and where meat, which contains an amino acid from which the body can make nicotinic acid, is also lacking. The disease is occasionally seen in this country in patients suffering from mental or digestive disorders. The main features of pellagra are dermatitis, gastro-intestinal disorders, commonly diarrhoea and mental symptoms, such as anxiety, depression and irritability. The rash is most marked on the backs of the hands, forearms, forehead and neck; it is made worse by exposure to sunlight and the exposed skin becomes pigmented. A red, sore tongue and inflammation of the mucous membrane of the mouth are also common symptoms.

The treatment is nicotinamide given by mouth and a liberal diet with a high protein value, 100 to 150 g daily. Brewer's yeast is a rich additional source of vitamin B.

Beri-beri is a disease resulting from a deficiency of thiamine and is common in Eastern countries where the diet is almost entirely rice, or other cereals, whose vitamin content has been reduced by bleaching or milling. Some of the symptoms of thiamine deficiency, such as polyneuritis or cardiac failure, may be shown by people whose diet is inadequate and largely carbohydrate, such as old persons living alone, the chronic alcoholic patient and patients suffering from sprue or other intestinal disorders which inhibit absorption of thiamine.

Polyneuritis due to thiamine deficiency is known as 'dry beri-beri'; the first complaints are usually of pain in the legs, which is relieved by rest, weakness of the muscles and loss of sensation. Cardiac symptoms, palpitations and breathlessness, with oedema, from the group of symptoms of the type known as 'wet beri-beri'. Both types may occur together, i.e. the patient with polyneuritis may also develop oedema and cardiac failure.

Treatment of severe beri-beri demands rest in bed, as there is always a danger of cardiac failure and the administration of synthetic thiamine, usually by mouth; in some cases intravenous or intramuscular injection may be needed in order to obtain a more rapid result. A well-balanced diet is essential but at first this may have to be given as a fluid or light diet with eggs and milk as the basis. Heat, in the form of radiant heat or hot applications, will relieve the pain in the limbs and physiotherapy may be needed to re-educate the affected muscles.

The relationship between vitamin B_{12} (cyanocobalamin) and pernicious anaemia is described in the chapter on 'Disorders of the Blood'. Folic acid may be useful in the treatment of other types of macrocytic anaemia, such as may be seen in patients suffering from sprue.

Vitamin C deficiency produces scurvy, a disease which for

many centuries has been recognized as due to lack of fresh fruits and vegetables. The opening up of new trade routes by sea in the seventeenth and eighteenth centuries meant that sailors had to live for long periods on such foods as hard biscuit and dried or salted fish and meat; the result of such conditions was a high rate of illness and death amongst the crews from severe scurvy. Infants also may suffer from scurvy if fed entirely on milk and a starchy diet; this risk is of course now well recognized and orange juice, blackcurrant or rose-hip syrup, given daily, will supply the needs of the bottle-fed infant. The importance of introducing fresh fruits and vegetables during weaning of infants is also emphasized.

The first signs of scurvy are commonly inflammation and bleeding of the gums; later, haemorrhages into muscles and under the periosteum of the long bones, such as the femur, cause marked pain and tenderness and may be mistaken for acute osteomyelitis. Anaemia also develops later, as well as rarefaction of the long bones and delayed healing of any wound.

Treatment requires rest in bed in severe cases, and the administration of vitamin C in concentrated form, such as synthetic ascorbic acid and in the diet, which must also be liberal in all other respects. Attention to the teeth and gums is necessary, but any cleaning must be carried out with the utmost gentleness. Light splinting will afford rest and protection for a painful limb and passive movements and exercises will be given when the pain and tenderness subside.

Vitamin D deficiency causes rickets, a disease in which normal metabolism of calcium does not take place, with resulting defective bone formation and other manifestations due to calcium lack, such as delayed dentition, lack of muscle tone and increased irritability of motor nerves producing a tendency to convulsions. Factors associated with lack of vitamin D in causing rickets are lack of calcium in the diet and lack of sunshine, which enables the body to manufacture the vitamin from a sterol (7-dehydrocholesterol) in the skin. Thirty years ago rickets was a common disease in the great industrial cities of this country where smoke and fog cut off the ultraviolet rays of the sun and the diet of the children of the poorer class was unlikely to contain such foods as milk, eggs and butter. Indeed it was so common that on the continent rickets gained the title of 'The English disease', a name now given to chronic bronchitis.

The pathetic picture of the child with rickets is now very rarely seen, although there are many adults in some of the great industrial cities in the northern part of the country whose shortened stature, spinal curvature and bowed legs are the results of rickets in childhood. The main features of the disease are deformities of the skeleton, poor teeth, flabby muscles, liability to respiratory infections, to muscular spasms of the hands and feet (carpopedal spasm) and spasm of the vocal cords producing attacks of respiratory difficulty known as croup. Overgrowth of cartilage, which does not get sufficient calcium to form bone, occurs at the ends of the bones, at the junctions of the ribs with the sternum and the forehead and produces bumps, known as 'bossing' of the bones. The long bones are incompletely ossified and unable to bear the weight of the body without bending; bowing of the legs, knock-knees, curvatures of the spine and deformities of the thorax and pelvis are common. The arms may become bowed from taking the weight of the body when sitting. Poor muscle tone leads to flabbiness of the abdominal wall and a 'pot belly'.

An adult form of rickets, osteomalacia, was at one time fairly common in Eastern countries amongst women who lived in purdah, whose bodies were not exposed to sunlight, whose diet was deficient in calcium and who lost calcium from the demands of repeated pregnancies. Rickets occurring after the growth period lead to softening and deformities of the bones and loss of muscle tone.

Treatment requires the administration of both calcium and vitamin D. The first is supplied in liberal quantities by milk and calciferol is given to supply the vitamin D. Skeletal deformities require orthopaedic treatment and physiotherapy.

Obesity (Over-Feeding)

Obesity is due to an intake of food which provides a larger number of joules (calories) than is needed for the energy requirements of the body and is one of the commonest nutritional disorders in this country at the present time. Over-feeding may be, and often is, associated with an unbalanced diet which contains too high a proportion of starches and sugars; this may be due to a liking for such foods or because economic circumstances make it necessary to buy the cheaper and less satisfying carbohydrate foods rather than the expensive fats and proteins. Considerable attention has been given recently to the effect of emotional disturbances on appetite and it appears that anxiety or unhappiness by no means always decrease the desire for food; many people find solace in eating and once the habit of over-eating is established it is not easily broken. Some parents express affection for their children by giving them sweets, chocolates or crisps and the over-weight schoolchild has now become a national problem. Obesity is often a contributory cause of many ailments in the middle-aged and elderly, such as osteo-arthritic changes in the joints, backache and muscular pains. Excessive fat is also a danger to the patient undergoing a surgical operation and predisposes to cardiovascular disease, gall-stones, bronchitis and diabetes.

Treatment simply by reducing the joule (calorie) value of the diet is usually successful. It is often noted that some people who put on excessive fat may eat less than a person who remains thin, but in every case the obese individual is taking more joules than are necessary for his or her particular needs. Dietary control needs to be supervised by a physician, as a slow steady loss of weight is more lasting and more beneficial than a sudden large loss. The help of the dietitian is sought in planning a diet with a low-joule and low-carbohydrate content, but otherwise adequate, and which satisfies the appetite. The nurse's part is to see that the patient understands all the directions and diet sheets, to encourage perseverance in the treatment and to reinforce the advice given by the physician and the dietitian. A sympathetic approach to the patient's problems may reveal some emotional difficulty for which help can be given.

Many patients find it easier to loose weight with the support of a group of fellow dieters; hence the success of clubs such as Weight Watchers.

9

Disorders of the urinary system

THE urinary system is concerned in helping to maintain the correct fluid and acid–base balance in the body fluids and extracting from the blood for excretion in the urine the end-products of protein metabolism chiefly in the form of urea. The main features therefore of disorders of this system are disturbances of fluid and electrolyte balance and other factors affecting the blood chemistry, the presence in the urine of abnormal substances or substances not normally excreted, and disorders of micturition.

Terms Used to Describe Abnormalities in the Excretion or in the Constituents of Urine

Retention. Urine is secreted by the kidneys but is retained in the bladder. The causes may be mechanical or functional.

Retention with overflow. There is a constant dribbling away of urine, but the bladder remains distended. This may occur in disease or injury to the spinal cord.

Anuria (suppression). The kidneys fail to secrete urine.

Incontinence. The patient cannot hold the urine in the bladder due to loss of control over the urethral sphincter.

Polyuria. The amount of urine excreted is increased.

Oliguria. The amount of urine excreted is decreased.

Frequency. Urine is passed at frequent intervals, but this is due to irritability of the bladder, as in cystitis, rather than to the secretion of excessive amounts of urine. A constant and urgent desire to micturate, accompanied by pain and the passage of only a few drops of urine, is described as *stranguary* and may occur in renal colic.

Bacilluria. Bacterial infection of the urine, commonly by *Escherichia (Bacterium) coli.*

Haematuria. The presence of blood in urine. This may be due to local causes, or it may be a symptom in such conditions as blood diseases, infective endocarditis and severe toxaemia.

The principal local causes of haematuria are acute nephritis, stones in the urinary tract, tuberculous disease of the kidneys, new growths in the kidney or bladder and acute hepatitis.

Proteinuria (*albuminuria*). The presence of proteins, albumin and globulin in urine, which may be found in such conditions as acute infections, cardiac failure, toxaemia of pregnancy and acute and chronic nephritis.

Postural proteinuria. This is a condition in which proteins are found in the urine of healthy individuals with no sign of renal or other disease. It occurs chiefly in young people at the end of the day. After the night in the recumbent position the urine passed next morning is free from albumin. Thus it seems that the erect position and exercise must be concerned. The condition usually clears up satisfactorily, is of no significance and therefore no treatment is indicated.

EXAMINATION OF THE URINE

Volume. In normal adults the amount of urine passed in 24 hr varies between 600 and 2000 ml (20 to 66 fl. oz.); the average is 1500 ml. The quantity will vary depending on such factors as the fluid intake, the diet and the atmospheric temperature.

Specific gravity. This ranges from 1003 to 1030, according to the concentration of the solids dissolved in urine. A high specific gravity is found in concentrated urine and in urine containing glucose; a low specific gravity is normally due to the excretion of a large volume of water; a persistently low specific gravity is one of the signs of renal failure.

Reaction. Normally urine has a slightly acid reaction, but may be alkaline immediately after a meal. Urine left to stand before testing becomes alkaline owing to the conversion of urea into ammonia.

Colour. This is described as pale amber, but will vary according to the concentration; very dilute urine is a light straw colour, more concentrated urine is a darker yellow. Abnormal variations include the red or smoky brown colour due to the presence of blood, a brownish-green colour due to bile, and colours due to dyes secreted in the urine, as for example indigo-carmine which colours urine blue, and phenolsulphophthalein which gives a pink colour.

Deposits. Urine usually shows a sediment if left standing in a specimen glass, due to the precipitating of urates and phosphates as the urine becomes alkaline.

Chemical Tests for Protein, Glucose, Ketone Bodies, Blood and Bile

There are many proprietary urine testing aids on the market. Many of these are strips of stiffened paper containing chemicals which exhibit a colour change when placed in the urine. Some strips contain bands of chemicals so that many substances can be tested at the same time. Tests given below are examples of methods that may be used:

Protein

'Albustix' test. Dip the test end of an Albustix strip in urine and remove immediately. Compare the colour of the dipped end with the colour scale provided. If no protein is present there will be no colour change. If the reaction is positive the dipped end turns green or blue green at once.

Salicylsulphonic acid test. Take two test tubes. Put 2·5 cm (1 in) of urine in each. To one add 1 ml salicylsulphonic acid 20 per cent. Any turbid appearance as compared with the control is due to protein. It is a delicate test showing the presence of small amounts of albumin.

Heat and acetic acid test. Take 1 cm ($\frac{1}{2}$ in) of urine in each of two test tubes, heat one to boiling and add 50 per cent acetic acid drop by drop down the side of the tube held in a sloping position. Shake as each drop runs into the urine. A flocculent turbidity which persists (compare with cold tube) indicates the presence of albumin.

Esbach's quantitative estimation for protein. If the specific gravity is over 1008 dilute the urine with water. This is important. Remember to multiply the final reading by the degree of dilution.

Filter the urine if it is cloudy. Add a few drops of acetic acid if it is alkaline. Fill the albuminometer with urine up to letter 'U'.

Add Esbach's reagent as far as letter 'R'. Replace the cork, gently shake the tube, and stand it upright for 24 hr. Read the height of the precipitate from the scale. This represents the number of grams of albumin per litre of urine. To estimate the percentage divide this figure by 10.

Glucose

If albumin is present filter the urine after boiling, as the precipitate may be mistaken for sugar.

'*Clinitest*'. This reagent, which is in tablet form, is particularly convenient for the diabetic patient who has to test his own urine at home. Place 5 drops of urine in a small test tube, using a pipette, rinse the pipette and add 10 drops of water and 1 Clinitest tablet; watch the reaction for 15 sec after the mixture has ceased to bubble in the test tube and then shake and compare the colour change with the colour chart provided.

'*Clinistix*'. Clinistix test strips are made of stiff, absorbent celullose; one end of each strip is impregnated with glucose oxidase and a colour indicator. Dip the test end in the urine and remove immediately. A positive result is shown by the test end changing from its original cream colour to blue within 1 min. This test is specific for glucose and the strips will not react with any other reducing substances which may be present in the urine.

Benedict's test. Place 5 ml of Benedict's solution in a test tube. Add 8 drops of urine. Bring to the boil. Boil for 2 min and allow to cool. The presence of a deposit, which may vary in colour from green to orange, indicates the presence of glucose.

Acetone

'*Acetest*'. The Acetest method is a convenient and accurate test for acetone and diacetic acid. Place 1 Acetest tablet on a clean surface, such as a white tile. Add 1 drop of urine. Note the colour at the end of 30 sec. A positive reaction shows a colour change varying from a pale to a deeper lilac mauve.

'*Ketostix*'. Dip the test end of the Ketostix strip in the urine and remove immediately. Exactly 15 sec later compare the colour of the test strip with the colour chart. A positive result is shown by the test end of the strip changing from cream to a shade of lavender mauve, or purple, within 15 sec.

Rothera's test. Place 2·5 cm (1 in) of urine in a test tube and saturate with ammonium sulphate crystals. Add a few crystals of sodium nitroprusside and shake well. Slant the tube and pour 1 cm ($\frac{1}{2}$ in) of strong solution of ammonia gently down the side. A purple colour developing at the junction of the fluids indicates acetone or diacetic acid.

Note: a yellowish or brown colour is *not* a positive reaction.

Diacetic Acid

Gerhardt's test. Take 1 cm ($\frac{1}{2}$ in) of urine in a test tube. Add drop by drop solution of ferric chloride. After precipitation has ceased add more ferric chloride. Port-wine colour appears if diacetic acid is present.

Urine of patient taking salicylates (including aspirin) also shows a purple colour. To exclude this possibility dilute a fresh portion of urine with an equal quantity of water. Boil down to the original volume. Cool and add solution of ferric chloride as before. Boiling drives off diacetic acid, hence any purple colour in the second test will not be due to diacetic acid.

Blood

'*Occultest.*' Place one drop of well-mixed urine in the centre of the test paper provided. Put one Occultest tablet in the centre of the moist area and place 2 drops of water on the tablet. A positive reaction is shown by a diffuse blue coloured area appearing on the test paper around the tablet within 2 min.

'*Hemastix*'. Dip the test end of the Hemastix reagent strip in a well-mixed specimen of urine and remove immediately. Compare the test end of the strip with the colour chart exactly 30 sec later. A positive result is shown by the test strip changing from off-white to blue within 30 sec.

Guaiacum test. Take 1 cm ($\frac{1}{2}$ in) of urine in a test tube. If the urine is alkaline add a few drops of acetic acid. Add 2 drops of tincture of guaiacum. Shake, slant tube and gently pour down the side a small quantity of ozonic ether. A blue ring appears at the line of junction if blood is present. This is however an unsatisfactory test. Urine of a patient taking potassium iodide, cascara, rhubarb, senna, aloes or phenolphthalein also shows a blue ring, but it appears more slowly. Pus also gives a blue ring, but this appears without addition of ozonic ether and does not appear if the urine has previously been boiled. (To clean the test tube, rinse with methylated spirit.)

Combined Strip Tests

'*Uristix*'. Uristix test strips are used for the detection of both glucose and protein in urine. The strip has two impregnated areas, the protein portion (coloured yellow) at the tip of the strip, and the glucose portion (coloured red) nearer the middle. Dip the test end of the strip in the urine and remove immediately. Compare the colour of the protein portion with the colour chart at once; a positive result is shown by the yellow area changing to a shade of green.

Compare the glucose area with the colour chart 10 sec after dipping; a positive result is shown by the red portion of the strip changing to a shade of purple within 10 sec.

'*Hema-combistix*'. Hema-combistix reagent strips are used to test urine for the pH value as well as for protein, glucose and blood. These multi-purpose strips have four impregnated areas. The area next to the printing on the strip (coloured orange) gives the pH value; the second area (coloured red) as the test for glucose; the third area (coloured yellow) for protein; the fourth area (coloured cream) for blood.

Dip the test strip in a well mixed specimen of urine and remove immediately. Holding the strip with the test end downwards compare the test areas with the corresponding colour blocks. The glucose (second) portion should be compared exactly 10 sec and the blood test (fourth) portion exactly 20 sec after dipping. For the pH and protein readings the time is not critical.

The pH reading ranges from pH 5 to pH 9, shown by varying colour changes from the original orange colour to blue. A positive glucose test is shown by the red colour of the second area changing to a shade of purple within 10 sec of dipping. A positive protein test is shown by the yellow colour of the third area changing to a shade of green. A positive blood test is shown by the fourth, cream-coloured area, changing to blue within 30 sec of dipping.

Bile

Bilirubin. '*Ictotest*'. Place 5 drops of urine in one square of the test mat provided and put one Ictotest tablet in the centre of the moist area. Place 2 drops of water on the tablet. A positive reaction is shown by a bluish-purple colour developing on the mat around the tablet. The amount of bilirubin present is proportional to the speed and intensity of the colour change.

Iodine test. Place some urine in a test tube and add a layer of 10 per cent iodine solution. A green ring indicates the presence of bile.

Bile salts. *Hay's test.* Put some urine in a test tube and sprinkle a little powdered sulphur on the top. The sulphur will sink if bile salts are present owing to the lowered surface tension.

Urobilinogen. *Ehrlich's test.* To 10 ml of fresh urine in a test tube add 1 ml of Ehrlich's solution. Invert the test tube several times to mix the fluids and leave for 5 min. The normal amount of urobilinogen will give a pink colour, abnormal quantities produce a cherry or darker red colour.

Bacteriological Examination of Urine

Specimens of urine for bacteriological investigations should be collected with aseptic precautions and in sterile urine jars. In the case of a woman patient this may entail obtaining a catheter specimen of urine. Since, however, catheterization carries some risk of infection in spite of careful aseptic precautions, a 'clean' specimen is often considered suitable. The vulva is first thoroughly washed and then the area around the urethral orifice is swabbed with a lotion, such as cetrimide, 0·5 per cent solution, and dried with a gauze swab. The patient is then asked to micturate and, when some urine has been passed, the mid-stream specimen is collected directly into a sterile jar. In male patients catheter specimens of urine are rarely required for bacteriological examinations and a mid-stream specimen collected with similar precautions into a suitable sterile container is usually satisfactory for this purpose. Such specimens should be properly labelled and sent to the laboratory without delay.

The presence of *Mycobacterium tuberculosis* in urine cannot be detected by routine bacteriological examination; this investigation requires a sample of urine collected over 24 hr, which need not, however, be sterile. At the time set for the beginning of the collection the patient empties the bladder, and the urine is discarded. Throughout the ensuing 24 hr all urine passed is saved in a large container; at the end of this period the patient empties his bladder and this urine is added to that already collected. A specimen of the 24 hr urine containing some of the sediment from the bottom of the jar is sent to the laboratory. A 24-hr specimen may also be required for certain chemical examinations; the entire amount may be asked for, or two specimens and a record of the total amount passed.

OTHER UROLOGICAL TESTS

Renal Function Tests

A number of tests can be used to estimate the extent to which renal function is impaired where disease of the kidneys is known or suspected.

The amount of urea present in the blood and in the urine and the ability of the kidney to excrete urea and to concentrate the urine can be investigated by one or more of the following tests:

Blood urea estimation. This is usually required as a routine test and also as a part of the urea concentration and urea clearance tests. The normal value for blood urea is 20 to 40 mg whereas the normal value for urinary urea is 2 to 4 g per 100 ml. Blood is collected from a vein, usually in the early morning, and food is withheld until the sample has been taken. Sterile test tubes containing oxalate to prevent coagulation must be provided for the blood sample.

Urea concentration test. The object of the test is to estimate the amount of urea excreted in the urine after giving a known quantity of urea. A blood sample is taken just before the test is started. The urine passed at intervals of 1, 2 and 3 (and sometimes 4) hours subsequent to taking the urea by mouth (usually 15 g dissolved in about 60 ml of water) is sent to the laboratory. A figure of 2 per cent urea or over in any one specimen is evidence of satisfactory renal function.

Urea clearance test. In this test the efficiency of the kidney is estimated in terms of the percentage of average normal function. The urine obtained at a stated time is required and also that passed at exactly 1 hr later. A sample of blood for urea estimation is also needed, and this should be taken after the first amount of urine has been collected. Fifteen grams of urea is sometimes given after the first collection of urine.

Urine concentration test. No fluid is allowed for about 16 hr before the test. At intervals of 1 hr for three successive hours the patient empties his bladder. The volume and specific gravity of each specimen is recorded. If renal function is normal a specific gravity of 1025 or over will be found in at least one specimen.

Water elimination test. The patient is required to remain in bed for this test. After emptying the bladder he drinks 1200 ml of water within the space of $\frac{1}{2}$ hr. He is then asked to empty his bladder at hourly intervals for four successive hours. The volume and specific gravity of each specimen is recorded. If the renal function is normal, in at least one specimen the specific gravity should fall to 1003 or less.

Renal Biopsy

Renal biopsy may be required as an aid to diagnosis. The specimen of renal tissue is obtained by puncture with a long and moderately fine trocar and cannula.

Before the procedure the patient's haemoglobin is estimated and his blood group must be known and his blood cross-matched in case a transfusion is necessary. An X-ray film is taken to show the size and position of the kidneys. The site of the biopsy is usually the lower pole of the right kidney. The patient lies in the prone position with a sandbag under the abdomen to fix the kidney against the dorsal surface of the trunk, a position which helps to reduce the risk of haemorrhage. After the injection of a local anaesthetic the position of the kidney is located by a fine exploring needle.

The patient must be under constant observation after the biopsy for any sign of bleeding as shown by haematuria. The urine passed immediately after the biopsy is usually blood-stained and the amount of bleeding may be slight, but it must always be reported at once.

X-ray Examination of the Urinary Tract

An X-ray film will show the outline of both kidneys unless they are obscured by the shadows cast by faeces and flatus in the colon. Some preparation of the patient is therefore necessary. An aperient such as Dulcolax is usually given about 36 hr before the examination and diet is restricted to fluids. If the patient is able to be up and to walk about, this helps to prevent accumulation of gas in the intestine.

If the examination is designed to show the outline of the renal pelvis (pyelography), an opaque medium must be used, and this can be injected into a vein or directly into the renal pelvis via a cystoscope and ureteric catheters. The contrast media used are complex organic iodine compounds; examples of these are diodine and iodoxyl.

Intravenous or *descending pyelography* is usually the method of choice. The opaque medium is introduced into the venous circulation and excreted by the kidneys in the urine, filling first the renal pelves, then descending via the ureters to the bladder. Radiographs are taken at intervals from 5 min after the intravenous injection, when the renal pelves begin to show the presence of the contrast medium. The films will demonstrate whether or not both renal pelves fill satisfactorily and whether the outlines are normal in each case.

Retrograde or *ascending pylegraphy* involves the injection of the contrast solution directly into the renal pelvis through a ureteric catheter. As soon as the renal pelves are distended and discomfort is felt, the injection of fluid into the ureteric catheter is stopped and the X-ray films are taken. If either ureter is blocked by a stone or other obstruction, this can be demonstrated as the radio-opaque ureteric catheter cannot be passed beyond the obstruction.

Outlines of the bladder and urethra are best obtained by injecting the opaque solution directly into the bladder via a urethral catheter. This examination is known as *cysto-urethrography*. Films are taken during the injection and during micturition. By this method reflux of urine from the bladder up the ureters can be demonstrated and the examination is also useful in the investigation of stress incontinence in women.

DISEASES OF THE URINARY TRACT

Acute Nephritis

This type of nephritis is associated with infection, usually a haemolytic streptococcal infection, this occurs, not in the kidneys but elsewhere in the body, frequently the throat and therefore probably an allergic reaction (compare Acute

Rheumatism, p. 208), causes the inflammation. There is usually a latent period of about 10 days before the signs of inflammation of the kidneys appear. The patient complains of headache and malaise, and his temperature is slightly raised, 38° to 39°C (100·4° to 102·2°F). Oedema appears first as puffiness of the face, especially the area around the eyes, and of the feet. Generalized oedema develops and the serous sacs of the peritoneum and pleura may fill with fluid. Examination of the urine shows the presence of blood and protein. The amount of urine is usually decreased (oliguria), and there may be complete suppression. The blood urea is usually raised and also the blood pressure.

The course of the disease depends on the degree of damage to the renal glomeruli; many patients make a complete recovery, a proportion of patients pass from the acute stage into a subacute or chronic nephritis.

Treatment

There is no specific treatment for this disease. Rest in bed is necessary; warmth and freedom from draughts should be ensured.

At first feeding is restricted to glucose drinks. If the output of urine is markedly diminished, then the quantity of fluid given in 24 hr must be no more than the previous day's fluid output plus an addition for the insensible loss of water through the skin and lungs, usually calculated as being about 500 ml in 24 hr. Fluids can be increased as the urinary output increases and the oedema lessens. As long as oedema is present the fluid intake must be regulated and no protein or salt is allowed. The addition of milk, bread, fish and eggs to the diet is made as the amount of urea in the blood diminishes.

The nurse's responsibilities include keeping an accurate fluid intake and output chart and the testing of specimens of urine daily for blood and protein. Specimens of urine for microscopic examination for the presence of blood cells and casts of the renal tubules will be sent to the laboratory.

The patient with generalized oedema should be nursed in any position in which he is most comfortable, his position changed regularly, and the skin watched for any signs of pressure. Otherwise the nursing care is on general lines. The period of bed rest depends on progress, often measured by the ESR (see

p. 74), but is usually required for several weeks, and convalescence is gradual. If there is any focus of infection, for example in the tonsils, this is treated by suitable chemotherapy, but chemotherapy has no effect on the inflammation of the kidneys.

In some cases of nephritis cardiac failure complicates the picture, and may be fatal. Digitalis therapy is usually begun at the first appearance of this condition. Severe headaches and convulsions due to cerebral oedema are other possible complications and are treated by sedatives, such as paraldehyde or barbiturates; intravenous magnesium sulphate may be given in the treatment of convulsions. This substance, by drawing water from the tissues into the colon, helps reduce the cerebral oedema. Acute renal failure with anuria and the treatment of this condition are discussed on page 200.

The Nephrotic Syndrome

The nephrotic syndrome may be caused by a form of nephritis (glomerulo-nephritis) or other renal diseases, for example, thrombosis of the renal vein, by degenerative changes due to amyloid disease resulting from chronic septic infection, or by the action of drugs, one example of which is troxidone (Tridione) used in the treatment of epilepsy. Examination of the urine reveals persistent massive proteinuria (albuminuria) and the presence of casts and epithelial cells; in contrast to acute nephritis there are usually no red blood cells in the urine. Oedema is marked and anaemia is also usually present (Fig. 22).

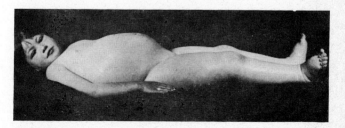

Fig. 22. The nephrotic syndrome causing gross ascites and oedema.

Treatment

Usually protein is not restricted in the diet in view of the need to balance the loss of protein in the urine. A high protein diet is given provided that the blood urea is not raised this will help increase the osmotic pressure in the blood vessels and thus draw the excess water from the tissues (see p. 20). Because of the oedema salt is restricted, and the patient will have to get accustomed to a diet containing very little salt and therefore lacking in flavour; fluids are however not restricted. Corticosteroids, prednisolone or ACTH, are used in the treatment of the nephrotic syndrome; these drugs lessen the excretion of protein and produce diuresis which reduces the oedema. Oral diuretics such as chlorothiazide are also used with added potassium. Anaemia is treated by the administration of iron; oral preparations may not be effective and intramuscular injections of Imferon are then given.

As far as possible the patient should lead a sheltered life, avoiding over-fatigue and exposure to infection. Chest complications, particularly pneumonia, are very liable to occur.

Chronic Nephritis: Chronic Renal Failure (Uraemia)

Chronic nephritis may be the end result of several different renal diseases, such as acute nephritis or pyelonephritis. Patients with long-standing hypertension may also develop chronic renal changes.

The blood urea is high, and also the blood pressure. The patient develops oedema as the condition progresses, and symptoms of renal failure with alterations in the electrolyte balance appear sooner or later. Sodium salts will be given in cases where the kidney is found to be unable to conserve these electrolytes.

The patient looks pale, his complexion is muddy, and a blood count reveals anaemia. He often complains of gastro-intestinal disturbances, hiccups, nausea, vomiting and diarrhoea; his breathing may be acidotic in type. The amount of urine excreted increases and the patient's night is disturbed by the need to pass urine. The urine is pale in colour with a low fixed specific gravity of about 1010. The blood urea is high. Signs and symptoms of hypertension such as raised blood pressure, headaches and dizziness, are usually, but not always present.

Treatment

The patient must follow strictly a low protein diet, with not more than 0·5 g protein per kg of body weight daily. Fluids by mouth should be increased to 3000 ml or more, and sodium salts given to help maintain electrolyte balance. The amount of sodium given may have to be reduced if the patient develops signs of cardiac failure. Hypertension, if present, is treated by drugs which reduce the blood pressure, e.g. methonium compounds, or mecamylamine.

In the terminal stage drowsiness and coma supervene.

The progression of this condition may be halted by the use of an artificial kidney which removes the toxic substances by haemodialysis and thus corrects the electrolyte distribution.

Haemodialysis is a diffusion of molecules in a solution through a semi-permeable membrane when the molecules in higher concentration on one side of the membrane pass through to the other side where the concentration is lower.

In the artificial kidney the patient's blood is dialysed against an electrolytic solution. This procedure does not treat the kidney condition, but by correcting the composition of the blood prevents the patient from dying. There are now many dialysis centres in the country into which patients are admitted for approximately 24 hr each week to have their electrolyte imbalance corrected, returning home working and living a normal life for the rest of the week.

An increasing number of patients have an artificial kidney at home and conduct their own haemodialysis but the equipment is expensive and therefore this method cannot be universally adopted.

Problems arising are primarily infection, especially of the veins in which permanent cannulae are fixed to enable the patient to be connected to the machine. These veins may also become thrombosed. Infected hepititis which is infection of the liver caused by blood-borne organisms, frequently viruses, may become a problem both in patients and in the people who staff dialysis centres.

A difficult problem is that of selection of patients for this treatment, as already stated these machines are costly and there are insufficient to treat all patients who might possibly benefit. This means that the doctor has to decide who should have this treatment and be returned to a degree of health and who must be left with the progressive condition.

Transplantation of kidneys is now an alternative method of treatment. The main difficulty is finding a suitable kidney to transplant. Kidneys may be taken from people who have just died (often as the result of an accident) providing permission can be obtained from relatives or else the person himself had previously signed a card indicating his willingness for his kidneys to be used in this way.

Acute Renal Failure (Anuria)

Anuria may result in any of the following circumstances:

(1) Obstruction of both ureters.

(2) Prolonged low blood pressure reducing the blood supply to the kidneys due to profound shock, particularly if combined with,

(3) Such factors as septic abortion, incompatible blood transfusion, severe crushing injuries.

(4) Damage by toxic chemicals such as sulphonamides, mercury, poisonous fungi.

The patient shows few if any symptoms for some days; then mental changes, muscular twitchings and cardiac irregularities occur and the patient is in danger of sudden death. Diminution in the amount of urine passed is likely to be followed by complete suppression.

Treatment

The principles of treatment of acute renal failure are:

(1) To relieve any obstruction blocking the ureters such as stones.

(2) To give no protein and to reduce breakdown of protein in the body tissues by a high carbohydrate intake.

(3) To limit the water intake to the previous day's fluid output plus 400 to 500 ml; this is given in the form of a 20 per cent glucose or lactose solution by mouth or by an intragastric tube.

If the patient is vomiting, a 40 per cent glucose solution is given intravenously, by means of a polythene catheter passed into the superior or inferior vena cava, since such a strong solution would cause thrombosis if injected into a superficial vein.

There is danger of cardiac arrest due to a high level of potassium in the blood; if this level rises to a figure higher than 7 meq/litre (normal 3·5 to 5) or if certain other biochemical features develop, the patient may be placed on renal dialysis. This treatment while not directly affecting the kidneys, may be

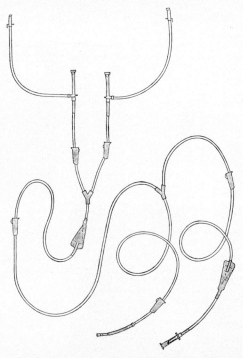

FIG. 23. Disposable polyvinylchloride 'giving set'. This is used with litre plastic bags of dialysing fluid; transfusion stand; warm bath (approximately 40°C)—a ward sink or a specially heated bath; lotion thermometer to measure bath temperature; serum syringes and No. 1 needles, spirit and swabs; heparin, 1000 μ to 1 ml strength; vials of tetracycline 250 mg; large container for return fluid; many-tailed bandage; and laboratory specimen jars.

preventing the patient from dying from severe electrolyte disturbance, allow sufficient time for the kidneys to recover naturally.

If treatment in a renal dialysis unit is not available, the same result may be achieved by the process of peritoneal dialysis. Figure 23 shows the disposable equipment used for this procedure. In this case the peritoneum is used as the semipermeable membrane through which the dangerous end products of protein metabolism are removed from the body. A special

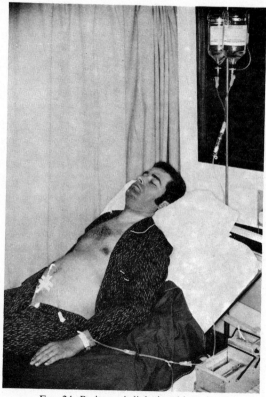

FIG. 24. Peritoneal dialysis taking place.

cannula is inserted into the peritoneal cavity and 2 litres of warmed fluid are run into the abdomen over a period of about $\frac{1}{2}$ hr. The liquid is left in the peritoneal cavity for $\frac{1}{2}$ to 1 hr, during which time urea is extracted from the blood. The empty transfusion bags are then removed from the transfusion stand and placed below the level of the patient's abdomen so that the liquid siphons off into them. In cases where kidney tissue is permanently destroyed and there is no hope of restoration of renal function, as for example in advanced polycystic disease of the kidneys, the patient may be kept in reasonable health for an indefinite period by repeated dialysis (Figs 23 and 24).

An anuric patient is very liable to develop infections, and therefore isolation nursing is important in order to provide as large a measure of protection as possible. If the patient survives the anuric phase this is followed by diuresis; in this phase the function of the renal tubules is poor and careful adjustment of the water and electrolyte balance must be made. In all stages of the management of acute renal failure most carefully kept fluid balance charts are essential.

Renal Calculus

Renal calculi, known as stones in the kidney are of many varieties, and may be present in the organ in numbers, or one only may be formed. The commonest types of stone are formed of uric acid, or oxalates, phosphates or cystine.

Any factors which produce concentration of the urine, e.g. diminished fluid intake with excessive sweating, urinary infection or obstruction, may lead to the formation of stones. Patients who are immobile for long periods, for example orthopaedic cases, may develop urinary calculi as a result of decalcification of the skeleton and the increase of calcium in the blood. The formation of calculi is sometimes associated with parathyroid disease, when again decalcification of bone increases the blood calcium.

Renal calculi often cause few symptoms unless the stone passes into the ureter, when an attack of renal colic occurs. The patient then suffers intense pain in the loin on the affected side, which radiates to the groin and the inner aspect of the thigh. Nausea and vomiting often accompany the attack. If infection is also present the patient may have a rigor and a sharp rise of temperature. Blood is usually present in the urine; frequency of micturition is common but the total output of urine is diminished.

Impaction of a stone may cause obstruction to the outflow of urine, with resultant dilatation of the pelvis of the kidney (hydronephrosis) and later suppuration (pyelonephrosis). Should impaction occur in the ureter of a solitary kidney, or in both ureters, renal failure and death will follow unless the blockage is relieved.

Treatment

In renal colic a hot bath sometimes gives relief, or the application of a hot-water-bottle or an electric pad, suitably protected. Morphine, 15 mg, is ordered for the very severe pain. An antispasmodic, e.g. atropine, 0·6 mg, may be prescribed 4-hourly to assist the passage of the stone through the ureter. The patient should be kept at rest and fluids, e.g. barley water imperial drink or fruit drinks, given liberally.

The stone causing the attack of colic may be passed down the ureter into the bladder and so voided in the urine, therefore all urine passed should be saved and carefully examined for the presence of a stone. The position of the stone can be checked by X-ray examination; if it is impacted in the ureter surgical removal is often advised in order to prevent hydronephrosis.

Large stones (staghorn calculi) fill the renal pelvis and are unlikely to cause acute attacks of colic, but are often accompanied by infection, blood and pus in the urine, pain and tenderness in the loin on the affected side. The treatment is usually surgical removal of the stone, and if the kidney is badly damaged this is also removed; obviously the situation becomes much more dangerous if the calculi are present in both kidneys.

In any condition which favours the formation of calculi, prophylactic measures should be taken. Persons who go from a temperate climate to live in tropical areas should be advised to step up their fluid intake to 2 to 3 litres (4 to 6 pints) a day in excess of the fluid normally taken at meal times. A high fluid intake is also necessary for the patient who is immobilized for any length of time, and if at all possible his position should be altered, or the bed tilted, at regular intervals.

Investigations, such as estimation of serum calcium level,

may be carried out, in order to exclude the presence of a tumour of the parathyroid glands.

Pyelitis

Pyelitis is an infection of the pelvis of the kidney which may be due to many organisms, e.g. streptococci or staphylococci, but is most commonly caused by *Escherichia coli* (colon bacilluria). The condition is much more common in women than in men.

The infection of the renal pelvis may spread to the renal tissue, giving rise to pyelonephritis which damages the kidneys, reducing their efficiency, and is therefore a more serious infection than a simple pyelitis.

Acute pyelitis has an abrupt onset, with rigor and a rapidly rising temperature, which tends to reach and maintain a considerable height. Other signs of fever may be present, e.g. increased pulse rate, furred tongue, vomiting and constipation. The urine is strongly acid and contains pus cells which give it a turbid appearance. Frequency of micturition with pain described as 'scalding', and pain and tenderness in the lumbar region are common symptoms.

After recurrent attacks of pyelitis the infection may become chronic, with persistent pain in the loin, frequency and urgency of micturition, and constitutional symptoms such as loss of weight, loss of appetite and anaemia. These symptoms may be less definite and fever and pain are often absent. Examination of the urine shows the presence of pus cells.

Treatment

This may need to be prolonged before a cure is effected, and some cases of chronic pyelonephritis are very intractable.

Rest in bed is necessary until the fever and the acute urinary symptoms have subsided. Fluids by mouth should be encouraged, 2 to 3 litres (4 to 6 pints) in 24 hr, and a careful record of the intake and output must be kept. The fluid intake should be sufficient to produce a urinary output of 1500 ml or more in 24 hr. A hypnotic such as butobarbitone may be required at night in order to ensure sufficient sleep.

A clean specimen of urine (see p. 192) will be required for bacteriological examination for the specific infecting organism.

When this has been identified the appropriate antibacterial drug will be given. Sulphonamides are effective against *Escherichia coli* infections, penicillin gives satisfactory results in a number of infections, and other antibiotics, e.g. tetraylines, chloramphenicol, polymixins, may be suitable in some cases. Co-trimoxazole (Septrin, Bactrim) or nitro-furantoin (Furadantin) may be ordered where the infection proves resistant to other chemotherapeutic agents.

X-ray examination of the urinary tract and cystoscopy with ureteric catheterization, in order to discover if any obstruction is present, may be undertaken when the acute symptoms have subsided.

Pyelitis tends to be a recurring infection, and measures to build up the patient's resistance, such as good nutrition, fresh air, adequate exercise but avoidance of over-fatigue and strain, may help to prevent further attacks.

Cystitis

Cystitis, inflammation of the bladder, is frequently associated with pyelitis, urethritis or urethral stricture and with paralysis of the bladder in the paraplegic patient, where inability to empty the bladder leads to stagnation of urine and infection. Cystitis can also readily occur as a result of frequent catheterization and it is a common complication of new growths in the bladder. Cystitis as a primary infection most commonly occurs in women and the infecting organism is usually *Escherichia coli*.

Frequent painful micturition is a marked feature of acute cystitis. The urine contains pus cells and red blood cells, it may have a distinctive unpleasant odour, sometimes described as 'fishy'. The patient's temperature is raised and rigors may occur. The treatment and investigations required for this condition are the same as those described for pyelitis. In addition tincture of nyocyamus is often prescribed to relieve the painful spasmodic contractions of the bladder.

Tuberculosis of the Kidney

Tuberculosis of the kidney is commonly a blood-borne infection, and is associated with tuberculosis elsewhere in the body. The urinary passages are bladder and involved in the late stages. The disease is at first unilateral, but the other kidney may become infected by upward spread from the ureter via the bladder.

There may be local pain and tenderness. The urine is usually acid and often contains pus and blood; there may be a deposit of debris from disintegrated tissues in which tubercle bacilli are sometimes found. Micturition is frequent and painful if cystitis is present. The general condition will show those signs typical of any form of chronic tuberculosis, lassitude, loss of appetite and loss of weight.

Bacteriological examination of the sediment of the urine collected over 24 hr is required (see p. 192) and a cystoscopic examination may be carried out to determine the presence of tuberculous ulcers in the bladder.

Treatment

Specific treatment with streptomycin and para-aminosalicylic acid combined with measures directed towards increasing the patient's resistance to tuberculous infection, i.e. a generous diet, fresh air and rest. Where the disease is unilateral, and other indications are favourable, nephrectomy may be advised and good results follow.

10

The rheumatic group and other disorders of bones and joints

DISEASES affecting the bones and joints are characterized by localized pain, often of a persistent and chronic nature, by varying degrees of limitation of movement and the development of deformities. They are therefore liable to be crippling diseases and to have serious implications in whatever period of life they may occur. In the child normal physical growth may be retarded and education interrupted; in adult life earning capacity may be seriously reduced, in the elderly patient increasing dependence on the help and good will of relatives and friends may present psychological and social problems.

THE RHEUMATIC GROUP OF DISEASES

Rheumatic diseases form one of the largest group of disabling conditions in this country and their prevention and treatment are rendered extremely difficult because the causes of the various conditions which come under this heading remain obscure.

Acute Rheumatism

Acute rheumatism, or rheumatic fever, is a disease of childhood and adolescence. It has long been known that rheumatic fever is associated with haemolytic streptococcal infection, but the organisms are never found in the rheumatic lesions and it is thought that the disease may be an immune reaction, or allergy, of the tissues to streptococcal infection. The disease often follows a few weeks after such an infection, most commonly tonsillitis; sometimes the rheumatic symptoms are very mild, or absent and subsequent rheumatic heart disease is found in a patient who has no recollection of having had rheumatic fever.

The characteristic features of a typical attack are fever, usually moderate, 38° to 39°C (100° to 102°F), but which may reach hyperpyrexial levels, with generalized symptoms of malaise, loss of appetite, furred tongue, constipation and pains mostly in the larger joints, such as knees, ankles, wrists and shoulders, which tend to move from joint to joint so that all joints are not similarly affected at the same time. The joints become swollen, hot and tender; on examination, nodules may be found in the subcutaneous tissues, particularly over the elbows, backs of the hands, the shoulders and on the back of the head. When these nodules are present it is an almost certain indication that carditis is also present. Similar structures, but microscopic in size, occur in the heart, and are known as Aschoff's nodes.

Treatment

The treatment is first and foremost complete rest in bed with the object of preventing cardiac damage. The patient is not allowed to wash or feed himself until all signs of active disease have disappeared. When this stage has been reached some activity is gradually introduced, but at least 6 weeks in bed will usually be necessary. The position in bed is that which is most comfortable and gives the greatest relief of the pain in the joints; any attempt to keep the patient lying flat on his back will defeat its own object if this position increases the pain and makes him restless. Some relief will also be given by supporting the painful joints on pillows, additional support can be given by light splinting or bandaging over a pad of cotton wool, which will restrict those movements which cause pain and protect the tender joints. A large bed cradle should be used to take the weight of the bedclothes off the feet.

Sweating is often profuse, sponging twice a day and frequent changes of nightgown and bedclothes are necessary. Considerable amounts of fluid may be lost in this way and therefore the patient must be encouraged to take fluids freely by mouth; this will also help to keep his mouth moist and clean. In the febrile stage the appetite is generally poor, but as soon as possible a generous diet should be given, because good nutrition is a valuable aid to recovery.

Temperature, pulse and respiration rate should be taken and recorded every 4 hr. The pulse rate during sleep is a useful guide; if the sleeping pulse is slowing satisfactorily, although the waking pulse rate remains somewhat high, this is evidence of improvement. Other signs of improvement are the disappearance of the joint pains and the return of the temperature to normal. Erythrocyte sedimentation rate estimations (see p. 74) are carried out periodically. The sedimentation rate is high during the active phase of the disease; a normal sedimentation rate denotes that activity has subsided.

Evidence of extension of the disease is shown by a persistent rapid pulse rate and fever, pain in the substernal region which may be due to pericarditis, and signs of cardiac failure such as increasing dyspnoea and an irregular pulse. The tissues of the brain may be involved and the manifestation of this is the appearance of jerky, restless, uncontrollable movements, the condition known as chorea.

Drugs used in the treatment of rheumatic fever are not specific but relieve the symptoms and reduce the severity and duration of the illness. Sodium salicylate in large doses can almost certainly relieve the joint pains and bring the temperature back to normal; indeed, it can be assumed that if this drug is given in sufficient dosage and is not effective, the condition is not rheumatic fever. From 1 to 2 g of sodium salicylate is usually given at 4-hourly intervals, and this may be increased to 2-hourly dosage. Large doses of sodium salicylate may cause toxic symptoms, nausea, headache, ringing in the ears and deafness, and if these symptoms develop the dosage will have to be reduced. Penicillin may be given as routine treatment at the onset of the illness; it does not directly affect the rheumatic inflammation, but combats any infection, such as septic tonsils, which may be the precipitating factor. In severe cases one of the cortisone drugs may be given, for example a course of prednisone in addition to sodium salicylate administered over a period of 6 weeks.

Convalescence must be gradual and prolonged: most patients, particularly town dwellers, will benefit by several weeks in the country or at the seaside if this can be arranged. It is noticeable that rheumatic fever and streptococcal infections are much less common in hot, sunny countries than in the damp, sunless conditions which tend to prevail for much of the year, particularly in the large industrial cities, in this country. When the child has recovered completely, removal of septic tonsils must be considered, since there is a liability to repeated attacks and almost inevitable cardiac complications if a septic focus remains active.

Chorea

The type of chorea known as Sydenham's chorea is included in the rheumatic group of diseases (see also p. 208), since it is also a manifestation of streptococcal allergy, which may complicate rheumatic fever but usually occurs as a separate illness. The disease attacks the central nervous system, and girls are more commonly affected than boys. It is insidious in onset, nurses and others in contact with children should be familiar with the earliest signs, such as grimacing and restlessness, clumsiness due to loss of muscle power and emotional disturbances, shown by a tendency to laugh or cry for inadequate cause.

Treatment at this stage may prevent further progress of the disease and a cure is comparatively easy. Rest is of first importance, both physical and mental. Plenty of sleep with early bedtime, good food, quietness in country air, freedom from lessons and all excitements are often sufficient to ward off further development.

In severe cases there are more or less pronounced general spasms of the muscles; these can be described as 'voluntary movements, involuntarily performed, without order or sequence'. These movements become exaggerated by excitement or if the child is aware she is being watched or commented on. Swallowing may be difficult or speech impeded. As a rule there is no rise of temperature and the erythrocyte sedimentation rate is normal; weight may be lost rapidly.

Treatment

The child is nursed in a room by herself, or in the quietest corner of the ward where there is little to attract the attention and as little noise as possible. Screens kept round the bed or cot are a further aid to isolation. The constant movements and friction will cause rubbing of the skin if care is not taken and the ingenuity of the nurse must be exercised to prevent this. An air bed or rubber mattress can be used, and padded bed-sides may be necessary if restlessness is so great that there is danger of the patient falling out of bed. If the patient is in a cot, pillows can be fastened to the sides and head of the bed. Sheets must be kept smooth, and those with seams or darns are not used for these patients.

The body should be sponged all over with hot water twice daily. This is refreshing and improves the action of the skin, which tends to be dry. The patient should not be left on the bedpan longer than is necessary, and this should be padded or, better still, a rubber one substituted. Pads of wool may be bandaged on to special areas (e.g. elbows or heels) to lessen friction. The mouth must be kept clean, and this requires a good deal of skill owing to the spasmodic movements. Forceps should not be used as the delicate mucous membranes may be injured; mouth sticks are less hard. Neglect results very rapidly in sores. The bowels are regulated by means of mild aperients as necessary. The temperature, pulse and respiration rate should be taken at least twice daily, and more often if complications are suspected. Observation of the pulse rate is especially important. The temperature must be taken in the axilla or groin and never in the mouth, nor must the patient be left whilst the thermometer is in position.

Food should be digestible and soft, meat being minced, potatoes mashed, and fluids should be taken in as large a quantity as possible. The nurse must always feed the patient; this requires patience and skill, and she must assure herself that the previous mouthful has been swallowed before giving another. It is more satisfactory in most cases to give fluids and medicines with a feeding cup, with a piece of rubber tubing attached to the spout. China cups and glasses are dangerous and should never be used, plastic utensils, including spoons, should be substituted. A diet cloth should be placed under the chin to protect the bedclothes, for it is often difficult to feed these patients in a cleanly manner, as spasms cause ejection.

Sedatives will be ordered, e.g. phenobarbitone. Corticotropin (ACTH) or cortisone may be prescribed.

These children require very special nursing care. They are often hypersensitive to their condition, and especially susceptible to emotional influences. The nurse must therefore shield them as far as possible and encourage and guide them back to health, and for these reasons it is highly desirable that the same nurse should care for the child throughout the acute phase of the illness. Convalescence is likely to be slow and recurrence common, even if no complications arise. Fresh air and a quiet country life free from emotional upset is the best way to re-establish the child's health.

Rheumatoid Arthritis

Rheumatoid arthritis is a very common and very crippling inflammatory disease of the joints which occurs more frequently in women than in men, usually between the ages of 20 and 45 years; there does appear to be a familial tendency to the conditions. The cause of the disease is unknown, but a number of precipitating factors have been suggested, particularly septic infection; but while an obvious source of infection, such as septic teeth or tonsils is usually best removed, this is not necessarily followed by any marked improvement. In a number of cases a lowering of the general state of health from lack of proper food and poor living conditions, which may be associated with emotional disturbances, such as long periods of anxiety and stress or a sudden bereavement causing both emotional shock and straitened financial circumstances, seem to be precipitating factors.

The onset is often insidious, with pain in one or two of the smaller joints, such as those of the fingers or toes, which progresses and involves the wrist, elbow, shoulder and knee joints. The ligaments and tendons around the joints become inflamed, and the synovial membrane and cartilages in the joints are also affected (Fig. 25). The changes lead to ankylosis,

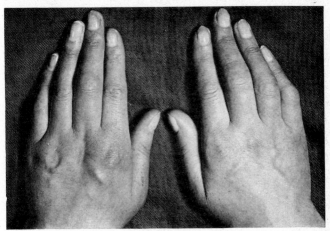

FIG. 25. Rheumatoid arthritis: early stages.

i.e. fixation of the joints, and the loss of movement, and deformity is further increased by wasting of the muscles (Fig. 26). The active stage may subside, leaving some residual damage, but the symptoms recur later, and pain, stiffness and loss of muscle power render the patient increasingly disabled.

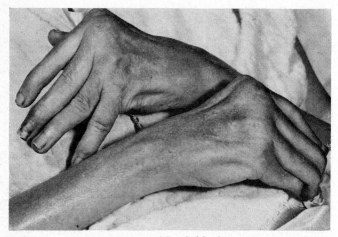

Fig. 26. Rheumatoid arthritis: late stages.

During an acute phase the temperature may be moderately raised, with malaise, loss of appetite and a moist, clammy skin. The erythrocyte sedimentation rate is usually raised, and anaemia may be marked. Occasionally enlarged lymph glands are found. Loss of weight is a common feature of rheumatoid arthritis.

Treatment

Rest in bed, with the affected joints supported in the most favourable position, using light removable splints where necessary, will be essential while the temperature is raised or in the acute phase of the disease. Warm, but light, clothing and bedclothes should be provided. A bed cradle is needed to take the weight of the bedclothes off the limbs, and the feet should be supported with the ankle joints fully flexed. If the patient is overweight a reducing diet may be ordered; usually, however, the patient is thin and ill-nourished, and requires a high joule diet rich in both first class proteins and all the vitamins. Iron in the form of ferrous sulphate tablets is often prescribed to treat the hypochromic anaemia which is commonly present in rheumatoid arthritis. Any possible source of infection is sought, and eradicated if found. If any operative treatment such as the removal of septic teeth or tonsils is contemplated, suitable antibiotic protective measures are instituted first to prevent an exacerbation of the disease.

As early as possible physiotherapy is given, in the form of heat, massage and passive movements of the joints. Heat may be applied in the form of radiant heat or as warm paraffin wax baths. Light splints should be worn while the patient is in bed and particularly at night; these will support the affected joints in the position which will best combat the tendency to deformity. For example if the wrist is affected, there is a tendency for the joint to get fixed in a position of flexion with deviation to the ulnar side of the arm; a bivalve plaster splint will then be applied to keep the wrist joint slightly extended and to correct the ulnar deviation. In cases where the knee joints are affected rest in bed is necessary in order to keep the weight of the body off the inflamed joints. Posterior splints which maintain the knee joints in a position of extension or slight flexion are worn to prevent tendency towards fixation in the position of flexion and subsequent disability. Bed rest is not continued for longer than is absolutely necessary, and the patient will need to continue with physiotherapy, taking a more active part in his own treatment, in the form of exercises, a certain amount of walking and some kind of occupational therapy, which is valuable psychologically and is also designed to exercise the affected joints and muscles as effectively as possible.

Drugs have a part in the treatment of rheumatoid arthritis in relieving pain and stiffness and controlling the progress of the disease. Sodium salicylate or aspirin is given to relieve pain and overcome muscular spasm, which is one of the factors in producing deformities. Sedatives such as Mogadon may be given in conjunction with analgesic drugs to provide adequate sleep and rest. Cortisone or the synthetic steroids, prednisone and prednisolone, have produced marked remission of symptoms when given in the acute stage of the disease, but the symptoms tend to reappear when the drug is stopped. At present these drugs are regarded as one of the measures that will usefully aid the arthritic patient, but not as a specific cure for the disease and if they are given over long periods, various side effects are produced, although these occur less frequently with the synthetic steroids. The side effects include the retention of salt and water, rounding of the face, 'moon face', hypertension, abnormal growth of hair, increased appetite, obesity, depression and fatigue. These drugs are also contra-indicated, or need to be given with extreme caution, to patients with myocardial damage, renal disease, tuberculosis or peptic ulcer. Hydrocortisone may be injected into large joints, such as the knee or wrist after aspirating as much fluid as possible. This procedure is carried out with full aseptic precautions.

Phenylbutazone and indomethacin (Indocid) may also be prescribed. Side effects include nausea, fluid retention, skin rashes and occasionally a fall in the number of white blood cells. Gold salts, in the form of 50 per cent solution of sodium aurothiomalate (Myocrisin) given by intramuscular injection, are sometimes prescribed in the early and acute stage of rheumatoid arthritis, but toxic reactions can occur very readily, and small doses given over a long period are now considered safer than a short course of fairly intensive treatment. Patients who suffer from skin diseases such as dermatitis or eczema, or who have impairment of renal or liver function, are not suitable subjects for gold therapy. The main toxic reactions are skin rashes, stomatitis, diarrhoea, nephritis, jaundice, purpura and a fall in the number of white blood cells (leucopenia). Frequent examination of the urine, skin and blood are therefore necessary throughout the course of treatment. Should toxic effects be produced administration of the drug is usually stopped; Dimercaprol (BAL) or corticosteroids may be given to counteract the toxicity of the gold salts.

One form of rheumatoid arthritis is commoner in men than in women; this affects the joints of the vertebral column and is known as spondylitis. The patient is frequently a young man, and the earliest complaint is of low back pain, often described by the patients as 'lumbago'. The joints of the spine and those between the ribs and the dorsal vertebrae become ankylosed, the spine is rigid, and the chest movements are limited. In progressive cases the cervical, dorsal and lumbar spine and also the hip joints are fixed and flexed, the trunk and neck are so bent that the patient is unable to lift his head, his chest expansion is much reduced and he is severely disabled. Such patients are also very prone to respiratory infections.

Treatment is on similar lines to that of rheumatoid arthritis generally, relieving pain and preventing deformities. A firm mattress over fracture boards, or a plaster shell, will help to prevent the development of curvature of the spine. One form of treatment which has proved effective in arresting the progress of the disease, particularly in the early active stage, is radiotherapy. So successful is this treatment in the majority of cases that although it is known that there is a definite risk of leukaemia following this treatment in a small percentage of the patients, this risk is still considered worthwhile. Radiotherapy relieves the pain and allows more effective physiotherapy, increased movements of the chest wall, thus lessening the risk of respiratory complications.

In those rheumatoid patients whose disease has produced disabling deformities much can be done by orthopaedic surgery, including manipulation and open operations on joints followed in some cases by a series of splints in order to gain the maximum effect. It will be obvious that, in addition to the medical and nursing care which these patients require, there are many members of the therapeutic team who have their part in preventing the development of the worst features of this very crippling disease, the dietitian, the physiotherapist, the occupational therapist, often the social worker, and not least the patient himself. Unless he can be helped to feel that his condition is by no means hopelessly progressive, that by his own efforts, and following the advice he is given, he has every hope of remaining independent, reasonably active and able to follow some interesting occupation or pursuit, he may well become a depressed, bedridden or chair-bound invalid, with little interest in life and no hope for the future.

Infective Arthritis

Infective arthritis, which may be due to a variety of causes, e.g. pyogenic or gonococcal or tuberculous infection, will produce symptoms in many ways similar to those of rheumatoid arthritis, joint pain, swelling, muscular spasm and deformities. Pyogenic and gonococcal arthritis are usually accompanied by a considerable degree of fever and constitutional disturbance; in pyogenic infection only one joint is usually affected. Tuberculous arthritis is commonest in children, and as a rule only one joint, often the hip or the knee, is involved.

Treatment

As in rheumatoid arthritis, treatment must include rest of the affected joints, splinting and physiotherapy. In addition the appropriate chemotherapy, once the diagnosis is established, will be given.

Osteo-Arthritis

Osteo-arthritis is a condition in which the articular cartilages covering the ends of the bones forming a joint degenerate and bony projections form along the edges of the joints, known as osteophytes. The disease occurs most commonly in middle-aged or elderly persons, and is in part due to the ageing process, but in most cases trauma is also a factor. The joints which have to take the weight of the body, such as those of the lumbar spine, the hip and the knee, are often affected, and often too the patient is overweight. Osteo-arthritic changes in a single joint may occur in patients of any age as a result of injury, such as a fracture of one of the bones forming the joint with some displacement of the joint surfaces.

The main features of osteo-arthritis are stiffness, aching and swelling of the joints. The general symptoms of an active inflammatory process which are seen in the patient with rheumatoid arthritis are not present. Movements in the joints are limited, and there is usually some degree of muscle wasting. Grating (crepitus) can be felt between the roughened ends of the bones.

Treatment

Painful joints need rest, and this is particularly important when the weight-bearing joints are affected. There is usually no risk of ankylosing of the joints such as occurs in the rheumatoid type of arthritis; damage is more likely to result from over-activity than from rest. Heat, in the form of hot pads, helps to relieve pain and overcome muscular spasm, and is usually combined with gentle exercises, but analgesics such as aspirin or codeine are also needed. Indomethacin (Indocid) may be useful in relieving pain.

If the patient is over-weight it is essential that his weight should be reduced. A low-joule low-carbohydrate diet, with sufficient protein and vitamins for adequate nutrition, is ordered. Once the weight has been reduced satisfactorily it is necessary for the patient to continue with his prescribed diet.

Orthopaedic surgery in the form of insertion of an artificial articulating surface in the joint or other type of prosthesis is now often used successfully whatever the age of the patient.

Gout

Gout is a disease which is thought to be due to an inborn error in metabolism, which causes the deposition of sodium urate in the joint tissues and in soft tissues elsewhere in the body. The chief feature of gout is the occurrence of repeated attacks of acute arthritis. A tendency to gout is known to be hereditary; it is uncommon in women, the patient is almost always a man over the age of 40. The first joint affected is usually the big toe; acute pain may wake the patient at night. The toe is red, swollen and extremely tender. A rise of temperature, vomiting, constipation and scanty urine often accompany the attack. A chronic form of gout may follow the acute phase, and a number of joints are eventually affected; this condition is sometimes called gouty arthritis.

At one time gout was ascribed to excessive intake of alcohol, and later to feeds with a high purine content, such as red meat, liver, kidneys, peas and beans. These views are not now generally held, although alcohol or a certain article of food may be found to precipitate an attack and in that case should of course be avoided.

Treatment

In the acute attack relief of pain is the first essential. Rest in bed with a bed cradle to take the weight of the bedclothes, hot or cold compresses, whichever are found to be most effective, applied to the affected joint, and analgesics such as codeine are the usual measures. Large quantities of fluid should be given;

fruit and fruit juices, milk and barley water form the main part of the diet for a few days.

The drugs which are most commonly prescribed in acute attacks are phenylbutazone (Butozoladin, 600 mg, indomethacin (Indocid), 200 mg, or colchicum in the form of colchicine tablets given by mouth. The drug is given at hourly or 2-hourly intervals until the pain is relieved or until symptoms of gastro-intestinal upset, diarrhoea and vomiting, occur. Other drugs used are corticotrophin by intramuscular injection, or prednis-one by mouth.

Treatment of chronic gouty arthritis is directed towards maintaining the general state of health, avoiding over-eating, alcohol except in very moderate quantities and over-exertion. If the patient is obese a reducing diet is followed. Otherwise a strict diet is not usually prescribed, although the amount of fatty foods is restricted and sometimes foods with a high purine content, such as liver, kidneys, sweetbread and meat extracts, or any other food which appears to provoke an attack, are forbidden. There is always a possibility of stones forming in the kidneys as a result of deposits of urates, therefore the fluid intake must be liberal, and at least 3 litres (5 pints) daily is advised.

Drugs used to promote the excretion of uric acid, and so to prevent acute attacks of gout, include salicylate and probenicid (Benemid).

Osteitis Deformans (Paget's Disease)

Osteitis deformans is a disease of unknown origin, in which the activity of both the bone-forming and the bone-absorbing cells is increased. The long bones, the pelvis and skull are most commonly affected. The bones increase in size; X-ray examina-tion shows patches of increased density and also patches of rarefaction where bone absorption has taken place. The disease is uncommon in patients below the age of 50, but as it may develop very slowly and cause no symptoms it is often difficult to determine the date of onset. As the condition progresses, however, deformities become obvious; the skull is enlarged, the long bones are curved, and this, together with a curvature of the dorsal spine (kyphosis), produces diminished stature. Some-times spontaneous fractures occur and so call attention to the condition. The patient may seek treatment as a result of persistent pains in the limbs and headache.

Treatment

The course of the disease will not be affected, although remissions often occur, but palliative treatment may be needed to relieve the pain. Aspirin or other suitable analgesics are usually ordered; where these have little effect radiotherapy may occasionally be tried.

11
Disorders of the skin

DISORDERS or abnormalities of the skin can arise from a variety of causes and in a considerable number of such conditions the cause remains obscure. The following factors are, however, involved in many of these diseases.

(1) Physical agents, such as pressure, friction, heat, cold, radiation from sunlight, X-rays or radioactive material.
(2) Chemical agents, such as acids, alkalies, drugs and dyes.
(3) Sensitivity to foreign proteins, either animal or vegetable.
(4) Bacterial and viral agents.
(5) Parasites, animal and vegetable.
(6) Disease of other parts of the body, such as neurological, vascular and endocrine disturbances.
(7) New growths.
(8) Congenital conditions.

Among the predisposing causes of skin disorders are heredity, race, climate, occupation and psychological factors.

Manifestations of Skin Affections

Among the manifestations of skin diseases may be found the following:

Blisters: elevations of the epidermis containing fluid.

Bulae: large blisters. On rupture they leave a raw surface.

Comedones: Blackheads formed of dried sebum which blocks the excretory ducts of the skin.

Crusts or *scabs:* dried serum, sometimes containing pus cells.

Ecchymoses: large purple blotches due to extravasation of blood. They do not disappear on pressure.

Erythema: redness, in many cases the skin will feel hot to the touch.

Excoriation or *erosion:* removal of an area of the epidermis, leaving a raw, red surface which exudes serum and is described as 'weeping'.

Fissures (*chaps*): cracks in the epidermis, which often involve the dermis, and are therefore painful.

Keratoses: thickening of the horny layer, which may appear as warty overgrowths or be more generalized—e.g. on the palms or soles.

Lichen: a collection of papules.

Lichenification: a condition produced by prolonged friction—e.g. in the creases of the skin. Thickening may occur, with flat-topped papules, and some scaling follows. The area irritates.

Macules: discoloration of small areas (spots) but with no alteration in surface level.

Papules: small, solid, raised spots.

Petechiae: small haemorrhagic spots.

Plaques: patches of skin harder than that which surrounds them, and sometimes raised above the normal skin surface.

Pustules: small swellings containing pus.

Scales: dried epidermis in flakes which may be small or large.

Ulcers: loss of surface tissue involving the dermis. They may be due to infection, vascular causes, new growths or physical agents, such as heat and friction or pressure.

Vesicles: small blisters. They may appear on top of a papule.

Weals: localized oedema in the dermis.

General Principles of Treatment of Skin Diseases

Investigation of the cause is in many instances the first step, since skin lesions may be a symptom of disease elsewhere and treatment of this underlying, possibly undiagnosed, condition will be required if success is to be achieved. For example, pruritus vulvae may be a symptom of diabetes, or urinary infection, or infection of the genital tract; it may also occur at the menopause unassociated with any disease. A rash may be the first symptom of an infectious disease such as rubella or chickenpox and this should be borne in mind particularly if the patient is a child.

Rest and sleep. In severe cases the patient must be kept in bed. The bedclothes should be light in weight and loose; the same applies to the patient's personal clothing whether he is in bed or not. Cellular cotton blankets are preferable to woollen ones; they are non-irritating and also are not damaged to the same extent as wool by frequent washing.

Most patients suffering from skin diseases experience continual irritation and discomfort and are quite unable to obtain adequate sleep without the help of sedatives. In some cases, if there is a marked degree of anxiety and emotional stress, one of the 'tranquillizing' drugs such as chlorpromazine (Largactil) may be ordered, but these are used with caution as one of the side effects of many of these drugs is a skin rash.

In addition the patient may, quite understandably, become depressed and anxious, particularly so if his disease is resistant to treatment or it tends to recur. Such patients need a great deal of help and encouragement, and the nurse must maintain a cheerful, optimistic attitude without, however, any suggestion that his complaint is trivial and his anxiety a form of self-pity. Many people firmly believe that all skin conditions are infectious, or due to dirt, or in some way rather disgraceful; this of course is far from true, but may cause the patient considerable distress, and if the nurse is able to correct such a misconception she will probably have helped the patient considerably. The place of local applications in allaying disturbing irritation will be discussed later.

Diet. Enquiry into the patient's history includes finding out the details of his customary diet. In general, special diets play little part in the treatment of skin disease but it may be necessary to make up deficiencies, for example lack of sufficient protein or vitamins C or B complex, or to supply a special diet if the patient is at the same time suffering from some disease necessitating this, such as diabetes or peptic ulcer.

It is, however, generally agreed that highly seasoned foods, excessive use of pepper and mustard, strong tea, coffee and alcohol in the form of spirits, are best avoided.

External applications. A bewildering number of lotions, ointments, creams, pastes and powders are used in the treatment of skin diseases, and it is impossible to give a comprehensive list of all the local applications that may be ordered. Some attempt has therefore been made to classify the types of preparations used and the indications for their use.

(1) Sedative applications are used where the lesions are inflamed, itching and oozing, as in acute eczema. Examples are calamine and coal tar lotions or creams, and starch baths.

(2) Stimulating applications, some of which are also employed for their action in dissolving the horny layer of the skin and are then described as keratolytics, are used in the treatment of chronic lesions, and examples of these include various sulphur, mercury and salicylic acid preparations. Dithranol is a keratolytic ointment used in the treatment of chronic psoriasis.

(3) Antipruritic applications for the relief of itching include phenol, calamine and lead and spirit lotions.

(4) Antiseptics, fungicides and anti-parasitics are used for their effect in bacterial or fungal infection and parasitic infestation, respectively. Examples of these are antibiotic solutions and ointments such as neomycin and tetracycline preparations, gentian violet paint used in the treatment of pyogenic skin lesions, Whitfield's ointment (benzoic acid and salicylic acid) in the treatment of ringworm, benzyl benzoate emulsion and Gammexane in the treatment of parasitic infestations.

(5) Hydrocortisone as a local application is used in a number of conditions, such as pruritus, eczema and contact dermatitis. One of 2·5 per cent hydrocortisone ointments, and hydrocortisone lotion in strength of 0·5 and 1 per cent, commonly applied as a spray, are available and also a combination of hydrocortisone ointment and lotion with various antibiotics and other local applications.

Methods of Using External Applications

Lotions are applied as wet dressings. Pieces of soft cotton or linen cut to suitable sizes are soaked in a cold or tepid solution and applied after wringing out excessive moisture. These dressings should be kept moistened and left uncovered. If necessary a light gauze bandage or a piece of cotton material pinned over the dressing can be used to keep it in place. Paints such as gentian violet and carbolfuchsin are applied with a swab and the area is left uncovered. Calamine painted on with a wide brush and left exposed to the air under open cradles is also most soothing in the acute stage.

Pastes are applied directly to the skin, using a wooden spatula, or spread on pieces of thin material, such as old linen or cotton sheeting, and then applied. Creams and emulsions are applied in the same way. Plastic 'squeeze packs' are convenient, particularly for the patient's own use at home.

Ointments may also be spread on strips of old linen or

cotton. Some ointments need to be rubbed into the skin, for example benzoic acid compound (Whitfield's) ointment used as a fungicide in the treatment of ringworm.

Keeping dressings in position is often a problem especially where large areas of the body are affected. Bandages should be as light as possible, and roller bandages are often unadvisable as many layers of bandage may be required to keep the dressing in place. If bandages are used they should be firmly applied; loose bandages rub the skin and entangle air making the part hot and irritable. Tubular gauze or elastic net is to be preferred; it can be used for limbs and trunk, and also for the face and scalp in the form of a mask or cap.

Poultices of boiled starch, containing boric acid powder, are useful for softening crusted lesions and scabs. Eighty millilitres (2 tablespoonsful) of starch mixed with 40 ml of boric acid powder is sufficient to make a pint of starch jelly. The dry starch is mixed with sufficient cold water to make a stiff paste, boiling water is added to this, stirring the mixture continually. When cool it should be 'set' but not too solid. The poultice is then spread on pieces of cotton or linen, applied, and kept in place by a bandage or tubular gauze.

Cleansing agents must be chosen to suit the particular condition and used with great care and gentleness. Water of itself is non-irritating but soap and water are harmful in most acute conditions. Cetrimide 1 per cent may be substituted. Arachis oil (groundnut oil) is a satisfactory cleansing agent for almost all cases.

Baths are on the whole not as commonly used in treatment now as they were at one time. Sodium bicarbonate baths may give relief in pruritus and sitz-baths may be used in pruritus of vulval and anal regions. Sodium bicarbonate, 0·25 to 0·5 kg, is required for a full bath of 135 litres (30 gallons), i.e. approximately 5 to 10 g per litre (1 to 2 oz per gallon) of water. The water should be warm but not hot. The time the patient spends in the bath should not usually exceed 20 min.

Drugs Which May Be Prescribed for Internal Use

Many drugs formerly prescribed in the treatment of skin diseases are now infrequently used. Hypnotics, sedatives and antibiotics have their place here as in so many other diseases.

One of the most important developments in drug therapy is

the use of steroids, cortisone, prednisolone and corticotrophin (ACTH). The use of hydrocortisone as a local application has already been mentioned. By parenteral injection or by mouth they exert a hitherto unobtainable effect on acute, extensive or fulminating skin diseases which formerly resisted treatment and might even endanger the patient's life: examples of such conditions are angioneurotic oedema, pemphigus, exfoliative dermatitis, and lupus erythematosus. The use of these drugs is not without risk, as they produce numerous and sometimes dangerous side-effects. The nurse should ensure that she knows which particular steroid is being used, the possible side-effects and the observations which should be recorded and reported.

Antihistamine drugs, which can be given orally, are also useful in the treatment of skin diseases due to allergic reactions. Examples of these drugs are promethazine hydrochloride (Phenergan), meclozine hydrochloride (Ancolan) and diphenhydramine (Benadryl).

Griseofulvin is one of the anti-fungal agents which is given by mouth.

CONGENITAL CONDITIONS

Ichthyosis ('Fish Skin')

In this condition the skin is deficient in sebaceous glands and is dry, scaly and often fissured. The skin should be lubricated with a lanolin preparation such as Hydrous Woolfat Ointment, B.P. or urea cream (Calmurid) which increases the hydration of the horny layer.

Naevi (Birth Marks)

A naevus is a localized patch of thickened and dilated blood vessels. Naevi may occur on any area of the skin but are commonly seen on the face. If extensive they are very disfiguring, and in certain cases, where the tongue is involved, the infant may be unable to suck. Some types will disappear without treatment. For those which persist various forms of treatment are employed, depending on the type of naevus and its position such as surgical excision, applications of radium or thorium X. For small naevi application of carbon dioxide snow may be successful.

BACTERIAL AND VIRAL INFECTIONS

Impetigo Contagiosa

Impetigo, as its name suggests, is a very contagious condition, both by direct and indirect contact. It is common in children, and the lesions occur where the skin is damaged by slight injury, for example grazed knees, or by constant discharge from nose or ear. Infection of the scalp is often associated with infestation with head lice.

The infecting agent is usually *Streptococcus pyogenes*. Poor hygienic surroundings and lack of personal cleanliness are contributory causes.

The micro-organism is likely to be present all over the skin, and is not confined to the obvious local lesions; therefore precautions must be taken to prevent spread of the infection by disinfection of articles of clothing worn, and of towels, bed-clothes, etc., used by the patient. Feeding utensils, brush and combs, and toilet requisites should be kept for his individual use.

The lesion appears first as a red area; this becomes a small blister which readily breaks and the exuding serum forms a crust.

Treatment

All crusts must first be removed by any of the following means: (a) cetrimide or warm oil; (b) starch poultices; and (c) bathing with normal saline solution.

When the area is clean either chlortetracycline 0·25 per cent or a solution of gentian violet 1 per cent may be used.

When the impetigo is associated with head lice the appropriate treatment for this type of infestation (see p. 233) must be the first step.

Sycosis. This is a form of impetigo due to staphylococcal infection of the beard and upper lip. The treatment is the same as for impetigo; the hair must first be clipped or shaved.

Pemphigus

Pemphigus neonatorum (or impetigo neonatorum) is a serious staphylococcal infection of the skin in new-born infants, in which eruption consists of large septic blisters (bullae); it was formerly a very fatal form of infection. Toxaemia is marked and the infant obviously seriously ill. The treatment is the systemic administration of a suitable antibiotic; chlortetracycline (Aureomycin) may be effective if the organism is resistant to penicillin. Another form of pemphigus which is seen in later life is not due to infection but is the result of the separation of the epidermis with the production of large blisters. This is also a serious disease as proteins are constantly being drained from the body in the exudate from the blisters. Furthermore the patient may develop some intercurrent disease, such as pneumonia, which, in combination with the skin disease, may prove fatal. Systemic treatment with one of the corticosteroids offers the best hope of success at the present time.

Lupus Vulgaris

Lupus vulgaris is an infection of the skin by *Mycobacterium tuberculosis*, which may be by direct inoculation or blood-borne. It is slowly progressive and destructive; the characteristic lupus nodules are present. The face and neck are commonly affected, but any part of the body can be involved. The typical feature is the *apple-jelly* nodule—i.e. a semi-transparent brownish lump, 1 to 2 mm in size, which is present in the dermis. The disease causes destruction of the skin and where healing occurs scar tissue forms. When it appears on the face, deformities of nose, mouth or eyelids may result. Malignant disease occasionally develops later.

Treatment

Lupus vulgaris treatment is on the same lines as that of other forms of tuberculosis, i.e. good food, fresh air, good hygienic conditions and the administration of isoniazid, or combinations of this drug with streptomycin and *para*-aminosalicylic acid (PAS).

Warts

A wart is a small growth arising from the horny layer of the skin occurring most frequently on the hands. The usual cause is a virus and warts are potentially infectious, although susceptibility to infection seems to vary very much from person to person.

Warts seldom cause trouble and often disappear spontaneously, but their removal may be sought because they are unsightly. Various methods are used, e.g. curetting with a sharp spoon or the application of caustics such as carbon dioxide snow or silver nitrate.

Warts on the sole of the foot, plantar warts, grow into the skin as a result of pressure and may require removal because they are painful.

Herpes

Herpes is an eruption of vesicles, which may occur on various parts of the skin surface.

Herpes Simplex

The cause of herpes simplex is a virus and the condition is mildly infectious. It is liable to manifest itself during an acute illness (e.g. pneumonia) or following a minor injury. Various foods or drugs, or strong sunlight, may cause an attack in some individuals, while in others anxiety is a precipitating factor.

Common situations are the lips, cheeks, nose, ears and genitals. A rather uncomfortable, slightly swollen, red patch first appears and after a few hours this becomes densely packed with small vesicles. These later become yellowish, then dry up and fall off. The redness clears entirely in a few days.

The area should be kept clean and dry by application of zinc powder or a spirit lotion.

Herpes Zoster (Shingles)

The cause is the same virus as that which causes chickenpox. Following an attack (clinical or sub-clinical) of chickenpox the virus remains dormant in the body until the patient's general condition is lowered when it may become active again. The eruption follows the distribution of a sensory nerve, and is characterized by preceding pain, with enlargement of the lymph glands. The associated posterior spinal nerve root is inflamed. The sensory nerves in the thoracic region are commonly affected, but any part of the body may be involved. Pain in the area is first complained of and mild febrile signs may be present.

Redness is then seen followed by the appearance of vesicles on the third and fourth day. These coalesce and may become purulent. At the end of a week the vesicles dry and fall off, leaving some scarring in many cases. Elderly patients frequently suffer afterwards from obstinate neuralgia in the affected nerve. Herpes involving the ophthalmic nerve may lead to eye complications, conjunctivitis and corneal ulceration with scarring which may result in blindness.

Analgesic such as codeine may be required to relieve pain. The vesicles can be protected by the application of calamine lotion and a light dressing.

Recovery is usually complete after about 2 weeks, except for the persistent neuralgia or eye damage that may occur in some cases.

Children may develop chickenpox as a result of exposure to an adult with shingles.

PARASITIC INFECTIONS

Ringworm (Tinea)

Ringworm affecting the hair and horny layer of the skin is caused by a species of fungus which infects man and man domestic animals. Certain types of fungus tend to occur in particular areas of the skin. The scalp is commonly the site of the infection in children under the age of 14 years; ringworm of the groin and the foot ('athlete's foot') are fairly common forms of the disease in adults. The fungus is acquired either directly from a human or animal source or indirectly from infected clothing, hairbrushes, combs, towels, bath mats or other toilet articles. Ringworm affecting the non-hairy skin is treated by the application of a fungicide in the form of an ointment; benzoic acid compound (Whitfield's ointment) is commonly used, or a paint such as Castellani's fuchsin paint.

The prevention of spread of infection or of reinfection entails boiling or disinfection of clothing and, where appropriate, disinfection of footwear, and ensuring that there is no communal using of such articles as towels, combs or hairbrushes.

When the fungus is present in the hairy skin of the scalp or beard, treatment is difficult because the infection spreads down the hair follicles and therefore surface applications are not usually successful.

Ringworm of the scalp is highly contagious amongst school-children and large numbers in a school may be affected. On examination of the scalp bald patches, which may be scaly, with a few broken stumps of hair are seen. The diagnosis is confirmed by examination of the scalp under Wood's light, a special type of ultraviolet lamp, when hairs infected with the fungus will give a green fluorescence. Microscopic examination of hairs from the affected area will also show the presence of the microsporon which produces this particular type of ringworm. For many years treatment therefore has been aimed at epilation of the scalp; the fungus is removed with the hair and a new growth of hair free from infection can then be expected. Superficial X-rays have been used to produce epilation, but this treatment is not without hazard; too small a dose is ineffective, and too large a dose may cause permanent baldness. Further, the view is now held that exposure to any form of X-radiation should, whenever possible, be avoided. An antibiotic, griseofulvin (Fulcin), given by mouth is effective against fungoid infections of the skin, hair and nails, which are resistant to surface applications of fungicides.

Scabies (The Itch)

Scabies is an infestation of the skin by a mite, *Sarcoptes scabiei*. The female burrows into the epidermis along the horny layer, deposing eggs in the track at intervals. These hatch in 6 days and the larvae come to the surface as the epidermis is rubbed off; the female is then fertilized by the male and, when full development is reached, the cycle starts again —i.e. in about 10 to 13 days from the egg stage.

The infection is not highly contagious and close contact is necessary for its spread. The burrows appear as grey or black irregular lines in the skin about 6 to 12 mm ($\frac{1}{4}$ to $\frac{1}{2}$ in) in length, at the end of which the mite can be seen as a minute speck. Scratch marks and excoriations of the skin are often seen. Common sites are the front of the wrist, ulnar border of hand, between the fingers, anterior axillary fold, lowest part of buttocks, around the nipples, on the penis, and in children on the inner side of the feet. The face and head are not affected. The irritation is extreme, especially at night when the patient becomes warm in bed. Secondary infection from scratching with pustules similar to those seen in impetigo, is not un-common.

One application of benzyl benzoate emulsion is nearly always successful in curing the condition. The patient should have a hot bath using plenty of soap and a soft brush; this will help to soften the skin and open up the burrows. After drying the skin the benzyl benzoate emulsion is painted on the skin covering the whole body from the neck to the soles of the feet. The emulsion must be allowed to dry before putting on the clothing which was being worn before bathing. Twenty-four hours later a fresh application of the emulsion, without the preliminary bath, is given. The following evening the patient washes thoroughly in a hot bath, and puts on clean clothes. The dis-carded clothing does not need disinfection but can be washed and ironed in the usual way. Some itching resulting from the chemical used may persist after the treatment and for this calamine lotion can be used. Gamma benzene hexachloride (Gammexane) 1 per cent emulsion, or cream, is also effective and simple to use. It is applied in a thin film covering the body from the neck down on three successive nights.

Where one member of a family is affected it is probable that others are also infested and will require treatment.

Pediculosis

Pediculosis is infestation with lice which are parasites that live by sucking the blood of the host through a proboscis. Many animals as well as man are the hosts for these parasites but the three types of lice that commonly infest human beings are:

(1) *Pediculus capitis*, the head louse which lives only on the scalp.
(2) *Pediculus corporis*, which lives on the skin of the body but lays its eggs in the seams of clothing.
(3) *Pediculus pubis*, which lives in the body hair particularly the pubic hair, but never invades the scalp.

Infestation with these parasites causes irritation which leads to scratching and subsequent infection. Impetigo of the scalp may be due to head lice and the posterior occipital glands are often enlarged and tender. Body lice can act as vectors of typhus fever, a disease which is rare in Great Britain, but which is endemic in some parts of the world. Gamma benzene hexachloride 1 per cent (Gammexane) kills all lice and can be used in the form of an emulsion or powder. Dicophane emulsion (Suleo) will effectively deal with infestation of the scalp, although the eggs, or nits, will remain attached to the hairs and need to be removed by combing with a fine-toothed comb. Thirty millilitres of dicophane emulsion is rubbed well into the hair and scalp which should then be covered for 24 hr. The treatment may need to be repeated at the end of 1 week. Gammexane is used in the same way. Thirty millilitres of an emulsion containing 0·1 per cent Gammexane is sufficient for one treatment.

OTHER SKIN DISEASES AND DISORDERS

Pruritus (Itching)

Pruritus, as might be expected, is a symptom of many skin diseases, as for example, eczema, urticaria and infestation of the skin in scabies. Local irritation of the skin of the vulva and peri-anal area is not uncommon and can be due to a number of causes, including vaginal discharge, urinary infection, or the irritating effect of sugar in the urine of the diabetic patient. Pruritus is also a symptom of such systemic conditions as uraemia and jaundice. Senile pruritus occurs in elderly persons whose skin has become dry and atrophic. Finally pruritus may arise without any discoverable organic background, and appears in these cases to be due to psychological factors. This type is included under the term 'neurodermatosis', a condition in which the skin lesions are a reaction to emotional disturbance and may be a manifestation of an anxiety state.

The cause of the condition must be sought and wherever possible removed or treated, and this includes psychotherapy where this is indicated. Soothing local applications include calamine lotion, or cream if the skin is dry, phenol 1 per cent solution, and hydrocortisone ointment. In generalized pruritus sodium bicarbonate baths may give relief. Any source of irritation or chafing of the skin, for example woollen clothing worn next to the skin, must be avoided.

Adequate meals are essential; some patients suffering from

intense pruritus may be so miserable that they have little interest in food. Some, on the other hand, may find solace in eating, and should be warned that very rich or highly seasoned foods may aggravate the condition. Obviously if the pruritus is part of systemic disease, such as diabetes or jaundice, the appropriate diet for the underlying condition will be necessary. A hypnotic may be necessary at night to enable the patient to obtain sufficient sleep.

Dermatitis and Eczema

Dermatitis simply means inflammation of the skin and eczema may be considered as a form of dermatitis, in that it is an inflammatory condition of the skin as a result of some irritant or of sensitivity to a substance harmless to normal people. Eczema therefore may be an allergic manifestation and may be associated with asthma and hay fever.

In acute eczema there is first erythema, due to dilatation of capillaries from which fluid escapes into the epidermis and forms minute vesicles which, increasing in size, push their way to the surface. The horny cells covering these become rubbed off, and a moist surface remains (weeping eczema). Later dried serum forms crusts, and healing may occur, although relapses are common at this stage. A frequent complication is a superimposed infection of impetigo. In chronic eczema the skin is dry, scaly and thickened. It is an intensely irritating disease with a burning sensation, aggravated by soap and water, and worse when the patient is hot and tired.

Infantile eczema is a type seen in young children, usually developing after the age of 3 months in infants with a family history of eczema, hay fever and asthma. These infants are particularly prone to other infections, such as bronchitis and gastro-enteritis, and need the most careful attention whether at home or in hospital. Irritation of the skin is intense, and light cotton tubular gauze gloves may be used to prevent damage from scratching. Woollen clothes and blankets are irritating and should not be allowed to come in contact with the skin. Exacerbations of the condition may follow emotional upsets, and this condition makes great demands on the mother who will have to exert great patience and also to avoid showing her anxiety in over-indulgence as the infant grows older.

Acute Eczema

Soothing applications such as calamine lotion or a thin calamine cream are dabbed on the area; aluminium acetate may be used, in combination or alone, especially in the weeping stage; later zinc cream is soothing. If a lotion is ordered linen can be soaked in this, applied and remoistened as it becomes dry without removal. A paint brush may be used for applying lotion.

Wet dressings should, if possible, be left exposed to the air; tubular gauze is excellent for the limbs. Hydrocortisone as a lotion or ointment is often effective in severe cases. Cortisone preparations such as prednisolone given orally may also be used.

For less acute cases zinc paste is applied, but before renewal all old paste must be removed with arachis oil or cetrimide. Chronic cases are treated with zinc paste to which tar has been added, or specially prepared coal tar may be painted on.

To prevent recurrence persons susceptible to eczema should avoid all exciting causes, especially those which individual experience shows are peculiar to themselves. Thus, washing with soap, bath salts, exposure to heat or bright sunshine, and cold winds are possible irritants.

The disease can be cured, but relapses are common and likely to occur if exposure to the exciting agent takes place. Chronic eczema is very resistant to treatment.

Other forms of dermatitis are contact dermatitis and exfoliative dermatitis.

Contact Dermatitis

This is caused by contact with a substance which is in itself irritant or to which the individual is sensitive. The latter group is very large and includes sensitivity of some individuals to antibiotics. The treatment is directed towards finding the cause and eliminating it and treating the dermatitis on the same lines as eczema.

Exfoliative Dermatitis

A severe, sometimes fatal, condition accompanied by constitutional disturbances such as fever. It is a possible complication of gold treatment, and is one of the reasons why this treatment is used cautiously. Exfoliative dermatitis may also complicate eczema or acute psoriasis. Erythematous patches coalesce and cover large skin areas; this is followed by desquamation resulting in large areas of raw skin.

General treatment includes the administration of corticoid preparation, plasma transfusion if necessary, and nursing the patient in a warm room protected as far as possible from any infection.

Acne Vulgaris

Acne is a very common adolescent affliction. It is one of a group of skin diseases described as 'seborrhoeic', associated with some abnormality of the sebaceous glands, and a tendency to develop skin eruptions on those areas of the body where the sebaceous glands are most numerous, such as the face, neck and back, and on the scalp to produce dandruff. The tendency to acne and other seborrhoeic conditions is often hereditary, but the immediate cause is probably hormone imbalance occurring at puberty, over-activity of progesterone in the female and testosterone in the male. Examination of the skin shows enlarged pores, blackheads, or comedones, red pimples and often pustules. In severe acne the scars of healed pustules can be seen.

The co-operation of the patient is an essential part of the treatment, which is likely to require both time and patience. However, as a young person's life may be completely disrupted by his consciousness of a disfiguring facial rash (Fig. 27), he is usually only too anxious to be given some help.

Fresh air, sunlight, the avoidance of late hours and of any foods likely to aggravate the condition are simple measures that should accompany the local treatment of the condition. Fried or fatty foods, chocolate and cocoa are commonly held to make an acne eruption worse. Treatment of the affected areas is directed towards counteracting the excessive greasiness of the skin by washing, always using a mild soap, and the application of stimulating lotions or pastes containing sulphur, salicylic acid or resorcinol. The application should be sufficiently strong to produce redness and subsequent mild peeling of the skin. Ultraviolet light can produce similar results. Dandruff of the scalp if present should be treated by frequent shampooing using

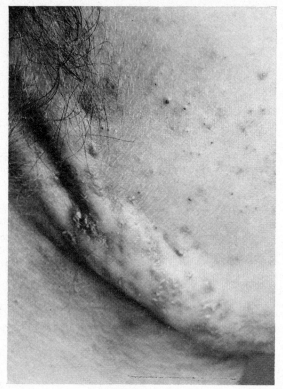

Fig. 27. Acne vulgaris.

a soap spirit shampoo. Blackheads can be removed by gentle pressure with a small metal instrument called a comedone extractor. The patient should be warned not to pick the pimples or to squeeze them with the fingers, as further damage and possibly scarring of the skin can be produced in this way.

Acne tends to disappear as the patient grows older, and in many cases disappears by the time he reaches the twenties.

Women patients may benefit by the administration of oestrogens, e.g. stilboestrol or oestradiol.

Acne Rosacea

Acne rosacea is a skin disorder of the seborrhoeic group mainly occurring in women of middle age. It affects the central area of the face, producing a red area with some raised red papules or pustules.

The cause of this condition is not known, although emotional stress may play some part. The treatment is on the same lines as that for acne.

Intertrigo

Intertrigo is a condition which may also, though not necessarily, be associated with the seborrhoeic state. Moist, inflamed areas of skin are seen in the skin folds, particularly under the breasts in female patients and in the groins and the anal region. Secondary infection is often present.

The inflammation is treated by soothing applications, such as zinc cream, applied on strips of cotton or linen, making sure that the skin surfaces are separated. Infection, if present, is treated by the application of an antibiotic ointment or lotion, e.g. neomycin. The patient must be warned of the danger of recurrence unless the skin is kept dry and free from chafing.

Psoriasis

Psoriasis is a disease in which there seems to be some hereditary element. It tends to recur, and sometimes has a seasonal incidence, sometimes nervous strain may influence its appearance. Injury to the skin seems to prepare the way in some cases and this may account for the elbows and knees being common sites (Fig. 28). Psoriasis is sometimes associated with rheumatoid arthritis. Acute exacerbations may occur in the course of a more chronic form of the disease.

The skin shows sharply defined patches, sheets, or rings of erythema covered with silvery scales, especially on the extensor surface of limbs; but some forms attack the face, nails, palms of hands, or soles of feet.

The lesions vary in size from minute spots to large patches. Discs may be several inches across, but the eruption is always

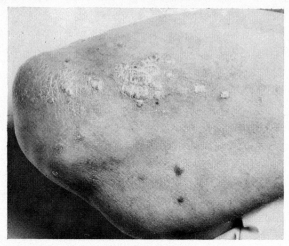

FIG. 28. Psoriasis.

dry, seldom infected. Itching is a symptom in some but not all cases.

During an acute phase the patient should be kept in bed, and soothing applications such as calamine cream are used. After the acute stage has subsided stronger applications with a stimulating and keratolytic action are used. Dithranol 0·5 per cent in Lassar's paste, combined with warm baths and ultraviolet light treatment, is usually successful but requires admission of the patient to hospital and careful observation of the response to the treatment. Complete clearance of the lesions can be expected but attacks tend to recur.

Lupus Erythematosus

Lupus erythematosus is not uncommon in women and shows a typically symmetrical distribution with scaly red patches on the nose and cheeks. Bright sunlight aggravates the condition. The cause is unknown but may be related to sensitivity to foreign proteins. Chloroquine or Atebrine daily for a considerable period, provided signs of toxicity do not appear, have given satisfactory results.

There is an acute disseminated form of the disease which is accompanied by fever, anaemia and serious symptoms such as nephritis and endocarditis, and may end fatally. The only treatment which has so far proved effective is the systemic administration of corticosteroids.

Pityriasis Rosea

Pityriasis rosea is a condition in which pink, oval macules occur on trunk and limbs, and tend to scale from the centre. One patch usually appears first ('herald patch'); then some days later the general eruption. Irritation is usually slight. The disease lasts 6 to 8 weeks, the macules fading, becoming wrinkly and brownish, and then peeling. The cause of this disease is unknown, and its course is not affected by treatment. If the rash is irritating a soothing lotion can be used.

Lichen Planus

Lichen planus is a chronic condition the cause of which is unknown. It appears to be associated in some cases with emotional stress.

The eruption is liable to occur along the line of a scratch, and consists of small, flat-tipped, shiny papules of a violet colour due to the nearness to the surface of the blood-vessels. These commonly occur on the anterior surface of the forearms, inner side of thigh and front leg, or round the waist in women. The affected area may have a mottled appearance, owing to variation in thickness of the superficial layers. Irritation may be severe or may be absent. In some cases dead white spots are present on the mucous membrane of the cheeks. The onset is insidious and is slowly progressive. When the papules fade a brownish pigmentation remains for months. It may manifest in several situations, and an acute generalized type is sometimes seen.

Acute cases should be kept in bed. Sedatives may be ordered for the irritation, and antipruritic lotions (calamine with phenol) for local application. Crude tar may be applied, or tar ointments or creams.

The duration may be long, and relapses are very likely.

Alopecia

Alopecia is loss of hair and may be local or generalized. Permanent loss of hair is part of the general process of ageing, premature baldness is commoner in men than in women and is associated with a hereditary tendency. Temporary loss sometimes follows an acute febrile illness, and some endocrine disorders affect the hair, for example under-activity of the thyroid gland in myxoedema.

Alopecia Areata

The hair falls out suddenly and in patches (Fig. 29) sometimes on top of the head, sometimes the sides, leaving the skin smooth

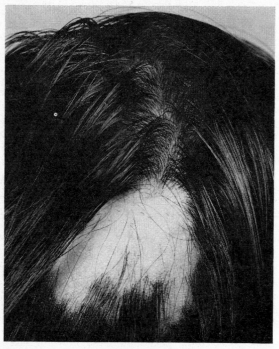

FIG. 29. Alopecia.

and shiny with broken hairs at the margins, causing the characteristic 'exclamation mark' appearance. The patches may
spread into each other. New hair starts to grow from the centre
of the patch, and may at first be white but regains its normal
colour later. The cause of this condition is unknown, but it is
thought that emotional factors are often present.

In most cases the hair grows again without treatment but a
stimulating application containing cantharides or localized
ultraviolet light therapy may hasten the growth. Any obvious
septic focus, such as infected tonsils or teeth, is treated.

Urticaria (Nettle Rash)

Urticaria is characterized by an intensely irritating eruption
which is a reaction to a great variety of sensitizing agents,
including toxins derived from drugs, infections, irritants such
as insect stings and nettle leaves. Emotional tension is often a
factor.

The rash is erythematous and may be papular, but often
appears as large wheals. In a severe attack the patient feels ill
and miserable, and the irritation is often intolerable. The most
effective treatment is adequate dosage of antihistamines, such as
promethazine (Phenergan) or diphenydramine (Benadryl).
Ephedrine or adrenaline, given hypodermically, are employed in
very acute cases particularly in the type known as angioneurotic
oedema or giant urticaria, in which large oedematous swellings
appear and, if the glottis is involved, may endanger life by
suffocation. In acute attacks one of the cortisone group of
drugs may be used effectively, if necessary as hydrocortisone by
intravenous injection.

12
Disorders of the nervous system

THE central system, consisting of the brain, spinal cord and peripheral nerves, is responsible for receiving and interpreting the messages which the body receives from its environment, for all conscious sensation and for the control of motor activity. The higher controlling centres are in the cortex of the brain; centres controlling reflex, automatic activities are situated in the lower levels of the brain and the spinal cord and these, although normally subject to some control from the cerebral cortex, can function independently if this control is removed.

Disorders of the nervous system therefore may be manifested by changes in motor control, in sensory perception, in consciousness, or awareness of the outside world, and in behaviour. The following brief description covers the main features of these manifestations.

Disturbances of Motor Control

Paralysis means loss of voluntary control over muscular movement. It may result from damage to the motor cells in the brain or spinal cord or to the fibres conveying the messages to the muscles. Damage to the motor tracts from the brain to the spinal cord produces the spastic or rigid type of paralysis, with increase of muscle tone and flexion of the joints, but no marked wasting (upper motor reverse disease). Damage to the motor cells in the spinal cord or to the nerve fibres to the muscles, produces the flaccid or limp type of paralysis with loss of muscle tone and wasting (lower motor reverse disease).

Hemiplegia is the term used to describe paralysis of cerebral origin affecting one half of the body vertically. The commonest type of hemiplegia is paralysis of the muscles of the face, neck, trunk and limbs on the opposite side of the body to that of the cerebral damage. In some conditions crossed paralysis is seen, the affected muscles of the trunk and limbs are on the opposite side of the body to the paralysed face and neck muscles.

Paraplegia describes paralysis of the lower half of the body resulting from injury to or disease of the spinal cord. Paraplegia is accompanied by loss of sphincter control.

Monoplegia is paralysis of one limb.

Paresis is the term used for loss of muscle power without actual paralysis.

Tremor is the term given to the shaking movements which the patient is unable to control. 'Intention tremor' is tremor which develops when the patient tries to perform a definite action demanding co-ordination of muscles, for example if he is asked to bring his finger to touch the tip of his nose.

Convulsions or *fits*, are violent, uncontrolled, generalized movements which may or may not be associated with loss of consciousness. The typical fit is seen in major epilepsy.

Disturbances of Sensation

Defects of vision, hearing, taste and smell may result from damage to the nerve paths or to the cerebral centres which interpret the messages received from the sense organs.

Anaesthesia is the term used for loss of sensation, and this is often an accompaniment of paralysis. Since protective sensations of heat and pain are absent there is constant danger of damage to the skin of the anaesthetic area.

Hyperaesthesia is increased sensibility to heat, cold and pain.

Paraesthesia is the term used for abnormal sensation such as tingling or 'pins and needles'.

Disturbances of Consciousness

Coma is a state of deep unconsciousness due to damage to or pressure on the brain cells, and may be caused by disease, injury or poisoning, e.g. by narcotic drugs. The patient in coma cannot be roused even by painful stimuli and this is always a serious condition.

Stupor, drowsiness or lethargy, are terms used to describe diminished awareness of and response to stimuli, although the patient can be roused to some degree of consciousness. Although a definition has been given for the above terms the boundary lines between them are not sharply defined and there are many degrees within each. For this reason, it is better for the nurse to describe the patient's condition under various headings, e.g.

Reaction to Stimuli:
Orientation in time and place.
Response to spoken word.
Response to touch.
Response to painful stimuli.

State of Pupils:
Response to light.
Right eye, left eye.

Syncope, or fainting, is a brief period of unconsciousness due to temporary anaemia of the brain.

Disturbances of Behaviour

Delirium is an acute mental confusion of short duration. The patient is unaware of his surroundings and often has very vivid hallucinations, i.e. he sees or hears things which have no reality. It is more often seen in toxic states such as alcoholic psychosis (delirium tremens) or accompanying the hyperpyrexia of an acute infection or heat stroke than in diseases of or injuries to the brain.

Other abnormal mental states which may be associated with disease of the nervous system include *delusions*, i.e. false ideas, such as the 'delusion of grandeur' in which the patient is out of touch with the realities of his situation and *dementia*, a form of mental deterioration in which the patient becomes progressively less and less able to exercise reasonable judgment or to follow a consecutive train of thought and at the same time is likely to show signs of emotional instability, being easily moved to tears or laughter and easily irritated.

Observation of the Patient

In few situations are careful observation and accurate reporting more important than in the nursing of patients suffering from disorders of the nervous system. The nurse has invaluable opportunities for observing the smallest details of the patient's behaviour, for example his mental and emotional state, his reaction to relatives and other visitors, any remarks that the relatives may make which would indicate recent personality changes. Bearing in mind that personality changes are often a part of the illness, the nurse will realize than an understanding and sympathetic approach is an essential step in gaining the patient's confidence and giving a feeling of security. The patient may tell her of some symptom which he considered too trivial or transient to mention, or some detail of his past medical history which he had forgotten. Complaints of pain, numbness or tingling, of double vision or other sensory disturbances, should be carefully noted, with details of the time of their occurrence and duration. Gait, posture and balance, tremor or uncoordinated movements are other signs that may be noted. Should a convulsion occur the nurse is likely to be the only person present, and she should note mentally, and afterwards record in writing, a full account of its onset, course and duration (see also p. 261).

The nurse should keep an accurate account of the hours of sleep at night; mental confusion and restlessness during the night may be associated with abnormal daytime drowsiness. In the case of a patient who is comatose the nurse should be able to give helpful information as to the level of consciousness. Failure to respond even to painful stimuli, such as pressure on the closed eyes or pinching the skin, small pupils which do not react to light, rapid weak pulse and shallow irregular breathing are signs of deep unconsciousness in which the state of coma may end in death. Diminishing depth of coma and some return to consciousness are shown by some response to pressure on or light slapping of the face, the return of reflex responses, spontaneous movements and improvement in the respirations. The return of the swallowing reflex can be tested by putting a moist swab or a spoon between the patient's lips, but until it is evident that not only does he attempt to swallow but can also hear and respond to a verbal instruction such as 'open your mouth', it is not safe to put any food or fluid into his mouth.

Terms Used for Various Signs and Symptoms of Neurological Disorders

Amnesia: impairment of memory.

Aphasia: impairment of the ability to form words or to name objects.

Ataxia: incoordination of voluntary muscular movements.

Athetosis: slow, writhing contractions of voluntary muscles.

Kernig's sign: inability to straighten the knee when the thigh is flexed, seen in meningitis and sciatica.

Nystagmus: oscillating movements of the eyeballs.

Papilloedema: swelling of the optic disc, the area where the optic nerve fibres leave the retina.

Reflex muscle responses: normal involuntary muscular responses to a nerve stimulus. Examples of these are:

(1) Patellar reflex, contraction of the quadriceps muscle of the thigh jerking the foot forward when the patellar tendon is tapped.

(2) Plantar reflex, plantar flexion of the toes when the sole of the foot is stroked. Babinski's sign is an extensor response of the big toe which occurs in disease of the motor tracts in the spinal cord.

(3) Pupil reflex; normally the pupils of the eye contract in response to a bright light, or when converging to focus on a near object. The Argyll Robertson pupil is a reaction to accommodation for near objects, but not to light.

Retinopathy: disease of the retina of the eye other than that due to inflammation, most commonly due to degeneration of or changes in the blood-vessels.

Vertigo: a sensation of rotating in space or of the rotation of objects in the environment. It is usually a symptom of disease involving the auditory nerve or the labyrinth of the internal ear.

Special Investigations and Examinations

Neurological examination. This detailed examination includes testing various reflex motor responses, the response to sensory stimuli, touch, temperature, pain, tests of balancing and posture, examination of the optic fundus and testing the fields of vision. The doctor will usually require the following items.

Patella hammer.
Tuning fork.
Ophthalmoscope, 2 per cent homatropine drops or other mydriatic to dilate the pupils of the eye.
Tape measure.
Skin pencil.
Pins.
Cotton wool mops.
Small soft brush.

Test tubes containing hot water and cold water.

Small bottles containing substances for testing sensations of taste and smell, e.g. sugar, salt, peppermint.

Stethoscope.

Sphygmomanometer.

Examination of the cerebrospinal fluid. A sample of fluid is usually obtained by lumbar puncture, occasionally by cisternal puncture at the junction of the skull and cervical spine, or by ventricular puncture.

Lumbar puncture is also used as a means of introducing drugs such as anaesthetics and antibiotics (see p. 338).

Two lumbar puncture needles and a glass manometer for registering the pressure of the cerebrospinal fluid, at least three sterile test tubes and a pathological examination form for the laboratory will be needed.

A local anaesthetic may be required and as this is a sterile procedure sterile towels, swabs and instruments should be supplied.

The patient should lie well over on to the left side with the knees so flexed that they are close to the chin; thus the spine is arched and the spaces between the vertebrae widen to their fullest extent. Marked stiffness and opisthotonos can be overcome by leverage applied by a bandage or roller towel passed under the knees and round the shoulders. The needle is introduced between the vertebrae at the level of a line drawn straight across between the two iliac crests. An alternative position for a patient who is not confined to bed is to have him sitting on a chair, facing the back, with his buttocks well out to the edge, his arms folded on the back of the chair and his head resting on his arms. After the procedure the patient may have a severe headache, but this can usually be avoided by keeping him lying flat and quiet for some hours.

Cerebrospinal fluid is clear and colourless, it contains chlorides, a trace of sugar, protein and a few lymphocytes. The pressure in the normal adult is from 80 to 180 mm of water.

The cell count increases in tuberculous meningitis, syphilis and other infections; pus cells are found in pyogenic infections. Protein content is increased in infective conditions and in spinal block. The normal amount of glucose is from 50 to 85 mg per 100 ml; this amount decreases in infective condition including tuberculous meningitis. Chlorides, normally 720 to 750 mg per 100 ml, are also reduced in various types of meningitis.

Smears for bacterial examination samples of fluid for animal inoculation for the Wassermann reaction test, and the colloidal gold test for syphilis may be needed.

X-Ray Examinations

X-ray films of the skull are useful in demonstrating the presence of fractures and also changes in the bony structure, such as enlargement of the pituitary fossa as a result of a pitui-

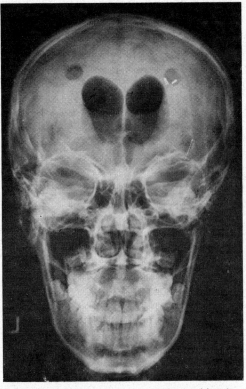

Fig. 30. Ventriculogram in antero-posterior position (normal).

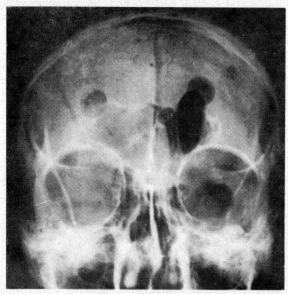

Fig. 31. Ventriculogram showing displacement of the anterior parts of both lateral ventricles to one side indicating a space-occupying lesion of the opposite cerebral hemisphere.

tary tumour. In the case of a female patient the nurse should be careful to see that hair pins, clips or combs, which might cast a shadow, are removed.

Ventriculography is an examination in which X-ray films are taken after the injection of air into the ventricles of the brain. Trephine holes are made through the parietal bones and a trocar is inserted into the lateral ventricle, cerebrospinal fluid is withdrawn, and air injected. The air-filled ventricles will give a dark shadow on the X-ray film, and the shape of the shadow may reveal displacement or blockage due to pressure from a tumour (Figs 30 and 31).

The prodecure is carried out in the operating theatre, and the patient is prepared as for operation, including shaving the scalp. The usual reason for ventriculography is to aid in the diagnosis and location of a cerebral tumour; if the X-ray examination confirms the diagnosis the surgeon will usually proceed straight away with the operation of craniotomy.

Air encephalography is another form of X-ray examination which outlines the ventricles. Cerebrospinal fluid is removed by lumbar puncture and air is injected into the subarachnoid space. This air being lighter than fluid rises into the communicating ventricles of the brain.

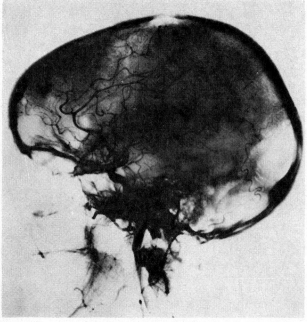

FIG. 32. A carotid arteriogram.

Carotid arteriography is an X-ray examination which will reveal changes in the cerebral blood vessels. Radio-opaque dye is injected into the carotid arteries and a series of X-ray films taken immediately (Fig. 32).

Electro-Encephalogram

The apparatus known as an electro-encephalograph amplifies and records the small electric discharges from the cells of the cerebral cortex. Normal patterns of these discharges are known, and the interpretation of an encephalogram is made by comparing it with a normal record.

DISORDERS OF THE BRAIN AND SPINAL CORD

Cerebrovascular Disorders

Cerebrovascular lesions may produce the dramatic symptoms of unconsciousness and paralysis that are commonly referred to as a 'stroke' or apoplexy.

Such an attack may be the result of cerebral haemorrhage, cerebral thrombosis or cerebral embolism. The predisposing causes of the first two are hypertension and atheroma, the patient is usually middle-aged or elderly. Cerebral embolism is a complication of heart disease, very commonly auricular fibrillation associated with mitral stenosis, but also occurring in myocardial infarct or bacterial endocarditis. Embolism occurs in patients of any age.

The symptoms of cerebrovascular disease depend on the extent and site of the damage. Coma is the result of sudden rise in intracranial pressure, and is not present in all cases. Paralysis is caused by damage to nerve cells in the motor area of the cerebral cortex or to the motor tracts forming the internal capsule at the base of the cerebrum. In the latter instance, since all motor fibres are gathered together in the internal capsule, complete paralysis of one-half of the body, hemiplegia, ensues. Damage to the cerebral cortex may interfere with some, but not necessarily all, of the motor paths, and the patient may escape with a weakness or possibly a paralysis of the face, hand and arm, but not of the leg.

Cerebral haemorrhage is often widespread; blood permeates the soft tissues of the brain substance and fresh bleeding is liable to follow. The patient may complain of violent headache of sudden onset, possibly following some mental or physical effort which has further raised an already high blood pressure. If the bleeding is extensive, coma and widespread paralysis-develop quickly, the patient falls to the ground in an unconscious state, the typical apoplectic fit, and may die a few hours or a few days later. In less severe cases the patient recovers consciousness and gradually some improvement in the initial widespread paralysis takes place.

Subarachnoid haemorrhage may be caused by the bursting of a small aneurysm in the arterial circle (the circle of Willis) at the base of the brain and bleeding into the subarachnoid space. The aneurysm is due to congenital weakness of the blood vessel (see p. 118) and therefore this type of cerebral haemorrhage frequently occurs in young adults. The initial symptoms are severe occipital headache and stiffness of the neck. A massive haemorrhage is usually rapidly fatal, but small recurrent leakages are fairly common. Carotid angiography may be carried out to localize the lesion, and surgical treatment is often successful. Craniotomy is also likely to be contemplated in cases of cerebral haemorrhage where a localized haematoma has formed.

Cerebral thrombosis is usually more gradual in onset than cerebral haemorrhage and is likely to occur when the patient is resting and the circulation is therefore slowed down. The course of events will vary according to the site and extent of the area affected. The patient may lapse into coma and death may follow, but the prospect of recovery from the immediate attack is often good and the degree of permanent paralysis may be slight. However, the underlying cause, which is almost always disease of the blood-vessel walls, is likely to remain and recurrent attacks are probable.

Anticoagulant drugs are sometimes given. Thrombosis of the internal carotid artery may be treated surgically by resection and anastomosis to restore the circulation to the brain.

Cerebral embolism, has a sudden onset, but unless a large vessel is occluded the patient is not likely to lose consciousness. The only symptoms in some cases are headache and a varying degree of paralysis. Anticoagulant drugs may be given as in cerebral thrombosis.

The history of the onset and development of symptoms and of the patient's previous medical history are important, as the treatment and prognosis in cerebrovascular lesions depend on the cause. It is therefore essential to obtain as much detailed information as possible, particularly in the case of an unconscious patient, from those present at the time and from his relatives.

Care of the Unconscious Patient

Lumbar puncture (see p. 249) may be carried out for diagnostic purposes. The fluid is commonly bloodstained in cerebral haemorrhage, always so if there is bleeding into the subarachnoid space. Venesection is performed if the blood pressure is high. Catheterization is usually required to obtain a specimen of urine for examination and to prevent overdistension of the bladder. Continuous bladder drainage with strict aseptic precautions is sometimes necessary, and this is described on page 268.

The patient should be placed in bed lying on his side, with a pillow to support his back or semi-prone. It is essential to see that a clear airway is maintained, if necessary the tongue must be held forward and suction may be needed to clear the mouth and pharynx of mucus and saliva. Increased intracranial pressure may make it desirable to raise the patient's head and shoulders. This can be done by lifting the head of the bed on an elevator or blocks. The patient should be turned from side to side every 2 hr and when so doing every care must be taken to move him gently and to ensure that his arms and legs are not under the trunk and that the paralysed limbs are supported in a normal relaxed position. Regular, frequent change of position is the best way of preventing the development of pressure sores and pneumonia, two of the dangers to which the patient in coma is exposed. Care of the skin by regular washing and special attention to pressure areas, and care of the mouth and eyes, are all part of the routine nursing of a helpless patient. Since an unconscious patient is heavy and gentle handling is essential, two and sometimes three, nurses will be needed in order to make the patient's bed and to change his position. Incontinence may complicate the picture, the use of an indwelling catheter and bladder drainage have been mentioned, faecal incontinence may be avoided by the use of glycerin suppositories.

Feeding is unimportant for the first 24 hr, and no attempt should ever be made to feed an unconscious patient by mouth. Intravenous fluids may be given if unconsciousness continues after 24 hr, or fluids may be given through an intragastric tube.

Continual close observation is essential, level of consciousness, pulse rate and respirations may be recorded at 2-hourly intervals, or if necessary more frequently. Temperature is taken 4 hourly in the axilla, a rapidly rising temperature in an unconscious patient is a grave sign.

Deepening coma is accompanied by failing, irregular breathing and a feeble pulse. Signs of recovering consciousness are spontaneous movements and some response to such stimuli as lightly tapping the face, shining a torch on the eyes or a distinct short question or instruction such as, 'Are you awake?' or 'Open your mouth'.

It must always be remembered that patients who appear unconscious and who are unable to respond can, nevertheless, sometimes hear and should therefore be informed as to the procedures being carried out. Their condition should not be discussed by their bedside. Relatives should be encouraged to touch them, perhaps hold their hand, and talk quietly to them.

Care of the Hemiplegic Patient

As consciousness returns the extent and degree of motor disturbance becomes apparent. In the acute phase of a stroke and while unconsciousness persists all the muscles are likely to lose tone and paralysis of the flaccid type is present. It may be noted that this is more marked on one side of the body. This indicates that the cerebral lesion is on the opposite side of the brain. Later, as muscle tone returns, it becomes obvious that there is spastic paralysis on the affected side. This may involve the muscles of the face, neck, upper and lower limbs or may be less widespread. Loss of sensation in the paralysed limb is an added danger, as the patient is unable to appreciate sensations of heat or pain. Hot water bottles or other forms of heat should not be used in the nursing of paralysed patients, not only is the skin in many cases insensitive and easily damaged, but even if the patient is able to feel he cannot move.

If the damage is on the left side of the cerebral cortex the speech area will be involved, and in addition to the loss of power in the limbs the patient will have speech difficulties (aphasia). He may understand what is said to him, but be able to use only a few words, or may be unable to name a familiar object successfully. The various areas of the brain concerned in the ability to describe by speech objects seen or heard and their link with the motor speech area are not accurately known, but from the point of view of nursing, the difficulties which the patient experiences have a practical application. Intelligent anticipation of the patient's needs, sympathetic understanding and interpretation of the sounds that he is able to make will do much to comfort and encourage him and relieve his frustration.

In many cases improvement in the paralysis may be expected, as the initial extent may be the result of cerebral oedema which will subside. However, the paralysis due to destruction of nerve cells and nerve fibres will be permanent. Paralysed limbs should be supported in the most favourable position for the prevention of disabling deformities. Passive movements of the joints and support or light splints are required to prevent contractures and deformities. Splints may be applied at night to prevent wrist and foot drop.

Rehabilitation is begun at the earliest moment possible, with a view to preventing complications and promoting the maximum degree of recovery. Exercises can be carried out in bed. the patient is encouraged to assist in movements required to change his position and to help himself in washing and feeding. Active leg movements, raising the trunk, movements in bed such as sitting and dangling the legs over the edge, are examples of exercises that may be prescribed. Obviously the patient will have to depend on the arm and leg on the unaffected side of the body for such movements. A firm mattress and a side rail and a trapeze hand grip will be of great assistance. As soon as possible the patient is allowed out of bed, and stands on his good leg using the good arm for support. He will need some support, such as a sling, for the paralysed arm. As progress continues stair climbing and walking with the support of a tripod stick are introduced. If there is no recovery in the muscles of the paralysed arm and leg, a light splint for the forearm and a leg brace are usually needed. The aphasic patient may be helped by by speech therapy which should also be commenced as soon possible.

Although re-education is largely the work of the physiotherapist and the speech therapist, the nurse has a part to play in rehabilitation. The patient's co-operation is an essential part of the process, and he may need much encouragement and explanation. He regains his feeling of independence as he finds that he is able to feed, wash and attend to his own needs, and this will be fostered by the nurse who understands the need to help him to believe that he will return to a reasonably normal life and is not a helpless burden for himself and his family.

There are a wide variety of aids for the disabled patient, e.g. elastic shoe laces, which should be utilized to aid this return to independence.

Cerebral Tumours

Cerebral tumours may be benign or malignant growths; the commonest type of primary growth in the brain is a malignant tumour arising from neuroglial tissue, the delicate supporting tissue of the brain, and known as a glioma. Secondary growths, or metastases, in the brain develop as a result of malignant cells from a primary growth in another organ, for example a carcinoma of the bronchus being carried in the blood stream to the brain. Examples of benign growths are a meningioma, arising from the membranous coverings of the brain, a neuroma of the auditory nerve, and an adenoma of the pituitary gland. Occasionally tumours are found to be tuberculous masses or syphilitic gummata.

A tumour in the brain will produce symptoms such as headache, vomiting and disturbances of vision which are characteristic of any space-occupying lesion within the skull, be it a growth, an abscess, a blood clot or a haematoma. The development of other symptoms, fits, paralysis, loss of sense of taste, smell or balance, deafness, blindness and mental changes, will depend on the size and site of the tumour. The commonest early symptom is intense headache which is described as 'throbbing' or 'bursting' and is at its worst when the patient first wakes in the morning.

Treatment

Since cerebral tumours, whether benign or malignant, eventually cause the death of the patient by pressure on and destruction of the brain, surgical removal is usually contemplated as the treatment of choice. Localization of the tumour is an essential preliminary to operation, and in addition to a full neurological examination the radiological investigations described on page 252 will be carried out. Tumours in certain positions are not easily accessible to surgery and some tumours, particularly gliomata, often cannot be completely removed. Radiotherapy may replace surgery in these cases or may be combined with surgery.

Where the disease has advanced to a stage in which palliative treatment is the only possible course burrholes may be made in the skull to relieve the intracranial pressure.

Nursing treatment, in addition to general measures aimed at promoting the patient's comfort and general health, includes accurate observation and recording of symptoms as described on page 245. If extensive surgery is to be undertaken it is probable that the patient will be transferred to a neurosurgical unit. What the patient and his relatives should be told about his condition and the probable prognosis is, of course, a matter for the doctor's decision and will be based on the assessment of all the factors in the individual case. The nurse should maintain a cheerful, encouraging attitude; provided that the patient does not get over-tired, visits by friends and relatives will help to pass the time and to interest him in matters outside his own illness. Treatment is wholly successful in some cases and, even in malignant growths where recurrence at a later date is probable, the patient may have several years of good health before symptoms again make their appearance.

In the advanced stage of a malignant growth the patient will eventually be bedridden; he may have fits and later become paralysed and incontinent. Skilled nursing care is essential to protect his skin from injury and to prevent such complications as bedsores, pneumonia and urinary infection. Scrupulous attention to the cleanliness of the patient, his clothing and bedding contributes to his comfort and a well-cared-for appearance will to some extent lessen his relatives' distress. If cerebrospinal fluid leaks continually through decompression holes in the skull, dressings will need frequent replacement. A tubular gauze skull cap is a comfortable, neat and convenient form of bandage; a woman patient may like to wear a light, pretty cap of nylon net or similar washable material over the bandage.

Epilepsy

Epilepsy is a condition in which disturbance of the cerebral cortex produces convulsive movements which may be accompanied by loss of consciousness and loss of control over the sphincters of the bladder and bowel. The epileptic fit may be a symptom of some cerebral lesion or of a toxic condition, as in acute infections and poisoning, or of a metabolic disorder such as uraemia or hypoglycaemia, or may be due to cerebral anoxia, as in heart block. The term symptomatic epilepsy is applied to fits due to such causes. Idiopathic epilepsy is a condition in which fits occur at intervals without any known organic lesion; abnormal electrical discharges in the brain can be demonstrated by encephalography, but the precipitating factor which causes the seizure is unknown.

The two main types of idiopathic epilepsy are described as major epilepsy or 'grand mal' and minor epilepsy or 'petit mal'. The condition is commonly manifested in childhood: if the first seizure occurs in adult life this suggests that it is symptomatic rather than idiopathic epilepsy.

Major epilepsy or grand mal, is characterized by convulsive movements involving the whole body, unconsciousness and often incontinence. The attack proceeds through definite recognizable stages; the first is the warning, or aura, a sensation which the patient recognizes as the precursor of the fit. It may be flashes of light, noises, epigastric discomfort or giddiness. He then falls to the ground unconscious and rigid, his face is congested and his teeth clenched. This is known as the tonic stage of the fit, and lasts about 30 sec. It is followed by the clonic stage, in which involuntary contractions and relaxations of the muscles produce the typical convulsive state. Saliva collects in the mouth, the tongue is alternately protruded and retracted and may be bitten, in which case the foam that forms around the patient's mouth will be bloodstained. This clonic stage lasts about 2 to 3 min as a rule, and during it incontinence of urine and sometimes of faeces may occur. Following the clonic stage the patient is relaxed and unconscious for a short period, and this may be followed by sleep. On waking he may have a headache or a slight degree of mental confusion, but otherwise appears to have recovered completely. Occasionally however, a dangerous condition known as status epilepticus supervenes, the patient passes from coma into another convulsion and one fit rapidly follows another. Unless this sequence can be interrupted the patient may die from exhaustion.

Minor epilepsy or petit mal, is a condition in which there are brief lapses from consciousness but no convulsions. The patient may fall down, but immediately begins to get to his feet again, he may stop talking in the middle of a sentence or drop any article that he happens to be holding. These attacks may occur with great frequency and may be associated with major epileptic fits.

Following both major and minor epilepsy there may be a period of mental disturbance during which the patient has complete loss of memory, or may show automatic behaviour, committing actions of which he afterwards has no recollection. Sometimes these actions are antisocial and will get him into trouble; for example he may attack another person for no apparent reason, or remove his clothes in the street. Because of the possibility of such behaviour and also because the patient may harm himself, he should be kept under observation following a fit and should be in the care of some responsible person.

Treatment

During the fit no treatment is required beyond protecting the patient from harm, unless status epilepticus follows. He need not be moved unless he is in a position of danger, such as near a fire, and no attempt should be made to restrain the convulsive movements. When the clonic stage begins a gag may be inserted into his mouth to prevent him from biting his tongue; for this purpose a piece of wood, or the handle of a spoon with a handkerchief wrapped round it, can be used. However if the jaw has become clenched nothing is to be gained by trying to force it open to insert a gag. Any tight clothing such as a collar or waistband should be loosened. If he is sleepy after the fit he should be allowed to rest.

Status epilepticus requires immediate treatment in hospital to interrupt the fits. Phenobarbitone or paraldehyde may be given intramuscularly, or thiopentone sodium (Pentothal) intravenously.

Accurate observation of the patient during the attack will help to establish its cause. Points to note are whether the convulsive movements involve the whole body from the onset, or whether they begin in one group of muscles, such as those of one arm, and spread from that area, whether consciousness is lost and whether incontinence occurs. The duration of the fit should be recorded and also whether a definite sequence of events such as is described under major epilepsy was noted.

Information regarding past attacks or any form of illness should be sought. Bearing in mind that a diabetic patient may be found in a hypoglycaemic state with coma and convulsions, it is worthwhile looking in the patient's pockets or handbag for a card stating that he is a diabetic and giving useful particulars such as instructions for emergency treatment, his name and address and the doctor's address.

General Management of Epilepsy

Epileptic patients require medical treatment and supervision for many years, often for their entire lifetime; the patient who discontinues treatment without the sanction of his doctor is in danger of developing status epilepticus. Regular administration of anticonvulsant drugs is the main line of treatment; examples of such drugs in general use are sodium phenytoin (Epanutin), phenobarbitone, primidone (Mysoline) and troxidone (Tridione).

In addition to such specific treatment the patient's life must be so organized that any factors likely to provoke a fit are avoided as far as possible and he is not exposed to situations which would be dangerous should he have a fit. Over-exertion, excitement and competitive pursuits should not be allowed, alcohol is forbidden, meals must be regular and not excessive in amount, although no special diet is required. The general health should be maintained; any source of infection, such as septic teeth or tonsils, will require treatment.

Steady employment, an interest in social activities and some suitable physical exercise, such as walking and dancing, are all part of the general management of the epileptic patient. The more his daily life conforms to that of normal people the lower the incidence of fits. Some occupations and activities are obviously dangerous and should be prohibited, for example work which involves being near fire, water or machinery, where a fall might cause injury, driving a motor-car or riding a bicycle. Some epileptics have fits at night; a low bedstead and no pillows, or one small firm pillow, should be advised in order to avoid injury from falling out of bed or suffocation by soft pillows.

Children can as a rule benefit by normal attendance at school, but in some cases mental subnormality or behaviour problems make it necessary for a child to be admitted to a special school or institution. Frequent epileptic fits may result in mental deterioration, and a small proportion of such patients require care in a psychiatric hospital.

Convulsions in Infancy

Convulsions in infants and young children may be due to the same causes as those occurring in later life, i.e. injury or disease of the brain and, as has been already mentioned, true epileptic attacks usually begin in childhood. Since, however, the nervous system tends to be somewhat readily disturbed in the early years of life, it is not uncommon for the onset of an acute infection or even a minor ailment to be accompanied by a convulsion.

In every case full medical examination is necessary in order to establish the cause of the fit. The treatment during the attack is to keep the infant quiet and warm in his cot, keeping his head turned to one side so that saliva runs out of his mouth and the airway is kept clear. The mother involved will need reassurance as fits in children are a frightening occurrence.

Paralysis Agitans

Paralysis agitans or Parkinson's disease, is a condition in which nerve cells in the collections of grey matter in the base of the brain known as the basal ganglia, degenerate and there is a partial loss of the ability to control and co-ordinate movement. This disorder is manifested by tremor, particularly affecting the hands and the head, muscle weakness, rigidity, slowing of some movements, a lack of facial expression described as the 'Parkinsonian mask' and a peculiar propulsive type of gait. The patient bends forwards and once he has started he moves with quickening steps, looking as if running to catch up with himself (festinating gait).

The disease occurs in elderly persons and is progressive, but relief of symptoms may be obtained by the administration of atropine, belladonna, hyoscine or one of the newer synthetic drugs, of which Artane is an example. Combinations of two or more drugs are commonly used. Some patients may be treated by destroying the globus pallidus or the ventral portion of the thalamus through which pass all the fibres from the globus pallidus. This destruction can be done by the injection of a chemical or by passing an electric current (stereotaxy) through the area. Recently similar destruction has been achieved by the use of hypersonic waves. This form of treatment is most effective if carried out early and if symptoms are confined to one side of the body.

General care of the patient is directed towards encouraging him to pursue as active a life as possible, while protecting him from stress, over-exertion or exposure to infection. His mental powers are not as a rule affected, but he may be very conscious of his altered appearance and his limited physical ability and therefore in need of continual sympathetic understanding as well as encouragement, if he is not to withdraw from all social interests and contacts.

Parkinsonism may also be a sequel to a type of epidemic encephalitis known as encephalitis lethargica, but in this case it is often accompanied by mental disturbance. Encephalitis lethargica is now a rare disease in this country, but epidemics occurred in the years from 1918 to 1930 and there is still a small group of patients who were attacked by the disease during those years, whose condition has never improved. Sporadic cases are occasionally seen.

Chorea

Chorea is a condition in which jerky involuntary movements, restlessness and often emotional instability are the main features. In severe cases the movements are continuous and sleeplessness and exhaustion may lead to death.

The commonest type is Sydenham's chorea, which is associated with streptococcal allergy, and is described under the rheumatic group of diseases (p. 208).

Other forms of chorea are hereditary, or due to degenerative changes in the brain; both these types are associated with mental disorder and the patients are likely to require care and treatment in a psychiatric hospital.

Cerebral Palsy

Cerebral palsy is a disease which is usually due to a congenital defect in the development of the cerebral cortex, but may be caused by intra-uterine disease or to injury during the process of birth. The most obvious symptoms are difficulty in carrying out co-ordinated movements, combined with stiffness and rigidity of the muscles, the typical picture of the 'spastic child'.

The degree of disability varies greatly, but in a number of such patients movements are limited and difficult. The gait is clumsy, stumbling and slow, the speech is often unintelligible because the child cannot co-ordinate the muscles necessary to form words; because he cannot use his swallowing muscles properly he dribbles saliva and food. In some cases there is associated subnormal mentality, in others the child is well up to average intelligence or even above it, but his physical disabilities which may also include hearing and visual defects, make it difficult for him to benefit by the normal school education.

Treatment

Treatment is aimed at developing the physical and mental potentialities of each child to the greatest possible degree. Physiotherapy to educate the control of muscles and to prevent deformities, orthopaedic treatment to correct deformities and speech training should begin as soon as possible. Assessment of the child's mental ability is carried out in order to decide how far he can benefit by a normal educational programme and what type of school he should attend. Parents will need to play a large part in the care and education of the spastic child, and should be brought in from the beginning as active members of the team with the doctor, physiotherapist, educational psychologist and teachers. Improvement may be very considerable as the patient reaches adolescence, and there is always room for hope. Some spastic children may have to spend their lives in a special institution, but a considerable number grow up to enjoy a useful if limited life, and to earn their own living in congenial employment.

Disseminated (Multiple) Sclerosis

Disseminated sclerosis is a disease whose cause is at present unknown, in which degeneration occurs of the myelin sheath of some nerves of the brain and spinal cord. The disease is usually first evident in early adult life, but many years may elapse before the patient is severely disabled. Remissions are common and may last for long periods; but the disease is progressive and at present there is no known cure.

The early manifestations of disseminated sclerosis are often transient, and vary depending on the site of the lesions; they include:

(1) Double vision or misty vision. These are often early signs as the optic nerve is frequently one of the first to be attacked.

(2) Sensations of numbness or tingling in a limb.

(3) Dragging of one foot, or clumsiness in carrying out fine movements of the hand, or loss of power in one arm.

(4) Weakened control of the bladder, with urgent micturition and slight incontinence.

As the disease progresses and more nerve fibres are affected disabilities increase, and the patient becomes more and more helpless. Co-ordination of muscular activity is impaired with the development of ataxia, intention tremor, nystagmus and staccato speech in which every word in a sentence is equally spaced and emphasized, in some cases speech becomes slurred. Mental changes are often manifested by emotional instability, the patient is easily moved to laughter or tears, and may develop a state of euphoria, a feeling of elation with little or no insight into his true condition.

The duration of the disease may be any period from 2 to 20 years from the onset, but eventually spastic paralysis develops and the patient becomes helpless, bedridden and incontinent. The actual cause of death is usually pneumonia or urinary infection.

Treatment

Treatment aims at maintaining activity as long as possible and the patient is encouraged to remain at work, provided that the type of work is not too strenuous and adequate rest periods can be assured. During an acute phase rest in bed will be necessary, but otherwise every effort is made to keep the patient mobile. Where there is loss of muscle power and inco-ordination, physiotherapy with re-educative exercises may be ordered. When spastic paralysis finally proves incapacitating he will require all the nursing attention that is essential for any paraplegic patient.

Pressure sores can develop very rapidly, probably due to the vasomotor paralysis affecting the superficial blood vessels and thus also affecting the nutrition of the skin. The patient should be nursed on a sheepskin pad or an air bed. A bed cradle will prevent pressure of the bedclothes on the feet, and pads and pillows will be needed to relieve pressure on various areas such as the ankles, knees and shoulders. If available, an alternating pressure pad (Ripple bed) may be a useful device; it is made of plastic and contains a series of air tubes. It is connected to an electric motor which works an air pump; when the motor is switched on, alternate sets of air tubes are inflated and deflated. The use of this apparatus, together with regular 2-hourly turning of the patient and also lifting him for a few moments every hour so that his back and shoulders are raised from the mattress, will do much to prevent the development of pressure sores. All areas subject to pressure should be treated at 4-hourly intervals, or more often if redness or discoloration of the skin develops, by gentle washing and drying to promote the circulation.

Whenever the patient is found to be wet or soiled the skin must be thoroughly washed, carefully dried and protected by an application of zinc and castor oil cream, or a silicone barrier cream. Damp or soiled bed linen and gown must be replaced by clean dry sheets and gown. At least two nurses will be required to turn or lift the patient for bedmaking and washing, in order to ensure that he is moved without dragging, as the skin is very easily damaged by the slightest roughness in handling.

If in spite of all care a pressure sore develops in the terminal stages of the illness, every effort should be made to prevent it from extending; large sloughing sores readily occur in the paraplegic patient and can be a contributory cause of death. A small break in the skin may be covered with Whitehead's varnish or an adhesive dressing; large sores must be dressed with the aseptic precautions required in dressing any wound. Short wave treatment by the physiotherapist may be ordered.

An enema or a rectal suppository on alternate days will usually prevent faecal incontinence. Urinary incontinence is often associated with retention of urine and is an overflow from a distended bladder. This distension can be detected by feeling the swelling of the distended bladder above the pubes, gentle pressure over the suprapubic area may help to empty the bladder more effectively. Catheterization may be needed, but if performed frequently almost inevitably leads to urinary tract infection. If all bladder control is lost continuous drainage is often needed. A suitable type of indwelling catheter for bladder drainage is a long fine polythene tubing, e.g. Gibbon's catheter (Fig. 33), which is introduced into the bladder with full aseptic precautions, Foley's self-retaining catheter is another type that may be used. The free end of the tube drains into a sterile receptacle containing antiseptic lotion or into a disposable plastic bag. A spigot may be kept in the open end of the catheter which is released periodically, e.g. every 3 hr, this encourages the development of an automatic emptying of the bladder.

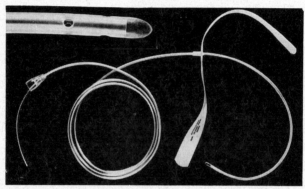

FIG. 33. Gibbon's polyvinyl in-dwelling catheter. Note tip of catheter with three side holes (*inset*); wings of soft material cemented 30 cm (12 in) from the tip of the catheter, which are strapped to the patient's abdomen; and graduated adapter (*left*) which fits the inlet tube of the collecting bag or bottle.

Spasticity of the legs is often accompanied by flexor spasms and contractions, the end result of which may be that the patient is in a permanent position of flexion, his knees and hips flexed on the trunk so that his knees are almost touching his chin. Regular passive movements of the joints will help to prevent contractures; some form of fixation by light splinting or by the use of roller towels placed over the joints held down by sand bags may be used, but the nurse must bear in mind that any form of pressure on the skin can easily cause damage. She should also remember that the skin of the paralysed limbs is insensitive to heat and that therefore hot water bottles or electrically heated pads should never be placed in the bed of a paralysed patient.

Diet should be nutritious and easily digested; very often the patient's appetite remains good until the final phase of his illness.

As the disease is chronic and progressive the nurse should be especially concerned in promoting an atmosphere of comfort and stimulation, so that the patient's life is as full and interesting as possible. In the late stages the mental powers fail, but until this happens some occupation should be provided.

Syringomyelia

Syringomyelia is a disease in which there is degeneration of tissue in the spinal cord and cavity formation. The cause is uncertain, although it is thought that it is probably a developmental abnormality. There is a loss of sensation of heat and pain, but tactile sense may be retained. Muscular atrophy develops particularly in the intrinsic muscles of the hands, but may also be seen in the arms and legs.

The disease is slowly progressive and may last for years and no specific treatment has so far been found. Radiotherapy has proved effective in halting the progress of the disease and relieving pain. The patient should be warned of the danger of burns, particularly on the hands; these can easily occur as he feels no sensation of heat or pain. In the late stages the nursing care of any patient with a spinal cord lesion will be required.

INFECTIVE DISEASES OF THE NERVOUS SYSTEM

Two infectious diseases which attack the nervous system, *meningitis* and *poliomyelitis*, are described in Chapter 14.

Encephalitis

Encephalitis, inflammation of the brain substance, may be a complication of such infections as influenza, mumps and measles and, very occasionally, may follow vaccination for smallpox. Headache, insomnia, possibly delirium alternating with lethargy and coma, are common manifestations. The epidemic form of encephalitis is now rarely seen, but when it does occur the prognosis is grave, as personality changes, with antisocial behaviour, lying, thieving and apparently purposeless cruelty, mental deterioration and Parkinsonism (see p. 263) are possible sequels.

During the acute stage of encephalitis the nursing care and treatment is similar to that of the patient suffering from meningitis. Analgesic drugs such as codeine may be given for the relief of pain, and a hypnotic such as nitrazepam (Mogadon) if the patient is unable to sleep.

Myelitis

Myelitis, inflammation of the spinal cord, may be acute or chronic; in the latter case the cause is frequently syphilitic infection. Acute myelitis is occasionally a complication of an infection such as typhoid fever or influenza; it may also result from tuberculous disease of the vertebral column, or injuries or tumours of the spinal cord. Acute widespread infection is usually fatal. Transverse myelitis, affecting one section of the spinal cord, has a more hopeful prognosis, and if due to syphilis or tuberculosis may give a good response to appropriate chemotherapy, if caused by injury or a new growth surgical treatment may be successful.

Careful and skilled nursing is necessary, and as in other lesions of the spinal cord every effort must be made to prevent pressure sores, urinary infection and pneumonia.

Neurosyphilis

Neurosyphilis may cause a chronic type of meningitis, myelitis or the formation of gummata which when occurring in the brain produce symptoms of a cerebral tumour. These manifestations of tertiary syphilis usually respond to antisyphilitic drugs. Forms of neurosyphilis which occur late in life and many years after the primary infection are tabes dorsalis, affecting the spinal cord, and dementia paralytica, where the lesions are in the brain.

Tabes Dorsalis

Tabes dorsalis (locomotor ataxy) is characterized by disorders of sensation resulting from lesions of the posterior columns and posterior nerve roots of the spinal cord, usually beginning in the dorsolumbar area. The disease is commoner in men than in woman; the patient is usually middle-aged, although the condition occasionally occurs in children as a result of congenital syphilis.

The symptoms that precede the more disabling manifestations of loss of muscle sense and ataxia, are acute transient pains in the legs, which the patient may ascribe to rheumatism, sensations of a tight constricting band around the waist and attacks of visceral pain known as 'crises', for example acute abdominal pain with vomiting, or renal pain which resembles renal colic. He may show some unsteadiness in walking and if in the dark, or when his eyes are shut, he sways and may fall. As the ataxic symptoms develop he will walk on a broad base, he lifts his feet well into the air with each step and brings them down to the ground with a stamping movement. He loses sense of the position of his limbs in space and has to keep his eyes on his feet and the ground as he walks. He may say that he feels as if he is walking on cottonwool. Bladder control is often lost or diminished, with consequent danger of urinary infection. Sensation of pain, heat and touch may be affected, but not as a rule to the same degree as muscle sense.

Trophic changes affecting the skin cause perforating ulcers, most commonly on the sole of the foot, trophic changes in the joint (Charcot's joints) cause a condition similar to osteoarthritis with gross swelling and effusion. Sight and hearing may be impaired. Examination of the eyes shows that the pupils react to accommodation for near objects, but not to light, (Argyll-Robertson pupil); ptosis, or drooping of the eyelids, is commonly present.

As the disease progresses the ataxic symptoms become more marked and the patient correspondingly more helpless. Eventually he is bedridden, incontinent, paralysed and likely to succumb to some intercurrent infection such as pneumonia or urinary infection.

Treatment

The treatment for this, as for other forms of syphilis, is a course of penicillin, or if the patient is sensitive to penicillin one of the tetracyclines may be substituted. Analgesic drugs may be needed for the relief of lightning pains and symptomatic treatment, warmth and sometimes morphine or pethidine is required for an abdominal or renal crisis. Physiotherapy may do much to re-educate muscles and to improve the patient's gait and balance.

In the late stages of this disease all the nursing care for a helpless, incontinent, paralysed patient will be required.

Dementia Paralytica

Dementia paralytica is also known as 'general paralysis of the insane' and is characterized by mental deterioration which often requires the patient's admission to a psychiatric hospital. Dementia paralytica may coexist with tabes dorsalis, when the syphilitic changes affect both brain and spinal cord.

The mental changes precede the physical ones and in the early stages may not be obvious to anyone except the patient's relatives and those persons who have known him over a period of years. He becomes forgetful, irresponsible, neglectful of his family, careless in attending to his business affairs and keeping appointments. A more obvious mental symptom is the curious behaviour that the patient exhibits later, known as 'delusions of grandeur'. He is quite sure, in spite of any evidence to the contrary, that he is extremely rich or occupies a very exalted position. When he begins to write cheques for astronomical sums and to sign himself 'Emperor' or 'Julius Caesar' it is very obvious that his mental state is abnormal. Later physical symptoms such as general weakness or paresis of the muscles, epileptiform fits and hemiplegic attacks, urinary and faecal incontinence, make their appearance. When the patient is bedridden, extensive bedsores may develop and an intercurrent infection, as in tabes dorsalis, is often the immediate cause of death.

Treatment

As in tabes dorsalis the treatment is a course of penicillin, which usually results in improvement and may be repeated later.

The mental state, however, may not benefit to the same extent as the physical symptoms, and these patients often require a period of care in a psychiatric hospital.

DISEASES OF PERIPHERAL NERVES

Lesions of the spinal or cranial nerves may be associated with disease or injury of the brain and spinal cord, they may be the result of direct injury to, or pressure on, the nerve tract, or may be attributable to toxic or nutritional disorders.

Neuritis

Neuritis literally means inflammation of a nerve, but the term is generally used to describe pain and impairment of function of a peripheral nerve.

Polyneuritis is a condition in which many nerves are affected at the same time and this can be due to a number of different causes, including infection, as in diphtheritic polyneuritis, poisons (e.g. arsenic, mercury), nutritional and metabolic disorders such as chronic alcoholism, beri-beri, diabetes mellitus and pernicious anaemia. An acute form of infective polyneuritis may closely stimulate poliomyelitis, the onset is sudden with headache, vomiting, backache and pain in the limbs, followed by paralysis affecting all the limbs and sometimes involving the muscles of the trunk, including the respiratory muscles.

The main manifestations of less acute types of polyneuritis are disorders of sensation, tingling, numbness, 'pins and needles', pain and tenderness in the muscles, loss of proprioception, i.e. the sense of the state of tension of muscles and tendons, so that fine movements become difficult, weakness of the muscles which may produce wrist drop or foot drop.

Treatment

In most instances this is mainly treatment of the cause. In acute infective polyneuritis corticosteroids, such as prednisone, may be given. If paralysis is widespread the treatment and nursing care will be similar to that required in poliomyelitis.

Rest in bed is necessary in most cases, with support for the affected limbs and a bedcradle to keep the weight of the bedclothes off the lower limbs and a support such as a footboard or sandbags to prevent foot drop. Analgesics, such as aspirin or codeine, will usually be needed in the acute stage. Passive movements of all joints should be carried out at regular intervals during the day, light splints may be applied at night.

Neuritis affecting individual nerves is usually due to trauma causing pressure on the nerve. Brachial neuritis is usually attributed by the patient to exposure to cold or sitting in a draught, but is often caused by prolapse of a cervical inter-vertebral disc, osteo-arthritis changes or the presence of an extra, 'cervical', rib.

Sciatica, pain in the sciatic nerve of the thigh, is often due to pressure and common causes are bony changes in the lower lumbar and sacral vertebrae, due to arthritis, prolapsed lumbar disc, secondary malignant growths, or new growths in the pelvis causing pressure.

The treatment is directed to removal of the cause if possible. Rest, analgesic drugs and the application of heat will relieve the pain. When the pain subsides massage and passive movements are usually ordered. A supporting collar of plastic material may help in cases of brachial neuritis, and a spinal jacket for a patient with sciatica is often helpful.

Bell's palsy, or facial palsy, is neuritis of the seventh cranial nerve and is due to compression of the nerve in the narrow bony canal through which it passes from the brain. The cause of the swelling of the nerve which leads to its compression is uncertain; it is often attributed to exposure to cold or sitting in a draught. The muscles of the face on the affected side are paralysed.

The patient is unable to close his eye on the affected side, he has difficulty in mastication and food collected between the teeth and the cheek.

In the majority of cases recovery takes place, beginning in 2 to 4 weeks, and is usually complete in a few months. Aspirin may be given in the early stages, the patient's face should be pro-tected from cold; hot applications or infrared treatment may help. A light wire splint covered with rubber in the mouth on the affected side and attached round the ear will prevent over-stretching of the paralysed muscles.

Neuralgia

Neuralgia means pain along a nerve path, the commonest form is trigeminal neuralgia.

Trigeminal neuralgia is an affection of the fifth cranial nerve which is manifested by transient but acute attacks of pain on one side of the face. The skin may also be very sensitive to touch and any slight stimulus such as chewing, exposure to cold, or washing the face may precipitate an attack, the patient may know the exact area of skin which will 'trigger' a spasm of pain. If the attacks are frequent the patient's life is almost unbearable, and adequate sleep is impossible. The condition tends to progress, and the pain may be almost continuous.

Treatment

In the first instance treatment aims at relieving the pain by analgesic drugs and avoidance of precipitating factors if possible. Investigations should be made in case there is a focus of infections, e.g. dental caries, as the pain may be referred to another part of the face and toothache denied. However, these measures are often unsuccessful, and interruption of the nerve fibres by injections of alcohol or by an operation dividing the fibres is then necessary. Although this relieves the pain, the affected side of the face is now insensitive and as this includes the cornea of the eye the patient may need to wear a shield whenever exposure to wind or dust might cause conjunctivitis or corneal ulcer.

Myasthenia Gravis

Myasthenia gravis is a disease of unknown origin which affects the neuromuscular junctions. The muscles become fatigued and unable to respond to nerve stimuli after a short period of exertion. The eye muscles are often the first to be affected and there is drooping of the eyelids and double vision. The muscles of mastication and swallowing are also involved, with consequent inability to chew and swallow food. If the respiratory muscles fail death may ensue.

Treatment

The main drug used to combat myasthenia gravis is neostigmine (Prostigmin), given every 2 or 4 hr by mouth, or if necessary by hypodermic injection. Atropine may be given with neostigmine. The patient's life should be regulated to avoid fatigue and excitement and he should be given an explanation of the condition and the need to take his medicine as ordered and to take adequate rest periods. If respiratory distress occurs, artificial respiration may be needed and the patient should be admitted to hospital, where tracheostomy, suction and a respirator should be readily available.

Thymectomy, removal of the thymus gland, may be considered; some patients, but not all, have considerable remission of symptoms following this operation.

13

Disorders of the endocrine system

THE glands forming the endocrine system secrete hormones, substances which are released into the blood-stream and either stimulate or depress metabolic processes. It is obvious, therefore, that the manifestations of disease of the endocrine organs will be many and varied. Furthermore, there is a close relationship between the various endocrine organs, and the abnormal function of one gland may in turn produce disturbed function in another. This is particularly true of the anterior lobe of the pituitary gland, which produces a number of hormones stimulating the activities of the thyroid, adrenal and sex glands.

The organs comprising the endocrine system are the pituitary, the thyroid, parathyroid and the adrenal glands, and the cells in the pancreas forming the islets of Langerhans. The gonads, the ovaries in the female and the testes in the male, in addition to secreting the germ cells, i.e. the ova and the spermatozoa also secrete hormones which are responsible for producing and maintaining the secondary sex characteristics in the female and the male respectively; disturbances of these glands are not included in this chapter.

DISORDERS OF THE PITUITARY GLAND

The pituitary gland, which lies in the sella turcica, a hollow in the sphenoid bone at the base of the skull, is formed of two sections, the anterior and posterior lobes. The anterior lobe produces a number of hormones of which six have been clearly isolated. It is possible, however, that there are more as an injection of a crude extract of the anterior lobe produces responses not covered by those listed below.

Anterior Lobe

Growth Hormone

This, as its name suggests, controls the rate of growth of the skeleton and the organs of the individual so that they progress in an equal manner. A deficiency in early life will result in a pituitary dwarf, a miniature person, perfectly in proportion and with normal mental capacity but usually underdeveloped sexually. If the condition is diagnosed early enough and the hormone administered, growth may be stimulated. Oversecretion in early life results in a pituitary giant, a person of

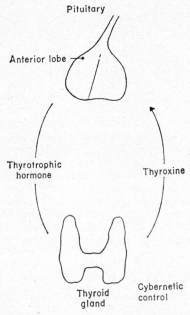

FIG. 34. Cybernetic control of hormones.

excessive height, often 7 ft or over. If however, the oversecretion occurs after the cartilagenous discs at the end of the long bones have become ossified, then the condition of acromegaly results. In this condition the bones grow thicker and this is most clearly seen in the hands which become wide and spade-like and the jaw which juts out due to its increased size. The skin also appears thickened and coarse in texture. Often this condition is due to a pituitary tumour and the patient complains of pressure symptoms, i.e. severe headache and loss of vision of the temporal half of the visual field. Treatment is either surgery or radiotherapy.

Thyrotrophic Hormone (Thyroid Stimulating Hormone)

This influences the growth and development of the cells of the thyroid gland and also the rate at which thyroxine is produced. In turn, it is influenced by the amount of thyroxine in the blood, and called a cybernetic or 'feedback' effect (see Fig. 34). Such a condition is usually treated at the level of the thyroid gland.

Adrenocorticotrophic (ACTH)

This has a similar effect on the suprarenal glands influencing the development of the cortex and its secretion of hormones (except aldosterone). Again treatment tends to be at the level of the suprarenal glands.

Gonadotrophic Hormones

These are two in number and are identical in both sexes. The follicle stimulating hormone (FSH) which causes the development of ova in the ovaries or spermatozoa in the testes, and the luteinizing hormone (LH) which controls the production of the sex hormones oestrogen and progesterone from the ovaries and testosterone from the testes. The presence of these hormones controls the onset of the development of puberty and secondary sexual characteristics and it is at this level that disorder of the gonadotrophic hormone is discovered and treated.

Prolactin

This hormone stimulates the breast to make milk after the child is born.

Simmonds' Disease

This is a condition which is due to destruction of the anterior lobe of the pituitary, usually by an infarct resulting from postpartum haemorrhage, or a tumour. As a result there is underactivity of other endocrine glands, with weakness, loss of weight, amenorrhoea in women patients, atrophy of the external genital organs and loss of hair in the axilla and the pubic area.

There is no available preparation to replace all the pituitary hormones which are lacking, cortisone is the drug commonly used with additional sodium chloride, or fluorohydrocortisone (fludrocortisone) which is a powerful salt retainer. Thyroid hormone in the form of l-thyroxine sodium may be given at the same time. If the disease is due to a tumour, radiotherapy or surgery may be successful.

Posterior Lobe

The posterior lobe of the pituitary gland secretes pitocin (oxytocin) a hormone which stimulates contractions of the uterus and allows milk to be released from the cells in the breast and to pass along the ducts to the nipples, and vasopressin, which causes contraction of involuntary muscles, raises the blood pressure, and also has an anti-diuretic effect.

Diabetes Insipidus

A rare disease in which there is failure in the production of the antidiuretic factor is known as diabetes insipidus. The tubules in the renal tissue are not able to reabsorb water and as much as ten litres of urine of low specific gravity may be passed in 24 hr; as a result of this large loss of fluid the patient has a continual thirst.

The treatment for this is to give vasopressin (Pitressin), the antidiuretic hormone, usually by intramuscular or hypodermic injection. The amount required by the individual patient is determined by trial. Administration of this hormone by mouth is ineffective but it is sometimes given in the form of snuff when it is absorbed from the nasal mucous membrane.

The effect of pituitary enlargement is to produce pressure on the optic chiasma which lies immediately above the gland. Because some of the optic nerve fibres cross only the outer half of the object can be seen. Continual pressure leads to blindness.

DISORDERS OF THE THYROID GLAND

The thyroid gland stores iodine in the form of thyroxine and this substance, which is released into the blood-stream under the control of the thyrotrophic hormone of the pituitary gland, profoundly affects the metabolic processes which convert food into new body cells and into energy. In childhood thyroxine is therefore one of the factors influencing growth and maturation. The main features of disorders of the thyroid gland will be a slowing down of metabolic processes if secretion of thyroxine fails, or a speeding up if too much is released. The defect may be in the production of the thyrotrophic hormone in the anterior lobe of the pituitary gland rather than primarily a disease of the thyroid gland. Two tests of thyroid function are: (1) the estimation of the basal metabolic rate, and (2) a test of the ability of the gland to take up iodine.

Basal Metabolic Rate (BMR)

At complete physical and mental rest a healthy individual consumes a definite volume of oxygen per minute, the actual amount depending mainly on the sex, age, height and weight.

During the test the patient lies quietly on a bed and breathes through wide rubber tubes into a special apparatus which records the respirations over a measured period of time, usually 6 min.

From the recordings so made the volume of oxygen used by the patient can be measured. This is compared with the volume used by a normal subject of the same sex, age, height and weight.

The BMR is considered normal if the figure obtained is within −10 to +15 per cent of the value predicted for the individual in question.

In a well-marked case of hyperthyroidism, a rise of 50 per cent or more may be observed; on the other hand, when the thyroid activity is diminishing, very low values for the BMR are usual.

Success in obtaining reliable results depends almost entirely on the patient being perfectly quiet and at ease; he must go without breakfast and should relax completely for about half an hour before the test is begun. This must be achieved without fuss about the test itself. In order to allay apprehension, the simple nature of the procedure and its object should be explained or, better still, demonstrated beforehand.

Radioactive Iodine

A tracer dose of radioactive iodine (^{131}I) is given orally or occasionally intravenously, and the amount of 'take up' or concentration of the radioactive material by the thyroid

gland is recorded by a Geiger counter sited over the thyroid
area.

The results of the test may be invalidated if the patient is
given radiological contrast media, food containing iodine, e.g.
fish, onions, watercress, thyroid preparations, perchlorates or
thiocyanates or radioactive isotopes. Some of these preparations may affect the result of the test even if a considerable time
elapses between their discontinuation and the test, as for
example Lugol's iodine and contrast media; it is therefore
advisable to have an interval of 4 weeks if at all possible before
carrying out the test.

Hyperthyroidism

Hyperthyroidism, also known as toxic goitre or Graves's
disease, is the condition in which the thyroid gland is over-
active and usually, though not always, enlarged. The metabolic
rate is increased, and the patient, while retaining a good
appetite, progressively loses weight. Toxic goitre is more
common in women than in men: the cause of the disease is not
known; sudden emotional shock or long periods of anxiety and
stress are thought to be predisposing factors in some cases.

Other manifestations of hypersecretion are seen mainly in the
cardiovascular and the nervous systems. The pulse is persistently rapid even when the patient is at rest, and a proportion of
these patients develop auricular fibrillation. The nervous
symptoms are emotional instability and irritability and a fine
tremor of the hands. A warm, sweating skin, protruding eyes
(exophthalmos), and retraction of the eyelids which gives the
patient a staring appearance, are also characteristic features
(Figs 35 and 36).

Treatment

Treatment aims at diminishing thyroid activity. This may be
attained by the administration of drugs, or, particularly in young
patients, by surgical treatment, removing the major portion of
the gland. Control of the symptoms by drugs precedes operative
treatment.

The anti-thyroid drugs are propylthiouracil, carbimazole
(Neo-Mercazole) and potassium perchlorate. If surgical
treatment is contemplated iodine in the form of potassium

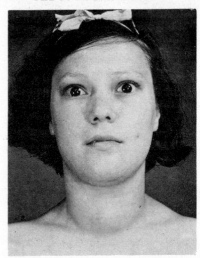

FIG. 35. A case of exophthalmic goitre, showing slight swelling in the neck, and also protrusion of the eyeballs and retraction of the lids.

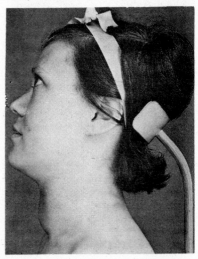

FIG. 36. Exophthalmic goitre. Side view of the same case as is shown in Fig. 35.

iodide or Lugol's iodine, is given for 10 to 14 days before operation, because it decreases the vascularity of the thyroid gland and temporarily controls the hyperthyroidism.

Treatment with radioactive iodine (^{131}I) gives good results, but owing to the technical difficulties in handling radioactive isotopes and the safety precautions needed, this treatment is only available at certain centres. The dose of radioactive iodine is given by mouth, and when it is absorbed into the circulation it is quickly taken up in the thyroid gland, where it will destroy the cells that concentrate it. The treatment of women patients with radioactive iodine is usually confined to those who have passed the reproductive period of life.

In addition to the specific treatment outlined above, the patient needs rest, a diet which has a high calorie and protein value and contains all the vitamins. Sedatives, such as pheno-barbitone 30 mg ($\frac{1}{2}$ gr.) twice daily, are often ordered. As the patient usually feels hot whatever the atmospheric temperature, a cool, well-ventilated room is desirable; if the patient is in a general ward the bed should not be near a fire or radiator. Bed-clothes should be light, and the patient will not as a rule like to have more than one blanket, or in some cases a sheet and light counterpane only will be appreciated. Mental rest is also needed and although visitors should not be excluded, they should be asked to make their visits short, not to talk about domestic problems or events of a worrying nature and to arrange to come to the hospital one at a time and not all on the same day.

The response to treatment is usually satisfactory, but occasionally complications occur. The development of auricular fibrillation or signs of congestive cardiac failure, such as breathlessness and oedema, requires treatment with quinidine or digitalis. Marked exophthalmos, with inability to close the eyes properly, is likely to produce conjunctivitis and possibly corneal ulcers. Therefore in these cases the eyes should be protected by an eye shield; sometimes stitching the eyelids together is necessary.

A 'thyroid crisis' is now rarely seen, but when it does occur it is an extremely serious condition. The patient's temperature rises to hyperpyrexial levels, 41° to 42°C (105° to 106°F), with a very rapid pulse rate, restlessness and delirium. Treatment must be started immediately if it is to be successful. Every means should be taken to reduce the temperature, e.g. by removing all clothing, by cold sponging (see p. 14) and the use of an electric fan. Drugs which may be ordered are chlorpromazine, Lugol's iodine and corticosteroids, such as hydrocortisone or ACTH (corticotrophin).

Simple (Non-Toxic) Goitre

Simple goitre is a condition in which the thyroid gland enlarges (Figs 37 and 38), but there are often no symptoms of either under- or over-secretion of thyroxine, although such symptoms may develop after middle age. It is common in areas far

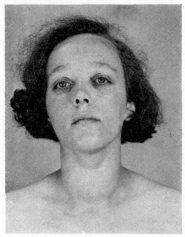

FIG. 37. A case of simple goitre, showing slight swelling in the neck only; front view.

removed from the sea, which is the source of all iodine, and where little sea food is obtainable and the soil contains no iodine. The Peak District in England and the Alpine valleys in Switzerland are examples of places where goitre was at one time endemic. The condition can be prevented by adding minute amounts of iodine to the diet, usually in the form of iodized table salt; as little as one part of iodine to 100 000 parts of salt is all that is required.

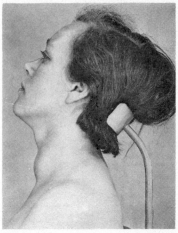

FIG. 38. Simple goitre. Side view of the same case as is shown in Fig. 37.

A large goitre may cause pressure on the trachea and oeso-phagus and may require surgical treatment, or the patient may ask to have an operation on account of the disfiguring appear-ance of the swelling. Enlargement without symptoms of hyperthyroidism is occasionally due to carcinoma of the thyroid gland. The treatment of this condition is either surgical or by radiotherapy, particularly radioactive iodine if the tumour is found to concentrate this from the blood-stream.

Hypothyroidism

Hypothyroidism, or insufficient secretion of thyroxine, may develop in adult life or may be a congenital condition. When the symptoms first appear in the adult the condition is known as *myxoedema*. The patient is usually a woman and usually middle-aged. In contrast to the picture shown by the patient with an over-active thyroid gland, the myxoedematous patient feels the cold and becomes physically and mentally inactive. There is no loss of weight, and the patient may in fact gain weight, although the intake of food is not increased. The term myxoedema describes a type of swelling which resembles oedema but which does not put on pressure. It is due to excessive deposits of mucin in the skin and subcutaneous tissue. The swelling is particularly noticeable as puffy eyelids and a thickening of the tissues of the face. The skin is dry, and the hair becomes coarse, brittle and falls out.

Treatment

In this case the treatment is to supply what the patient lacks, namely thyroxine. For many years the standard preparation has been dried thyroid gland extract, and these tablets are still frequently prescribed. The pure hormone is now available as L-thyroxine sodium (Eltroxin) tablets, 0·1 mg of which is approximately equivalent to 60 mg of the dried thyroid extract. Small doses are given at first, and gradually increased until the symptoms of myxoedema disappear; then the dose is adjusted to the optimum maintenance dose necessary in the individual case.

A special problem associated with this condition is that of hypothermia. Some elderly people with a degree of myxoedema become so inactive that they neglect to eat or keep a fire alight in the house. As the environmental temperature falls, so does the body temperature. The individuals become drowsy and eventually unconscious behaving in much the same way as a hibernating animal. They are frequently found curled up with an indetectable pulse and a temperature so low that it does not register on a normal thermometer. Such people may be thought to be dead. However, it is possible to detect electrical activity of the heart and brain. Treatment consists of very gradual warming of the patient and administration of hormones.

The infant who is born with a defective thyroid gland is known as a cretin. He begins to show symptoms of the condition shortly after birth; he is lethargic, not showing any signs of hunger, seldom moving in his cot or crying. Without treatment his growth is mentally and physically retarded and if he survives the hazards of childhood and liability to infections his eventual state is that of a mentally subnormal dwarf. However, as in myxoedema, supplying the missing hormone is the key to treatment although some permanent mental retardation is usual unless the hypothyroidism is diagnosed very early.

Autoimmune Thyroiditis

Autoimmune thyroiditis is a condition in which the patient is producing antibodies which are harmful to his own thyroxin-producing cells. The thyroid gland in these cases becomes enlarged, nodular and tender. The patient is most commonly a woman of menopausal age and she complains of aching pains in the limbs, that she is always cold and that her hair is falling out. Lymphocytic deposits and fibrosis of the gland lead to a state of myxoedema. The treatment is, therefore, the administration of appropriate dosage of L-thyroxin sodium.

Malignant Disease of the Thyroid Gland

Malignant disease of the thyroid gland is usually a primary carcinoma which may produce secondary deposits, or metastases, in the bones. Radioactive iodine may be used in the treatment of this condition, or alternatively a combination of surgery and radiotherapy.

DISORDERS OF THE PARATHYROID GLANDS, AND TETANY

The four small parathyroid glands lie very close to the thyroid gland, usually resting against its posterior surface, sometimes included within the capsule of the thyroid, but their function is entirely separate. The parathyroid glands control the level of calcium in the blood serum. Hypersecretion causes excessive release of calcium from the bones into the blood-stream, and hyperparathyroidism is one cause of renal calculi. Loss of calcium in the bones may be revealed by X-ray examination, or spontaneous fractures may occur. The commonest cause of over-activity is a parathyroid tumour, and the treatment is surgical.

Under-activity of the parathyroid glands results in a lowering of the level of calcium in the blood, and the chief manifestation of this is tetany, a condition of muscular spasms and cramp. Spasm of the hands with flexion at the wrist and at the metacarpal phalangeal joint and extension at the phalangeal joints, accompanied by acute flexion of the ankle joints, is character-

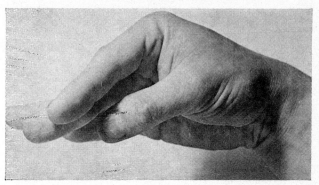

FIG. 39. Tetany: the typical position of the hand, produced by muscle spasm.

istic of tetany and is known as carpopedal spasm (Fig. 39). In children carpopedal spasm, convulsions and spasm of the larynx (laryngismus stridulus) often occur together. Hypoparathyroidism seldom occurs as a primary condition; it is more often a sequel to thyroidectomy, when the parathyroid glands, which are sometimes buried in the thyroid tissue, have had their blood supply damaged, or been inadvertently removed, or following an operation for removal of a parathyroid tumour.

Since other factors are concerned in the maintenance of the serum calcium, tetany can occur without any abnormality of the parathyroid glands. The calcium intake may be insufficient or vitamin D, which is necessary for the absorption of calcium, may be deficient. Before the role of vitamin D in calcium metabolism was known, rickets was a very common condition, and tetany in children was most often due to rickets, now a very rare cause of the condition. Deficient absorption of vitamin D, and therefore of calcium, also occurs in steatorrhoea and similar conditions, referred to under 'the malabsorption syndrome' (p. 152).

Another cause of tetany is alkalosis, which can result from the continued vomiting of acid gastric juice, from taking excessive quantities of alkalies, or overbreathing, which lowers the carbonic acid in the blood; this latter condition is sometimes a hysterical manifestation.

Treatment

Where the symptoms are due to lowered blood calcium the immediate treatment is to give intravenous injections of calcium gluconate. A parathyroid hormone preparation is available but is seldom used. Maintenance doses of vitamin D will usually be required, in addition to ensuring that this substance is also adequately present in the diet. Milk and milk products are good sources of both calcium and vitamin D.

Laboratory tests which are likely to be required are estimation of the blood calcium, phosphorus and alkaline phosphatase, and calcium balance estimation. The latter test involves a weighed and analysed diet which is prepared by the dietitian, the substitution of distilled water for tap water for drinking, cooking and mouth washing and the separate collecting of all urine and faeces for laboratory examination during the period of the test. Full instructions for this somewhat complicated test will be issued by the laboratory and dietetic department and must be carefully followed.

DISORDERS OF THE ADRENAL GLANDS

The adrenal glands, which are two small bodies lying over the upper pole of each kidney, are in fact two glands in one. The outer layer of cells or cortex, produces at least three types of steroid hormones. One group influences the retention of water, sodium and chloride and the loss of potassium from the body. A synthetic preparation, deoxycorticosterone acetate (DOCA), has the same effect as the naturally occurring steroid, which is known as aldosterone. A second group, the cortisone hormones, are concerned in the metabolism of proteins and carbohydrates, the production of glycogen and its storage in the liver. Thirdly, the adrenal cortex produces hormones influencing the development of the sex characteristics at puberty and sexual activity. Stimulation of the adrenal cortex is brought about by the adrenocorticotrophic hormone (ACTH) secreted by the anterior lobe of the pituitary gland. In general it can be said that the adrenal cortex regulates and maintains the essential chemical functions of the body and protects the tissues in times of abnormal conditions of stress. The medical use of cortical hormones in a wide variety of disorders and in grave emergencies is based on this conception of the conserving and defensive role of the cortex, enabling the body cells to gain time in which to combat the crisis and to benefit by whatever specific treatment is appropriate.

The inner part of the adrenal glands, the medulla, secretes the hormones adrenaline and noradrenaline, which are closely associated in their action with activity of the sympathetic nervous system; indeed in the embryo they develop from the same group of cells. These hormones are liberated immediately there is a call for extra energy to meet some urgent danger or a situation which excites such emotions as fear, anger or excitement. Their effect is to contract the superficial vessels and increase the heart rate, thus raising the blood pressure and the blood supply to the muscles, the brain and the lungs. Respiration quickens, so that more oxygen is obtained, the liver releases its stores of glycogen so that more fuel is available for muscular activity. Bearing in mind, therefore, the extremely complicated and important functions of these two distinct groups of cells in the adrenal glands, their connection with the activity of the sympathetic nervous system and with the anterior pituitary gland, it is not surprising that disorders of their function can produce a wide variety of symptoms.

The two most distinctive syndromes, or groups of symptoms, resulting from disease of the cortex of the adrenal glands are Addison's disease and Cushing's syndrome.

Addison's Disease

Addison's disease is described as 'adrenocortical insufficiency' and results from atrophy of both adrenal glands; this is in some cases caused by tuberculous infection, in others the cause is unknown. The main features of this condition are weakness, often accompanied by feelings of giddiness, fainting attacks, loss of appetite, diarrhoea and vomiting. On investigation the patient is found to have a low blood pressure (hypotension) and various changes in the blood chemistry, including a low fasting blood sugar level and disturbances of the electrolyte balance of the blood plasma, in particular a lack of sodium. Sudden exacerbations of the symptoms may occur, with vomiting, dehydration and collapse; unless treatment is promptly available the patient may die. These attacks are known as Addisonian crises.

Treatment

The treatment of Addison's disease is much more hopeful than it was in days when little was known of the adrenal hormones and their functions, since it is now possible to correct the insufficiency by the administration of corticosteroids. Cortisone or hydrocortisone is given daily; the maintenance dose required will need to be assessed in each case. Some patients will also need supplementary administration of salt and water-retaining hormone, usually given in the form of fludrocortisone given by mouth. Additional salt with food or as sodium chloride tablets may be ordered, particularly in a hot climate where salt is freely excreted in sweating. If an adrenal crisis occurs, hydrocortisone is given intravenously. Immediate treatment of the severe collapse which accompanies the crisis includes keeping the patient lying flat with the foot of the bed raised on high blocks, plasma and saline infusions and the injection of vasopressor drugs such as noradrenaline (Levophed).

Although the patient can feel well and remain well once he has regained his lost weight, appetite and energy, his disease is only controlled by hormone therapy and he needs to lead a somewhat protected life. His diet should contain plenty of protein and carbohydrate, small frequent meals are best, and long periods of fasting are harmful. As far as possible exposure to infection should be avoided and the patient is advised to call his doctor at once if he does contract any infection, however mild.

Cushing's Syndrome

Cushing's syndrome results from over-activity of the adrenal cortex, which may be caused by an overgrowth of cortical cell sometimes stimulated by increased pituitary activity or by a tumour. The main features of this condition, which is more common in women than in men, are obesity, amenorrhoea, growth of hair on the face and coarsening of the skin, with the development of acne. Accumulation of fat is mainly seen in the face and trunk; the limbs are often thin. Although the patient gains weight, at the same time muscle weakness and wasting occur; inability to keep the spine erect produces a hump-backed deformity, kyphosis (Fig. 40). Diabetes with

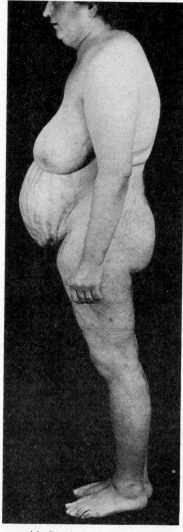

FIG. 40. A woman with Cushing's syndrome, showing shortening of the trunk due to collapse of the vertebrae, flabby abdomen accentuated by lumbar lordosis and wasted buttocks.

raised blood sugar and glycosuria is a common feature of this disease.

Treatment

Treatment may be surgical—even if both adrenal glands are affected, since replacement therapy by the administration of corticosteroids can be given successfully—or medical, by irradiation to the pituitary gland.

DISORDERS OF THE PANCREATIC HORMONE

The pancreatic hormone, insulin, is produced by the cells of the islets of Langerhans in the pancreas. Insulin has the function of regulating the level of sugar (glucose) in the blood within narrow limits. The condition associated with failure of this function is diabetes mellitus.

Diabetes Mellitus

Diabetes mellitus is caused by failure of insulin action, either as a result of deficient production of insulin by the islet β cells of the pancreas or by resistance to its action. Thus diabetes is a syndrome which can result, for example, from destruction of the pancreas or from resistance to its action as a consequence of other endocrine disturbances such as is seen in Cushing's syndrome. In the majority of cases, however, diabetes mellitus is a disease in which the exact role of deficient insulin production on the one hand and resistance to its action on the other hand, are at present obscure. Failure to secrete or to use insulin results in an inadequate metabolism of glucose and fat, which leads to excess glucose in the blood (hyperglycaemia), and also to an increased production of ketone bodies (and products of inadequately metabolized fat) which are acidic and by their accumulation in the blood produce acidosis. Both glucose and ketones will be excreted in the urine; therefore the first diagnostic tests required in a suspected case of diabetes are examination of the urine (see p. 189) and of the blood. These tests may be followed by a glucose tolerance test.

Estimation of the blood sugar. The blood specimen for the test should be obtained in the early morning before food is taken. The blood is collected into a small test tube which contains a special preservative mixture of sodium fluoride and thymol.

The great majority of normal fasting blood sugar values will be between 80 to 120 mg of glucose per 100 ml of blood. Almost without exception values of 130 mg or over are found only in those cases where a diabetic curve is found when the glucose tolerance test is done (Fig. 41). Low values are found after large doses of insulin have been given or in the rare condition of hyperinsulinism. Where repeated observations are needed during the adjustment of diet and insulin dosage, all specimens of blood must be collected at the same time of day in relation to meals and insulin administration.

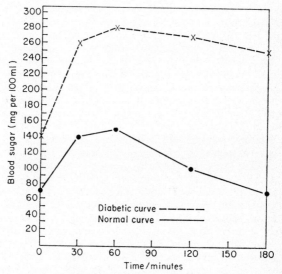

FIG. 41. Blood sugar curve.

Glucose tolerance test. If possible the test should be carried out in the morning before food has been taken, and smoking should be forbidden. Before the first sample of blood is taken the patient should empty the bladder and a specimen of this urine is saved in a bottle marked 'A'.

A known quantity of glucose solution, usually 50 g of glucose in 100 ml of water for an adult, is given by mouth, and five more samples of blood are taken at ½-hourly intervals. The patient must empty the bladder 1 and 2 hr after the administration of the glucose solution. These two specimens are placed in bottles marked 'B' and 'C'.

The normal result of a large dose of sugar is a rise in the first hour, and a return to the fasting level in 2 hr. The maximum reading should not exceed 180 mg per 100 ml of blood, and no glucose should be present in any of the urine specimens.

In the diabetic patient the initial blood sugar level may be normal or raised; the level rises above 180 mg after the administration of glucose and remains above the fasting level for more than 2 hr. In most cases the first urine specimen does not contain glucose, but this appears in the later specimens.

In a few cases the renal threshold for sugar is lower than normal, while it is rare in these instances to find glucose in the first specimen it will appear in the second specimen of urine although the blood sugar remains within the normal range. This has no pathological significance and no other signs of diabetes are present. Hypersecretion of the thyroid gland and disturbance of the pituitary gland are occasional causes of abnormal results in this test.

The main features of diabetes are polyuria (passing of excessive amounts of urine), causing dehydration and consequent thirst, loss of weight, lack of energy, genital pruritis from the irritating effect of glycosuria. In children the onset is often acute and the symptoms are severe; in the adult the onset is often insidious and sometimes relatively symptomless, the condition being discovered during the course of a routine medical examination. Attention may be drawn to the diabetic condition as a result of the appearance of one of the many complications that can occur. Boils or carbuncles may sometimes occur, as resistance to pyogenic infection is lowered; recurring infections may be particularly troublesome if due to antibiotic-resistant strains of staphylococci. Other complications are diabetic cataract and retinopathy (i.e. damage to the retina of the eye caused by haemorrhages), pulmonary tuberculosis and peripheral neuritis. Where the disease has been present over a long period, vascular changes in the kidneys occur with proteinuria and oedema and in the peripheral and coronary blood vessels leading to gangrene of the toes and ischaemic heart disease.

Hyperglycaemic (diabetic) coma is due to excessive ketone bodies affecting the brain cells and may be an initial manifestation of diabetes of acute onset, especially if this is accompanied by an acute infection or the administration of a general anaesthetic to a patient who is not known to be a diabetic. It is seen more commonly in a known diabetic patient who for some reason has not had his usual insulin dosage, or who falls victim to an acute infection. In the pre-coma stage the warning signs are thirst, nausea abdominal pain or discomfort, constipation and vomiting. The patient, if untreated, gradually becomes, drowsy and eventually lapses into unconsciousness, with deep 'acidotic' respirations, low blood pressure and a rapid pulse rate. Signs of dehydration quickly appear, with a dry tongue, dry skin and low intra-ocular tension, the eyes feel flaccid if gentle pressure is exerted on the closed eyelids. The sweetish smell of acetone can often be detected in the patient's breath.

Hypoglycaemic coma is due to an inadequate level of glucose in the blood. It is usually the result of the patient having a dose of insulin and not following it by a meal. Onset is rapid, the patient may appear disorientated, possibly mistaken as drunk, and quickly becomes unconscious. Respirations and pulse remain normal or raised. There are no signs of dehydration and the skin remains moist to touch.

Treatment

Treatment can be considered under three main headings.

(1) Control of the diabetic state by diet and insulin or anti-diabetic drugs.

(2) Treatment of complications.

(3) Education of the diabetic to maintain control of his diabetes and to avoid complications.

(1) Control of the Diabetic State

Aim of treatment is first of all achievement and maintenance of a satisfactory body weight and ability to carry out normal activities by controlling the bio-chemical inbalance. Secondly, it is important to prevent complications. The patient is recommended to take a diet which has a restricted carbohydrate intake to reduce glycosuria and avoid ketosis. This diet is varied according to the weight of the patient and his occupation.

Having determined the number of joules required to maintain weight and the amount of carbohydrate to abolish ketosis, then the amount of insulin which will metabolize this amount of carbohydrate is determined, and given by hypodermic injection.

Blood sugar estimations and frequent testing of the urine for ketones and glucose are therefore important factors in determining the dosage. In the stabilizing stage the urine is usually tested three times a day before the main meals, later once daily is as a rule sufficient.

Various types of insulin are available; the more recent of these are the result of a search for insulin which will exert an even control over carbohydrate metabolism over a reasonably long period in order to avoid sudden changes in the blood sugar level and the inconvenience of frequent injections.

Soluble, or regular, insulin is the type which first became available for the treatment of diabetes in 1922 as a result of the work of Banting and Best in Canada. It is quick-acting, reaching its maximum effect in 2 to 3 hr, but then rapidly decreases in activity. It is therefore useful in an emergency such as ketosis or threatened diabetic coma, and also may be given with the longer-acting types of insulin in order to cover the blood sugar rise following the first meal of the day.

The long-acting insulins have the advantage of exerting their effect over 24 hr or longer and one injection in the morning is all that is needed in most cases. Examples of long or intermediate acting insulin are the insulin zinc suspensions prepared in three forms, semi-lente (IZS amorphous), lente (IZS) and ultra-lente (IZS crystalline); of these semi-lente has the shortest period of action and ultra-lente the longest. Other insulin preparations in use are globin zinc insulin and isophane. Protamine zinc insulin has a very long action, and is often combined with soluble insulin.

Insulin is measured in units; the standard preparations are 'single strength', 1 ml containing 20 units; 'double strength', 1 ml containing 40 units; and 'quadruple strength', 1 ml containing 80 units.

Insulin, or hypoglycaemic, reactions occur if an overdose of insulin is given or if the maximal effect of the insulin injection is reached at a time when the carbohydrate intake is at its lowest, i.e. at night if the last meal has not contained sufficient carbohydrate, or if for some reason the patient has not taken a meal, or if he has undertaken some unexpected strenuous exertion. The manifestations of the condition are sweating, hunger, weakness, irritability, quick pulse, tremor, dizziness. These symptoms are quickly relieved by taking sugar or glucose, but unless treatment is prompt the patient may develop convulsions and become unconscious. Should this condition ensue, intravenous infusion of glucose 50 per cent solution will be needed, and an injection of 0·5 ml of 1:1000 adrenaline solution may be given.

If the patient is in hospital the signs of hypoglycaemia should be easily detected, and the condition dealt with before it becomes serious. In fact a mild hypoglycaemic state may be deliberately induced while the patient is in hospital so that he will in future be able to recognize the onset of symptoms. If he is an out-patient he must be warned to have lumps of sugar or glucose sweets always with him and to take some at once if he feels hungry, weak or dizzy.

Some middle-aged or elderly and overweight patients with mild diabetes become free from symptoms on a reducing, carbohydrate restricted diet and do not need insulin. If, however, the condition is not completely controlled by diet alone, one of the oral antidiabetic drugs may be given. The fact that daily injections are not needed is an obvious advantage, particularly if an elderly patient, possibly disabled by arthritis or blind, cannot give his own injections. Two preparations of the sulphonylurea group of drugs are tolbutamide (Rastinon) and chlorpropamide (Diabinese). These drugs are chemically similar to the sulphonamides, but have no antibacterial effect: it is thought that they act by stimulating the islet β pancreatic cells to produce more insulin.

(2) Treatment of Complications

The complication which calls for the most urgent treatment is coma. Hyperglycaemic coma is treated by the administration intravenously of fluid, electrolytes and eventually glucose. Soluble insulin is also administered intravenously at regular intervals initially of 1 to 2 hr. A catheter specimen of urine is required for examination, and the catheter may be left in the bladder so that specimens can be obtained every hour. Blood samples are taken for laboratory examination before treatment commences and at hourly intervals to check the level of glucose in the blood. When the patient recovers consciousness small amounts of fluids, glucose drinks and milk are given. A light diet with a relatively high carbohydrate content is often ordered for 2 or 3 days following recovery from coma.

Pyogenic infections will usually require treatment with anti-biotics, and the tendency to such infections lessens when the diabetes is controlled. Where degenerative changes have taken place in the peripheral blood vessels, special care of the feet is necessary, as gangrene of the toes is always a danger. Such patients should be told to avoid the risk of trivial injuries such as may occur in cutting toe nails or corns, and should have their feet attended to by a chiropodist. After washing the feet should be dried carefully; very hot water should not be used, particu-larly if the feet are cold. Hot water bottles are also inadvisable; woollen bedsocks are safer. Wool stockings or socks are best for day-time wear, and should never be too tight-fitting; the same caution applies to shoes.

Eye complications require the attention of the ophthalmic surgeon; diabetic cataract can be treated surgically, but there is little that can be done to improve diabetic disease of the retina. Peripheral neuritis and pulmonary tuberculosis associated with diabetes will receive treatment on the usual lines for these diseases.

(3) Education of the Diabetic Patient

Education of the diabetic patient begins while he is in hospital when he learns from the nurse how to give his own injections of insulin and to test his urine, and from the dietitian how to manage his diet. The best type of syringe for the patient's own use is the syringe which is graduated in units. Although the graduations are intended for single strength insulin this is seldom used, but it is an easy matter to explain how many units to draw up with either double or quadruple insulin. Each division representing one unit of single strength insulin will represent 2 units of double strength or 4 units of quadruple strength insulin. The patient should also be familiar with the standard system of coloured labels on the insulin phials, buff for single strength, blue for double and green for quadruple strength. He should be shown how to clean the top of the phial, insert the needle and draw up the dose; also how to clean, sterilize and care for his syringe.

The use of 'disposable' syringes has made life less complicated for many patients just as urine testing has been made simple for the patient by the introduction of test tablets and test sticks (see p. 190). He should carry out the tests a few times under the supervision of the nurse before he leaves hospital. He will be told by his doctor how often he is expected to test his own urine and what to do should he find a positive glucose reaction.

The dietitian explains to the patient how to use the skeleton diet sheets, what substitutions are allowed, and what exchanges can be made in the distribution of carbohydrates should he be instructed by his doctor to take a larger proportion of the starch and sugar foods at any particular time of the day. Usually he will need to weigh all his food for a time but when he learns to judge amounts fairly accurately some weighing may be omitted. When he is at work he may have to have a midday meal out and it is very helpful if he has learnt to know the value of average helpings and what foods to select.

A diabetic diet is often a more expensive way of eating than the normal meals of many families, where the cheaper, starchy foods provide most energy requirements, particularly where children are concerned. If the nurse has any reason to believe that home circumstances may make it difficult for the diabetic patient to follow his prescribed diet, the help of the social worker should be sought in securing some assistance for him.

The importance of carrying sugar at all times has already been mentioned. All diabetic patients should also carry a card stating their name, address, doctor's name and address, their usual dose of insulin, and also a note on the treatment for an overdose of insulin. A diabetic patient who develops an acute infection such as influenza or a gastro-intestinal upset should be told to call in his doctor without delay.

Child patients are particularly liable to become 'unbalanced', and insulin reactions or diabetic coma may occur with very little warning. If these dangers are explained, and the ways of avoiding or treating them should they occur, there is usually no reason why a diabetic child cannot attend school and join in the normal activities of his age group. As soon as possible the child should become independent and be able to give his own insulin injections and manage his own diet. Co-operation of the parents and their understanding of the condition is essential;

they should also be taught how to give insulin injections and to test urine.

Diets for the Diabetic Patient

Specimen diets for the diabetic patient are shown on the following pages. Weights of food are as eaten unless otherwise stated and the amounts of carbohydrate, protein and fat are given in grams.

The first diet is arranged for an intake of 10 500 joules (2500 Calories) with one injection of Lente Insulin before breakfast. The second is a restricted carbohydrate diet to be used only on doctor's orders.

With the skeleton diet sheets the patient is given a list of alternative foods which can be exchanged for one or more items in any meal, provided that the full quantity of the alternative is eaten and the directions followed as to any adjustment needed in any other component of the meal. For example, 28 g (1 oz) of white bread equals 15 g of carbohydrate, 21 g (¾ oz) of un-cooked oatmeal and also equals 15 g of carbohydrate. Therefore if the patient wished, he could replace 28 g of bread at breakfast by porridge made with 21 g of oatmeal. One medium sized potato also equals 15 g of carbohydrate; 15 g of carbohydrate is called 'one carbohydrate exchange' (written 1 Ch ex.) and in the skeleton diet sheet each helping of a carbohydrate food is given its exchange value. Many diabetic patients are allowed a free choice of protein foods.

Diabetic Diet 10 500 joules (2500 Calories). Total weights for each meal are shown in bold.

	Carbo-hydrate	Protein *(grams)*	Fat
Breakfast	**44·0**	**22·5**	**25**
14 g (½ oz) cornflakes	12·5	0·5	—
2 eggs	—	14	14
42 g (1½ oz) bread	24	3	—
7 g (¼ oz) butter	—	—	6
150 ml (5 fl oz) milk, for tea and cereal	7·5	5	5
½ grapefruit, if liked	—	—	—
Mid-morning	**20**	**6**	**18**
120 ml (4 fl oz) milk for coffee	6	4	4
2 water biscuits (18 g)	14	2	2
14 g (½ oz) butter	—	—	12
Lunch	**68·5**	**30**	**20**
85 g (3 oz) lean meat	—	21	15
226 g (8 oz) potatoes	40	4	—
Green vegetables as liked	—	—	—
Banana custard			
7 g (¼ oz) custard powder	6	—	—
150 ml (5 fl oz) milk	7·5	5	5
85 g (3 oz) banana	15	—	—
Afternoon tea	**54**	**10**	**22**
85 g (3 oz) bread	48	6	—
21 g (¾ oz) butter	—	—	18
Salad, paste or marmite if liked	—	—	—
120 ml (4 fl oz) milk for tea	6	4	4
Supper	**50**	**19**	**32**
56 g (2 oz) cheese	—	14	20
Salad	—	—	—
70 g (2½ oz) bread	40	5	—
14 g (½ oz) butter	—	—	12
1 orange (141 g, with skin)	10	—	—
Bed-time	**14**	**7**	**6·5**
180 ml (6 fl oz) milk	9	6	6
7 g (¼ oz) Ovaltine	5	1	0·5
Daily total	250.5	94.5	123.5

10 466 joules (2492 Calories).

Diabetic Diet 4200 joules (1000 Calories). Total weights for each meal are shown in bold.

	Carbo-hydrate	Protein (*grams*)	Fat
Breakfast	**15·0**	**11·4**	**13·5**
Tea or coffee	—	—	—
Milk, fresh, skimmed, 90 ml (3 fl oz)	4·2	3·0	0·3
Bread, 18 g (⅔ Ch ex.)	10·8	1·6	0·2
Butter, 7 g (¼ oz)	—	—	6
1 egg, *or* alternative from list	—	6·8	7·0
Mid-morning			
Drink of diabetic fruit squash or Marmite, Oxo or Bovril	—	—	—
Lunch	**15·6**	**21·2**	**18·6**
Lean meat, 56 g (2 oz)	—	14	10
Carrots, 170 g (6 oz) (½ Ch ex.)	7·2	1·2	—
Green vegetables, a liberal helping	—	—	—
Margarine, 9 g (⅓ oz)	—	—	—
Milk, fresh, skimmed, 180 ml (6 fl oz)	8·4	6·0	0·6
Tea	**15·0**	**4·6**	**6·5**
Tea	—	—	—
Milk, fresh, skimmed, 90 ml (3 fl oz)	4·2	3·0	0·3
Bread, 18 g (⅔ oz) (⅔ Ch ex.)	10·8	1·6	0·2
Butter, 7 g (¼ oz)	—	—	6
Salad when available	—	—	—
Supper	**15·0**	**18·6**	**20·5**
Cheese, Cheddar type, 56 g (2 oz)	—	14	20
Bread, 18 g (⅔ oz) (⅔ Ch ex.)	10·8	1·6	0·2
Milk, fresh, skimmed, 90 ml (3 fl oz) in tea or coffee	4·2	3·0	0·3
Salad when available	—	—	—
Bed-time			
Drink as mid-morning	—	—	—
Daily total	**60.6**	**55.8**	**59.1**

14

Infectious diseases

THIS chapter deals with some of the commoner infectious diseases in this country. Many of them have, happily, now ceased to be the menace to life and health that they were a few decades ago, but it would be most unwise to assume that they could never again become so if the measures necessary for their control were relaxed.

Two important infective diseases, tuberculosis and syphilis, are mentioned in this chapter, but some of their manifestations will more appropriately be described in other sections of the text. Many diseases due to bacteria, viruses and protozoa are major health problems in tropical countries, but these, for the most part, are outside the scope of this book, and for information about them the nurse should consult an appropriate textbook of tropical nursing.

In describing the course of the common infectious fevers, the following terms may be used:

The incubation period. This is the period that elapses between the time of infection and the onset of symptoms. This period varies according to the disease and even for one specific disease it is rarely constant; for example, as will be seen in the table below, it may be between 2 and 7 days in scarlet fever, while in mumps the incubation period, though rarely less than 18 days, may be as long as 24 days.

Incubation Periods of Specific Fevers

One week

Diphtheria	1 to 4 days
Influenza	2 to 4 days
Scarlet fever	2 to 7 days

Two weeks:

Whooping cough	7 to 10 days
Typhoid fever	10 to 14 days usually (extreme limits 7 to 21 days)

Measles	10 to 14 days
Chickenpox	14 to 16 days
Smallpox	7 to 16 days (usually 12 days)

Three weeks:

| German measles | 18 to 21 days |
| Mumps | 18 to 24 days |

The prodromal period. This is the period between the onset of symptoms and the appearance of the typical signs of the specific fever, such as the rash, and it is usually during this period that the patient is most infectious. Again this varies considerably in different fevers; for example in measles the rash appears on the fourth day of the illness; in German measles the rash is often the first sign of the infection, so that there is virtually no prodromal period.

The fastigium. This is the period during which the illness is at its height.

Defervescence. This means that the acute symptoms are subsiding and the temperature is returning to normal levels.

Nursing Care in Infectious Diseases

When nursing a patient who has an infectious disease the nurse has a two-fold responsibility: the care of the patient and the prevention of spread of the infection.

Prevention of Spread of Infection

The danger of spreading the infection to other patients or to members of the hospital staff is not the same in all diseases; it depends on the route by which the particular micro-organism gains entry to the body and also on the type and virulence of the organism and the immunity of the population. Therefore, if the organism is present in the alimentary tract, as in typhoid fever and dysentery, infection can be spread only by contamination of hands or articles by excreta or vomit. In such cases the patient may be nursed in a ward with other patients if the necessary precautions are taken; this practice is termed bed isolation or 'barrier nursing'. If, however, the disease is airborne, as is the case with such infections as whooping cough, measles and smallpox, then the patient should be completely isolated from others who are not infected and nursed in a single room or in a cubicle. In most isolation units, and also in paediatric wards, the partition walls of cubicles are made of glass for ease of observation by the nursing staff; these partitions should extend to the ceiling if isolation is to be effective.

If the carrying out of the necessary precautions against the spread of infection is to be effective, attention at all times to all the details of the appropriate techniques is essential. Due allowance must be made when planning for the care of the patient for the fact that nursing treatments will take a longer time than would be required were the complicating factor of infection not present. The use of disposable articles such as paper towels, masks, handkerchiefs, and of disposable 'incontinent' pads and infant's napkins, provided facilities are available for the prompt burning of used material, is an aid in the prevention of cross-infection, and can also save the nurse's time.

The following rules for the prevention of spread of infection should be observed:

Rules for Isolation Nursing

Masks

Masks are usually worn for isolation nursing in order to protect those attending the patient. They are also frequently worn by the nurse while she is attending to surgical dressings, spinal or thoracic punctures, obstetric deliveries, and when looking after premature babies to protect the patient. One mask should be worn for attending to one patient only, or for a maximum period of 30 min, or 20 min if it is a disposable mask. Should the mask become wet due to the nurse coughing or sneezing it should be discarded immediately as a wet mask is no longer impermeable.

A mask which is worn incorrectly is more dangerous to the nurse than if one is not worn at all. Because of this some hospitals do not use masks except in areas such as the operating theatre.

Gowns

Gowns must be worn for the same procedure as masks with the addition of maternity nursing. The following rules must be observed:

(1) In open wards the gowns are kept inside the screens on pegs beside the bed.

(2) In cubicles or isolation rooms the gowns are kept in the rooms.

Only the contaminated outer surface of the gown should be handled when removing it, care being taken that the hands do not touch the inside. The inside is regarded as being clean and for hanging must be folded inward. The word 'inside' may be marked in red on the inside of the collar band as a reminder of the importance of this point.

Hands

The hands are scrupulously washed with soap and running water, before donning the gown and after removal of it, and before any other object is touched. Hands should be washed thoroughly before preparing or giving drinks, meals or infants' bottle feeds and before examining a patient; also after attending to the patient, dealing with excreta, changing napkins, handling used crockery or soiled linen, cleaning or dusting the room or collecting specimens, and after examining a patient.

Many hospitals are now using a soap containing hexachlorophane in wards and departments because of its effectiveness against Gram-positive cocci, and pHisoHex cream in the theatres.

Screens

Screens are regarded as clean and must be handled only with clean hands. In bed isolation, glass screens may be kept around the patient's bed, and when he is receiving attention ordinary screens are set up outside the glass ones.

If curtains are used round beds these should be touched only with clean hands.

Utensils

Utensils are treated according to their composition and use:

(1) All used crockery and cutlery are boiled in a special sterilizer in the kitchen.

(2) Washing bowls are kept separate from others when bed isolation is being carried out, and in the room or cubicle for isolation patients, and must receive terminal disinfection.

(3) Bedpans and urinals should, if possible, be disposable. If not they are boiled in a special sterilizer after use or are kept separate in all isolation techniques. When heat disinfection is not possible they should be placed in a disinfectant solution after sluicing, and then rinsed before use. One of the cresol disinfectants, such as Jeyes' Fluid, 1:80, is suitable for this purpose.

Disposal of Excreta

Stools, urine, discharges and vomit from infectious patients are mixed with lysol 1:20 and left for 1 hr.

Sputum should be collected in waxed disposable cartons with lids. When used these are placed in a strong paper bag which is sealed and then burnt in a closed incinerator.

Infected Linen

The following rules apply to all isolation techniques:

(1) Unsoiled linen is sent in bags to the laundry for disinfection and laundering.

(2) Soiled linen is placed in dry pails with lids, which are brought to the bedside, and covered. Pails are taken to a tank containing one of the white fluid disinfectants, e.g. lysol strength 1:160 (i.e. 7 g to 1 litre), in which they are placed for 12 to 24 hr. Sometimes a tank on wheels is provided and this can be taken to the bedside. The tank is then transferred to the laundry intact; alternatively, lysol 1:40 may be used for 2 hr soaking, but this is more extravagant. In other cases special plastic bags are provided into which the linen is put and it is then disinfected in a similar manner in the laundry.

(3) Paper handkerchiefs which can be burnt are ideal and these, after use, should be placed in destructible paper bags and not under pillows or in pockets. If linen ones are used these should be kept in a bowl at the bedside, soaked in disinfectant (white fluid 1:80, or chloroxylenol 1:80) when soiled, and sent to the laundry for boiling.

(4) Napkins should be discarded into a sanitary bin containing white disinfectant, strength 1:160, in the ward, and dealt with in the laundry.

(5) Face masks should be discarded into a bowl of chloroxylenol solution, strength 1:80, Milton, strength 1:80, or a similar disinfectant, washed, boiled, ironed and autoclaved, or discarded and burnt if paper.

Bedding

The following rules should be observed for all infected bedding:

(1) Blankets, mattresses and pillows are sent to the steam disinfector or autoclave after use. They are disinfected by steam at 105·8°C (228°F) with 2·25 kg pressure for 30 min.

(2) Mackintoshes or waterproof sheets, air rings and rubber mattresses are soaked in lysol 1:20, Roccal 1:10 or cetrimede 1:20 (5 per cent), for 2 hr, and are then scrubbed with soap and water and dried. Oxygen tents are treated in the same way, and are aired after drying.

Books and Toys

Books and toys either should be cheap so that they may be destroyed after use, or they should be capable of being washed and disinfected. They should be tied to the bed or cot so that they do not fall on the floor—which, as a rule, is grossly contaminated. Washable toys, belonging to the ward, are best for hospital use. Pencils and crayons should not be passed from child to child and should, therefore, be reserved for older children who can understand the order not to lend them to others.

Floors

Floors contaminated with infected material should be disinfected with a white disinfectant, such as lysol, strength 1:10, with a mop and pail.

Terminal Disinfection

The following rules are applied:

(1) Thermometers are placed in phenol 1:80 or Roxenol or Roccal 1:40 for 1 hr.

(2) Stethoscopes are mopped with phenol 1:20 or Roxenol or Roccal 1:10, and are then washed with soap and water.

(3) Lockers, bedsteads and other furniture are scrubbed with soap and water after first being mopped with phenol 1:20 or cetrimide 1:100 or Savlon 1:200. (Mopping is done only to remove extraneous debris; it does not disinfect. Scrubbing and washing with soap and water ensures thorough cleansing, which is the most important part of disinfection.)

(4) Disposable oxygen masks should be used.

(5) The cubicles and contents are sometimes subjected to a special spraying process with formalin or other bactericide and left for 12 to 24 hr. If the room and its contents are dirty, they should be washed with cetrimide 1:20 solution.

Measles (Morbilli)

Measles is a highly infectious disease, which occurs in epidemics and is caused by a virus. It is especially prevalent in the late winter and early spring months, January to March. In infants and young children it is a serious disease because of its liability to produce chest complications; in older children and adults complete recovery and lasting immunity is the rule. Immunity can be given by injections (see p. 38).

Measles is spread mainly by droplet infection from person to person, but infected toys, clothing or other articles may play some part. The incubation period is usually 10 or 11 days. The disease is most infectious in the prodromal stage (i.e. the period between the onset of illness and the appearance of the rash) although infectivity remains for about one week after this. The initial symptoms are fever, the temperature rising to about 38·3°C (101°F), upper respiratory catarrh with watery discharge from the eyes and nose, sore throat, sneezing, coughing, and possibly laryngitis. Conjuctivitis is often especially marked at a later stage of the illness. The nervous system is hypersensitive, and a miserable, crying child, with a strong dislike of light (photophobia), is the typical picture of this disease.

On the second and third days the fever tends to subside somewhat and typical spots in the mouth, known as Kiplik's spots, may be apparent. These should be looked for on the mucous surface of the cheek in a line with the upper or lower molar teeth and show as white spots surrounded by an area of hyperaemia; the presence of these spots is diagnostic. On the fourth day the temperature again shoots up, and the respiratory signs increase as the rash appears (Fig. 42). This is a dusky red, maculo-papular eruption, which can be first seen at the margin of the hair and behind the ears. It spreads, involving the whole

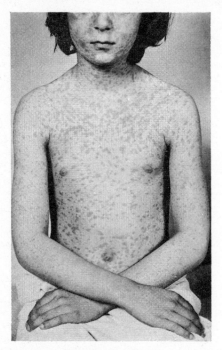

Fig. 42. Measles.

body, including the face; the blotchy rash on the face, together with the conjunctivitis, gives the patient a characteristic bloated, bleary-eyed appearance. The rash tends to appear in crescent-shaped groups, and once it is fully out the fever and other symptoms, including the rash begin to subside. The temperature returns to normal in about 6 days, or less in a mild attack. A fine, branny peeling follows.

Treatment

The patient must be nursed in bed while febrile, he should be kept warm and guarded against draughts, but ventilation must be adequate. One of the sulphonamide drugs or penicillin may be given to prevent infective complications in the lungs, ear or other sites; alternatively it may be withheld until the first sign of any such complication appears. The mouth and lips must be kept clean and moist. Conjunctivitis may be severe and require frequent irrigation of the eyes and treatment by systemic antibiotics.

If laryngitis or bronchitis threatens, or is present, the patient is propped up in bed with pillows and is encouraged to spit out any sputum, but with very young children this is often difficult, as they more frequently swallow it. A steam kettle and tent may be used to moisten the air. Tracheostomy (see p. 324) may be needed for acute respiratory obstruction resulting from inflammation of the larynx.

The commonest serious complication of measles is bronchopneumonia and, apart from the liability of this disease to be fatal in young children, it can produce fibrosis of the lung with the later development of bronchiectasis. Immediate and adequate chemotherapy is therefore important both as a means of saving life and preventing future disablement. In infants enteritis sometimes occurs with bronchopneumonia and increases the gravity of the situation. Encephalitis is a much less common complication, but it can be fatal and can produce residual defects such as spasticity, speech defects and retarded mentality.

As with other febrile conditions, fluids should be given freely and as nutritious a diet as can be taken. Complan, a proprietary food containing all the essential food factors and additional predigested protein, is often useful. Good feeding, appropriate to the patient's age, is important during convalescence from measles as the child's resistance to other infections is lowered by the disease.

German Measles (Rubella)

German measles is a mild fever caused by a virus; it is distinguished from true measles by its longer incubation period, by the earlier appearance of the rash (it is the first sign of the disease), and the absence of the definite respiratory symptoms. The rash consists of raised pinkish papules; it somewhat resembles the measles rash but is less blotchy. The incubation period is 2 to 3 weeks and the period of infectivity is probably from the onset of symptoms to the disappearance of the rash. There is slight fever for two or three days. Enlargement of the glands of the neck is characteristic and helps in the diagnosis. Complications are not likely to occur and no special nursing treatment is necessary. Infection is spread before the rash appears, so that isolation is now considered useless. In adults there may be aching in the joints.

Pregnant women, if exposed to this infection, should be protected by the injection of gamma-globulin, as there is a risk in the early months of pregnancy that the toxins may affect the foetus and cause congenital defects such as blindness, deafness, heart malformations and mental subnormality (see also p. 38).

Chickenpox (Varicella)

Chickenpox is a highly infectious but mild disease due to a virus akin to the virus of herpes zoster. The incubation period is about 17 days. The patient is infectious for about 6 days after the onset of the illness, but if pustular crusts form infection may remain until these have separated. The disease is characterized by a rash which is the first sign. There is usually slight fever, about 37·7°C (100°F) which soon subsides. The rash is first papular and then becomes vesicular; it appears first on the trunk, and then spreads to the limbs (Fig. 43). Pustules may form and occasionally permanent scarring, 'pitting', results. This rash appears in crops, therefore papules and vesicles are seen at the same time. There are no complications as a rule and no special treatment is needed. As previously mentioned, its chief importance lies in the danger of its confusion with smallpox, but in chickenpox the spots are mainly found on the trunk, are never umbilicated and are of varied types at the same time. Scratching the spots is likely to lead to secondary infection and subsequent scars and this should be prevented by allaying the irritation, for example by the use of carbolized petroleum jelly or an antihistamine drug, such as promethazine (Phener-

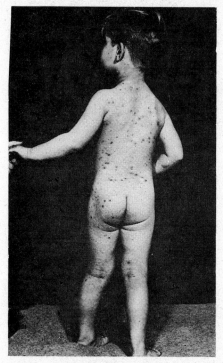

Fig. 43. Chickenpox.

gan) may be given by mouth. If sepsis occurs an antibiotic drug may be ordered.

Smallpox (Variola)

Smallpox is a highly infectious disease due to a virus. A recent statement by the World Health Organisation indicates that it has almost been eradicated as a result of preventive vaccination. However sporadic cases or small epidemics are liable to occur anywhere in the world if infection into an otherwise protected area is carried by travellers. If those protected by vaccination do contract the disease it is in a much less severe form so that a mild case of smallpox can be mistaken for chickenpox. For this reason if smallpox should occur in a district it then becomes usual to notify also cases of chickenpox.

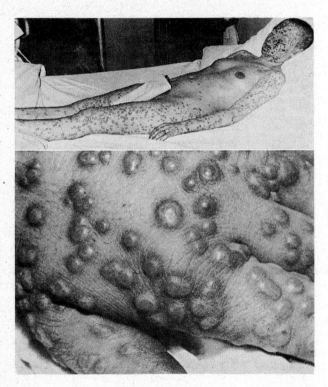

FIG. 44. Smallpox.

The incubation period is usually 12 days but may be as long as 14 days. The period of infectivity extends from just before the onset of symptoms until the last crusts have separated from the skin. Quarantine measures may be enforced for a period of 16 days; more commonly contacts are vaccinated, or revaccinated and kept under observation, and children are excluded from school. The infection is transmitted by droplets or dust carried in the air, the virus has been shown to withstand drying for long periods. The onset of the disease is acute, with fever, intense headache and backache, sore throat, often vomiting and prostration. The rash appears from 2 to 4 days after the initial symptoms, but a transient erythema over the lower abdomen, the 'bathing pants area', may appear during the prodromal period. The true rash of smallpox is at first papular, the spots being red, raised, and hard, often described as 'shotty'. It is present in greatest profusion on the face and the limbs; the trunk may be affected but to a lesser degree (Fig. 44). Mucous membranes, particularly of the mouth and fauces, are usually involved. At this stage the temperature falls several degrees and may reach normal; the patient then feels better. Later, vesicles or small blisters develop. These vesicles tend to become depressed at the apex and are described as 'umbilicated'. At about the end of the first week the vesicles become pustular and a further rise of temperature occurs, the typical secondary fever of smallpox. The eruption may remain as separate spots (discrete), or these may become massed and run together (confluent) later. Haemorrhage may occur into the vesicles (haemorrhagic rash) in very severe cases. The rash gradually subsides, becomes dry, and scabs form which later scale off. A peculiar odour is given off from the skin and acute irritation always occurs. With the fading of the rash the general signs of illness decrease. If the pustules have penetrated to the true skin, permanent scarring results, the 'pitting' which used to disfigure so many victims of smallpox. Haemorrhagic cases are generally fatal even before the pustular stage.

Treatment

Strict isolation is necessary to prevent the spread of infection. Treatment is not specific, but consists of general nursing and hygienic care as already laid down for fevers. Fluids and soft solids are given liberally; if vomiting is troublesome intravenous fluids may be necessary. The intense irritation can be allayed by swabbing the skin with a soothing antiseptic lotion, e.g. 1 per cent potassium permanganate solution or applying compresses of this solution. The unpleasant odour from the skin can be lessened by the use of deodorants such as sodium hypochlorite solution. When crusts are forming frequent permanganate baths may be given and petroleum jelly applied to the lesions. The mouth must be cleansed frequently, and, if conjunctivitis is present the eyes are bathed regularly and paroleine or other oily drops instilled. Delirium may be present in severe cases, and sedatives such as barbiturates will be ordered.

Chemotherapy is used to combat the secondary infection which is responsible for skin sepsis, septicaemia and pneumonia, and treatment is usually started on the fourth day of the illness. In most cases penicillin is successful, but if resistant organisms are present some other suitable antibiotic will be used.

Mumps (Epidemic Parotitis)

Mumps is a virus infection which affects the salivary glands, most commonly the parotid glands, but it may also cause inflammation of the testes, ovaries and pancreas.

The incubation period is usually 18 to 21 days and the infectious period lasts from the first appearance of symptoms until the swelling has disappeared. Usually both parotid glands are infected, but one only may be and occasionally the other salivary glands are involved. There is some rise of temperature at the onset, the patient does not feel well and vomiting may occur. There is considerable pain and swelling at the side of the face and difficulty in opening the mouth, mastication and swallowing are painful. Rarely suppuration occurs, but usually the swelling subsides in the course of 1 or 2 weeks.

The patient is kept in bed for the first week. Heat in the form of kaolin poultices may be applied to relieve the pain if necessary and hot mouth-washes given frequently are comforting. Until the swelling has subsided the diet will consist of fluids and soft, easily swallowed foods, and it is well to remember that appetizing dishes and acid fruit drinks by stimulating salivary secretion add considerably to the pain. For the patient who cannot open his mouth, sucking through a drinking straw is helpful. Inflammation of the pancreas, ovaries or testes if it occurs usually subsides without specific treatment. Analgesics are ordered where necessary for the relief of pain. Supporting the scrotum with a suspensory bandage or other form of support gives relief in orchitis.

Meningo-encephalitis is a rarer manifestation which may be suspected if the patient complains of severe headache, this usually responds to treatment with analgesics and repeated lumbar puncture.

Mumps is highly infectious and owing to its long incubation period, is difficult to get rid of in communities of children, such as schools; therefore, those who have been in contact with the infection should endeavour to avoid carrying it into susceptible communities.

Whooping Cough (Pertussis)

Whooping cough has a seasonal incidence in the months in which respiratory diseases are most common, i.e. during the winter, and especially the late winter months. If untreated it causes a high mortality in the very young owing to the chest complications which are common. The cause of the disease is a bacillus, *Haemophilus pertussis*. Immunization with pertussis vaccine is widely practised and appears to check complications even if the disease develops. The antibiotic drugs now available have also reduced the mortality of the disease.

The disease is transmitted by droplet infection and has an incubation period of from 10 to 14 days.

The chief symptoms are those of upper respiratory infection and bronchitis. There is some fever, and the pulse and respiratory rate are increased. The paroxysmal cough is characteristic. A series of violent coughs is succeeded by a prolonged inspiration which, drawn through the glottis which is partially closed by spasm, produces the typical 'whoop'. In patients who have been immunized this characteristic 'whoop' may be absent making diagnosis difficult. Marked cyanosis and vomiting are likely to follow a coughing fit. Considerable sputum is also ejected when this occurs. A small ulcer may appear on the fraenum of the tongue due to pressure of the lower incisors on it during the bouts of coughing, this is common in children of about 2 years of age. Conjunctival haemorrhage and umbilical hernia may also be seen as the result of increased pressure caused by coughing. In infants convulsions are a possible complication.

Treatment

The patient is kept at rest in bed while any fever is present, and, if possible, is best nursed in the open air. When there is no rise of temperature he may get up and should go out into the fresh air, provided he is protected by warm clothing. In the acute stage, if laryngitis is marked, steam inhalation by means of a kettle and tent are useful. Early treatment with one of the broad spectrum antibiotics, e.g. tetracycline, prevents the chest complications, particularly bronchopneumonia, which have frequently been the cause of death in infants in the past. Sedation with barbiturates or chloral may prove help in producing rest and diminishing the spasmodic attacks.

As vomiting so frequently follows a paroxysm of coughing, the child should be fed shortly after an attack as soon as he has quietened down. This gives a better chance for the feed to be assimilated before the next bout of coughing. Adequate nourishment must be given and frequent small feeds are usually advisable. In the case of infants, in whom dehydration can develop quickly, parenteral fluids may be necessary. Expectorant drugs may be ordered to assist in the removal of sputum but often have little effect.

Infectivity is highest in the early stages of the illness. In most cases there is little fear of infection at the end of 4 weeks, although the patient may still have a troublesome cough and whoop.

Diphtheria

Diphtheria is not now the killing disease of childhood that it was even after the introduction of treatment with antitoxin, but before the days of wide scale immunization with toxoid. There is, however, little doubt that serious outbreaks could easily reappear in a susceptible community, and therefore the danger to their own children and to others, if active immunization is neglected, should be a matter of concern to all parents.

The causal organism is the *Corynebacterium diphtheriae* (Klebs-Loeffler bacillus), which most commonly affects the upper respiratory tract, nose, throat and larynx, but occasionally attacks the conjunctiva of the eye or the vagina; rarely the organism infects wounds. At the site of the infection the bacteria produce a greyish-white membrane. From this local infection the bacterial toxins are absorbed into the bloodstream and cause a toxaemia which in severe cases can be fatal. A test known as the Schick test can be used to show susceptibility to diphtheria; this consists of the intradermal injection of a small dose of diphtheritic toxin into the left forearm. If the individual is susceptible, an area of redness appears after 24 hr and reaches its maximum by the third or fourth day. A control injection, containing no active toxin, is given at the same time into the skin of the right forearm, which may produce an area of redness but is less marked than the positive Schick reaction and is more transient. This test is useful in detecting susceptible persons in the case of an outbreak of diphtheria, and also in indicating whether children immunized in infancy need a 'booster' dose.

Diphtheria is spread by droplet infection, the organisms are expelled into the air in the moisture exhaled by an infected person; carriers are a common source of infection. More rarely fomites, i.e. infected articles, may be responsible and outbreaks have been known to occur in schools as a result of communal pencils being constantly sucked and passed from child to child.

The incubation period is 2 to 7 days and the infectious period lasts until cultures from throat or nose prove negative. Full clearance is not usually given until three successive swabs, taken at intervals of at least 3 days, have been negative.

The patient is usually a child between the age of 2 and 12 years, although infection can occur at any age. The most usual site of the infection is the nasopharynx or the pharynx, laryngeal diphtheria is almost always due to spread of infection from the pharynx. At the onset of the illness the patient feels unwell, listless, is disinclined to eat and may vomit. In this pharyngeal type of diphtheria the patient complains of headache and sore throat, although in many cases the soreness of the throat is slight, there is a moderate degree of fever, not as a rule higher than 38·8°C (102°F) and the pulse rate is high in proportion, 120 per min or more. On examination the throat is seen to be red with a greyish-white membrane on one or both tonsils, spreading to the fauces and the pharynx. This membrane is adherent and cannot be swabbed off readily, if removed it leaves a bleeding surface. In very mild cases, however, no membrane forms and the diagnosis may be in doubt until the bacteriological examination of a throat swab reveals the presence of the diphtheria organisms. In severe and moderately severe cases there is swelling of the neck and enlargement of the lymph glands.

Diphtheria occurring in a patient who has not been effectively immunized can be a fatal disease, the cause of death is as a rule due to the effect of the diphtheria toxin on the heart muscle. Asphyxia from the spread of the diphtheritic membrane to the larynx was also a cause of death in young children in the days when epidemics of this disease were common in this country, although the discovery of diphtheria antitoxin at the beginning of this century reduced the mortality rate very considerably.

Treatment

The patient is isolated and the necessary precautions taken against the spread of infection (see p. 307). Swabs used for mopping up discharges from the nose and mouth are highly infectious and should be burnt at once. Antitoxic serum is given, usually without waiting for the bacteriological confirmation of the diagnosis, the dose depending on the severity of the attack and the age of the patient. In severe infections very large doses are given, up to 100 000 units, in moderate cases the dose may vary between 15 000 and 40 000 units. Penicillin is generally given in addition to antitoxin to help control the infection by preventing the multiplication of the diphtheria bacilli although it has no direct action on the exotoxins produced by the bacilli.

In order to minimize the risk of serious myocardial damage the patient is nursed lying flat and at complete rest for the first 3 weeks. All effort on his part is forbidden, he must be fed, washed, lifted on to and off the bedpan and carefully turned from side to side for bedmaking and attention to pressure areas. By the fourth week a slightly more upright position in bed is allowed and one or more pillows are added. Sudden changes of position must be avoided as fatalities can occur as a result of cardiovascular failure. Myocardial failure is a particular danger which may occur at any time in the course of the illness, warning signs are pain, which may be referred to the abdomen, nausea, vomiting and an irregular pulse. There is little specific treatment for this condition but oxygen given by a mask or in a tent may be helpful. Rest in bed is likely to be required for 2 or 3 months in those cases where there is evidence of cardiac involvement.

While the patient is feeling ill and his throat is sore, a fluid or soft diet will be needed. Milk in any form, eggs, sugar or glucose and liberal fluids will usually be acceptable, as soon as he feels better the patient can be encouraged to take such food as bread and butter, puddings, fish and chicken, until he is eating a normal diet with the addition of milk and sweetened fruit drinks.

The usual nursing measures for the care of the mouth (see p. 13) will need to be carried out at frequent intervals and hot saline mouth washes may be comforting. If there is a nasal discharge the nostrils will require constant, gentle cleansing and a protective application of petroleum jelly, or other ointment.

Complications

In addition to the effect of the diphtheria toxin on the cardiovascular system, which has already been mentioned, the toxin may also affect the nerves supplying certain muscles, thus causing paralysis. This is a comparatively late complication which does not often occur before the second week of the illness and may be much later, 6 weeks or more after the onset of the illness. The muscles most commonly affected are:

(1) The muscles of the eye, causing squint or loss of power of accommodation, which is shown by an inability to focus on near objects and therefore the patient is unable to read.

(2) The muscles of the soft palate, shown by regurgitation of fluids when the patient attempts to swallow and by a nasal tone to the voice with inability to form labial sounds, such as 'b'. If the patient is asked to say 'Billy' he will say 'Milly'. The difficulty in swallowing may be overcome by giving thickened fluids with a spoon, this being less likely to produce regurgitation than thin fluids drunk from a cup. In some cases feeding by an intragastric tube passed through the nose may be necessary and this procedure is usually well tolerated by children.

(3) The muscles of the limbs, shown by loss of power, as for example the dragging of one leg or inability to walk. Passive exercises and in some cases light splinting to prevent deformities may be needed.

(4) The intercostal muscles and diaphragm, shown by respiratory difficulty. This is not a common complication, but if it does occur it may necessitate nursing the patient in a respirator (see p. 333).

Whatever form this toxic neuritis takes, complete recovery in a comparatively short time can be expected.

Laryngeal Diphtheria

The larynx is occasionally seen as the primary site of the disease but diphtheria here more often results from infection spreading from the pharyngeal type. The diphtheritic membrane forms in the larynx and obstructs the breathing, a condition which is particularly dangerous in young children in whom the airway of the larynx is small. The signs of laryngeal obstruction are increasing dyspnoea, cyanosis and stridor. Young children will show a marked sucking in (recession) of the chest wall in the intercostal spaces.

Tracheostomy

Early treatment with antitoxin and penicillin will in many cases prevent development of the diphtheritic membrane, if it does form it can sometimes be removed by suction with direct laryngoscopy. Tracheostomy is, however, now commonly performed as soon as signs of obstructed breathing are seen whatever the cause without waiting for the condition to become desperately urgent. Occasionally an emergency will occur in which opening the trachea and keeping it open with any instrument to hand, such as a pair of scissors, is the only possible way of preventing immediate death from asphyxia, but as a general rule the instruments for tracheostomy are kept ready for use in any situation where this operation is likely to be necessary. The following list gives the usual requirements.

Suitable tracheostomy tubes, e.g. two sizes of Durham's inner and outer tubes, with pilots.

Scalpels, one for the skin and one small tenotomy type knife, for opening the trachea.

Short, toothed and non-toothed, dissecting forceps.

Fine curved dissecting scissors.

Six pairs of fine haemostats.

Two blunt-ended double hooks.

One sharp hook.

Tracheal dilators.

Stitch scissors.

Curved and straight cutting-edged needles.

Ligatures and sutures, e.g. thread size 90, plain catgut size 3/0, and silk size 3/0.

Local anaesthetic, amethocaine or cinchocaine hydro-chloride, 10 ml syringe and needles.

Catheter and tubing to be connected to suction apparatus.

Oxygen apparatus.

Cetrimide or Hibitane, 0·5 per cent solution for cleaning the skin.

Sterile towels, swabs and dressings will also be needed. A key-hole gauze dressing is cut to fit round the tracheostomy tube, a tulle gras or Carbonet non-adherent dressing may be used to protect the skin. Firm support is needed under the shoulders so that the head falls back and the trachea is stretched, a square sandbag is suitable for this purpose. When the tracheostomy tube has been inserted it is kept securely in position by tapes fastened round the neck.

When the patient is returned to his bed he is nursed sitting upright and a warm jacket may be needed round his shoulders; a humidifier or a steam kettle and half tent are often used to moisten the air. Constant nursing care must be provided both day and night to ensure that the airway is kept clear. Oxygen, suction apparatus and a trolley with all the requirements for the care of the tracheostomy should be at the bedside. On the trolley the nurse keeps sterile gauze swabs, dressings, a sterile pair of tracheal dilators and a second tube which is identical with the one which has been inserted. A bowl of sodium bicarbonate solution, a small bottle brush or strips of narrow ribbon gauze and a pair of sinus forceps are required for cleaning the inner tube when it is removed. The tube must be kept clear by the frequent use of the suction apparatus with a suitable size soft rubber catheter attached, at first suction will be needed at 15 min intervals. If no suction apparatus is available any material coughed through the tube is gently swabbed with a moistened swab and a sterilized pipe-cleaner can be used to clear the tube. The inner tube is removed and washed in the bicarbonate solution at about hourly intervals, or more frequently if bubbling noises in the tube shows that it is partially blocked, or if the patient is having difficulty in expelling the secretions. Should the outer tube become displaced, as sometimes happens during a coughing fit, the doctor must be informed at once and the trachea kept open with the dilators. The dilators must be inserted from the side with the blades closed and the handles resting flat against the neck. The handles are then raised and turned to the midline and the blades opened gently. Meanwhile the nurse must assure the patient that he is in no danger and point out that he is breathing quite well even though the tube has slipped out. To prevent soreness and excoriation of the skin around the opening a protective application, such as sterile petroleum jelly or Carbonet dressing, is used, although if the dressings are changed as soon as soiled and the skin kept dry, soreness is less likely to occur. A patient with a tracheostomy is unable to speak, or in the case of a child to cry, so a writing pad and pencil should be give to the patient if he is able to write. A small handbell is useful for attracting attention if help is required. It may be necessary to splint the arms of a young child to prevent interference with the dressing or pulling at the tube. Where a tracheostomy is required as a temporary measure only, as in diphtheria, an attempt may be made to remove the tube at the end of 48 hr, but if the patient's breathing is distressed it will be reinstated and another attempt made, probably after a further 24 hr. A small cork may be inserted into the opening of the tube for short periods in order to accustom the patient to normal breathing.

Feeding does not as a rule present much difficulty, liberal fluids should be given, with a spoon at first; later the patient will drink easily from a feeding cup. If there is any difficulty in swallowing, an intragastric tube will be passed through the nose and fluid given by this route for the first 1 or 2 days.

When nursing a patient with laryngeal diphtheria the nurse must remember the danger of infection to herself from the material which is expelled through the tube with considerable force when the patient coughs. She should, as far as possible avoid standing immediately in front of the patient, as infection of the conjunctiva of the eye can occur if he coughs directly into her face. Wearing spectacles or goggles will also give protection to the nurse's eyes.

Intubation is sometimes performed in laryngeal diphtheria as an alternative to tracheostomy. A metal tube with an introducer is passed through the glottis into the larynx, and a stout ligature threaded through the outer end of the tube is fixed to the cheek by a piece of adhesive strapping. Should the tube become dislodged the doctor must be sent for at once to replace it; a mouth gag, tubes and introducers are kept at the bedside ready for such an event. The patient may be able to swallow fluids given with a spoon or feeding cup, but if he has any difficulty, feeding by an intragastric tube will be required. The same constant attention of a nurse as that following a tracheostomy is needed.

Nasal Diphtheria

Nasal diphtheria is often a chronic condition and is not accompanied by the toxaemia which is so marked a feature of the other forms of this disease. The patient has a purulent, often blood-stained, nasal discharge which is highly infectious. The skin of the nostrils and upper lip is excoriated and these sores are commonly the feature that draws attention to the condition. The usual treatment is penicillin and diphtheria antitoxin injections.

Diphtheria Carriers

Carriers are unfortunate people who, having had the disease or possibly having been infected without developing any clinical symptoms, harbour the organisms in their nose or throat and so infect others. Carriers should be isolated until they are free from infection, which will be demonstrated by negative results from three successive swabs. Tonsillectomy may effect a cure, and penicillin and erythromycin are two antibiotics which may be successful in eradicating the carrier state.

Scarlet Fever

Scarlet fever is a specific fever due to infection with a haemolytic streptococcus and associated with streptococcal tonsillitis. Streptococcal tonsillitis is the result of the invasion of the tonsillar area by the bacteria; and sometimes the infection includes the nasal sinuses and middle ear. The rash and certain other symptoms characteristic of scarlet fever are caused by absorption of the toxins manufactured by the haemolytic streptococcus. The disease is most prevalent in this country in the autumn and spring, but has become a mild infection compared with the position in the latter half of the last century when it was one of the severest and often the most fatal of the infectious diseases of childhood.

The spread of infection is most commonly by direct contact, or by droplet infection, but may also be transmitted by infected milk, food or fomites. Carriers of haemolytic streptococci are responsible for some outbreaks.

The incubation period is short, from 2 to 7 days. Infectivity is probably highest during the acute stage of the illness, but a patient who, though convalescent, still has a nasal discharge can spread infection.

Diagnosis is made by clinical signs and confirmed by the appearance of the rash 24 hr after the onset of the symptoms. The onset is sudden, with marked chill, or convulsions in the case of children, fever, with a temperature rising to 39·4° or 40°C (103° or 104°F), and an increase in pulse-rate, vomiting, headache and sore throat. The throat has a typical fiery red oedematous appearance. The tonsils are swollen and may show a whitish exudate somewhat similar in appearance to the false membrane of diphtheria; this exudate however, unlike diphtheritic membrane, can easily be swabbed off and the surface does not bleed. The tongue is thickly coated and white, the fur tends to peel off at the edges and after 2 days the coating has disappeared, leaving the tongue brightly red with the papillae abnormally prominent—the characteristic 'strawberry tongue'.

Twenty-four hours after the patient first becomes ill the rash appears. It shows as a red blush first on the chest and neck. This spreads and involves the whole body, except the face, head, palms and soles, small pin-point spots appear in the red areas and the rash is described as a punctate erythema. The face is very flushed save for an area around the mouth and nose giving the typical circumoral pallor.

The temperature remains high for a day or so after the rash appears, but gradually declines until, if no complications occur, it is normal on the sixth day. The other signs of fever gradually subside, and the soreness and redness of the throat disappear. The rash starts to fade as the temperature falls, and at the end of the first week peeling of the skin begins. This occurs first on the chest, where the rash started, and follows the order in which it spread. Where the skin is thinnest a fine desquamation occurs, but from the hands and feet, which peel last, large flakes and sometimes a cast of the entire part are shed.

The isolation period is usually 2 to 3 weeks, though shorter periods of isolation in hospital have been introduced as a result of modern treatment. Isolation is usually enforced until all signs of inflammation have disappeared from the throat and all discharges from the nose and ears have ceased; patients with a nasal discharge are particularly likely to be carriers of the haemolytic streptococcus.

Treatment

Sulphonamides and penicillin are specific remedies given to treat the disease and they also lessen the danger of complications. Penicillin is suitable for non-resistant strains of streptococci; oral penicillin V may be preferred for young children. Sulphadimidine is the usual form of sulphonamide chosen in streptococcal infections.

The patient is kept in bed until the temperature has been normal for at least a week, but no special treatment is needed other than that for febrile conditions. If the throat is very sore and the tongue furred, it may be difficult at first to persuade the patient to take sufficient fluids, iced drinks may be found the most acceptable fluids. Mouth-washes should be given regularly, and the usual measures taken to ensure good oral hygiene (see p. 13). The temperature, the pulse and respiration rates are taken 4-hourly for the first few days, and the urine must be measured and tested for blood and albumin daily until the danger of the development of nephritis is past. Since the discharges from the upper respiratory tract are a source of infection, special care is needed in the disinfection of mouth or other swabs, and feeding utensils particularly must be kept separate from others. As with other infectious diseases, fresh air and sunlight are valuable aids in preventing spread of the infection.

Special watch should be kept for the onset of complications, which will, if they occur, need specific treatment. Complications due to infection include cervical adenitis, rhinitis, sinusitis, middle ear infection, pneumonia and possibly septicaemia and a pyaemia with septic arthritis. Early and effective use of antibiotics has greatly reduced the incidence of secondary infections.

Acute glomerulo-nephritis is a complication that can arise as a sequela of any streptococcal infection and is evidenced by haematuria, puffiness of the face, particularly round the eyes, malaise and fever. Rheumatic fever is another possible complication of scarlet fever, and of streptococcal tonsillitis, but with effective antibiotic treatment of the initial infection, this is now less common.

Influenza

Influenza is a highly contagious virus disease mainly spread by droplet infection. One attack, as most people are only too well aware, does not confer immunity and this is probably due to the fact that there are several strains of influenza virus. For this reason also active immunization is difficult, although a polyvalent vaccine may afford temporary immunity.

The disease varies greatly in its severity; it can be so mild that there is difficulty in distinguishing between influenza and a 'febrile cold', or so virulent that many succumb to a fulminating and frequently fatal influenzal pneumonia. Since the Middle Ages there are records of world-wide (pandemic) outbreaks with many deaths. The worst recorded pandemic was in 1918 to 1919, when it was estimated that over 500 million people were affected and over 20 million died. Such outbreaks appear to occur at long intervals, perhaps once in a century, but more restricted epidemics varying in their severity appear about every second year. In this country influenza outbreaks usually occur during the winter months, although an epidemic of Asian-type influenza reached this country from the East in the late summer of 1957.

Chill, rising temperature, malaise, headache and general pains are the common initial symptoms and are usually accompanied by catarrh, laryngitis and tracheitis. In the most virulent types of infection the patient rapidly develops signs of a fulminating bronchopneumonia, with dyspnoea, cyanosis and pain in the side due to pleurisy. In milder infections bronchopneumonia may develop as a secondary infection and this is a serious complication in elderly persons and young children.

In some patients, especially infants and children, vomiting, abdominal pain and diarrhoea may be more marked than respiratory symptoms.

Treatment

In most cases rest in bed, warmth, analgesics such as aspirin or codeine, with liberal fluids and such food as the patient feels inclined to take will be all the treatment needed. The patient should remain in bed until the temperature is normal and the symptoms have subsided, and for the next 2 or 3 days he should be up for only short periods. Depending on the severity of the attack a period of convalescence is advisable, as relapses are not uncommon and also most patients feel weak and often depressed under an attack of influenza. The danger of pneumonia is greatest in young children and elderly patients and will require immediate treatment with antibiotics and possibly oxygen therapy.

Poliomyelitis

Poliomyelitis is an infection which particularly attacks motor nerve cells in the spinal cord and the brain. The cause is a virus of which three distinct strains, types 1, 2 and 3, have been identified. From the time when outbreaks of the disease were first reported in the last century until some 50 years ago, those affected were mainly in the under 5 age group; hence the disease was given the name 'infantile paralysis'. Although it is now rare for cases to occur in the U.K., in the epidemics in the 1940s and '50s, adults were also affected.

The mode of transmission of the disease has been the subject of much research; the live virus has been repeatedly found in the faeces of patients and therefore faecal contamination of food and flies acting as vectors are probably mainly responsible for outbreaks. The virus is also present in the pharynx of infected persons and therefore may be spread by droplet infection. Infection of human beings with poliomyelitis virus is thought to be very prevalent, and healthy carriers of the virus are probably the source of infection in a number of cases. Many of those infected never develop any sign of the disease, others may have a very mild illness of which little, if any, notice is taken.

The incubation period is uncertain and as wide a range as from 3 to 30 days has been given, with the probability that in most cases incubation is between 7 and 14 days. The period of infectivity is also doubtful; the virus may be found in the stools of the patient for a number of weeks. It is probable that the infectious period begins a few days before the onset of symptoms, and in practice infectious precautions are seldom continued for more than 3 weeks. These precautions are mainly concerned with prevention of faecal contamination, thorough hand-washing on the part of the nurses and all other persons concerned after any attention to the patient must be conscientiously observed. Sanitary utensils should be kept solely for the patient's use and disinfected. There is, however, usually no point in disinfecting excreta, since it can be assumed that the virus is already present in the local sewage.

Reference has already been made to the use of poliomyelitis vaccine (p. 37). The first extensive use of Sabin live virus oral vaccine to give immediate protection during an epidemic in a highly populated urban area in England was carried out in Hull in October 1961.

The onset of poliomyelitis is sometimes marked by general mild febrile symptoms from which there is apparent recovery, but which is followed by a return of fever with backache, vomiting, headaches and stiffness of the neck, i.e. meningeal symptoms. If the disease does not progress beyond the initial febrile symptoms this is described as an abortive attack; meningeal symptoms may not be followed by paralysis and the attack is then termed non-paralytic. In paralytic poliomyelitis the symptoms are usually apparent within a day or two of the onset of the febrile meningeal stage and will vary according to the severity of the attack and the level of the greatest damage in the spinal cord and brain-stem. In the *spinal type* the muscles of the limbs are most commonly affected, although the trunk can be involved and in severe infections with rapidly extending paralysis, respiratory failure threatens life if immediate resuscitation is not available. Weakness and paralysis of the skeletal muscles has usually reached its maximum by the end of the febrile stage of the illness and considerable muscle recovery may be expected in most cases. However, those muscles whose nerve supply has been completely killed cannot recover. Where all the main muscle groups of a limb are permanently paralysed the limb will be smaller than normal, due to muscle atrophy (in children this will be all the more marked because the growth of the limb will be affected), and it is cold and blue. Later, deformities such as club foot and spinal curvature may develop.

Where the greatest damage is in the brain-stem bulbar paralysis develops and this type is responsible for most of the deaths from poliomyelitis. The muscles of speech, mastication and swallowing are affected; attempts at swallowing are often followed by regurgitation through the nose, and secretions which the patient cannot swallow collect in the pharynx causing respiratory obstruction and are likely to invade the lungs. In addition vasomotor and respiratory centres are likely to be involved.

Treatment

In the acute stage of the illness rest is obviously essential and a careful watch must be kept for signs of the onset or extension of paralysis. Local hot packs, radiant heat and aspirin may be used to relieve the muscular pain and tenderness. Weak muscles should be supported by sandbags or light splints to prevent over-stretching and deformities. A firm mattress is needed for support and a foot board is useful to prevent foot drop, bed cradles will prevent pressure by the weight of the bedclothes. Passive movements of the joints through their full range are carried out during the acute stage; later active movements are introduced. If the patient has retention of urine catheterization will be necessary. Constipation, which may lead to faecal impaction, will if present require treatment with enemas or rectal suppositories such as Dulcolax (bisacodyl) or glycerin. Ample fluids should be given, and such light diet as the patient feels able to take. Lumbar puncture is usually carried out for diagnostic purposes and also for the relief of meningeal symptoms.

Difficulty in eating or swallowing, change in the voice, respiratory impairment, rising pulse rate or rapidly extending paralysis, are all danger signs indicating that immediate emergency measures are needed. While preparations are being made for more effective treatment the patient should be placed in the semi-prone position and the foot of the bed raised to drain secretions away from the lungs.

Obstructed airway and pharyngeal paralysis require tracheostomy and suction apparatus to drain pooled secretions. This measure is usually combined with artificial respiration, which may be carried out at first by a Radcliffe type of resuscitator (Fig. 45) attached to an oxygen supply. The face-piece of the apparatus is fitted with a hand-controlled spring valve. When

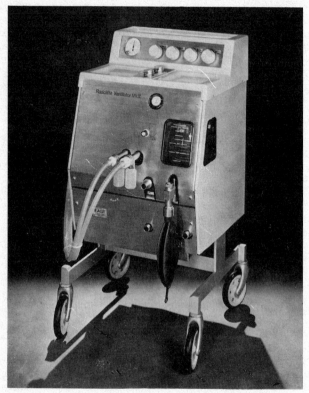

FIG. 45. East–Radcliffe positive–negative pressure respirator.

the spring is closed oxygen is forced into the lungs and inflates them; when the spring is released the flow of oxygen is cut off and the lungs deflate. For continued artificial respiration with positive pressure the Beaver type of apparatus is useful. A cuffed rubber tube is passed through a tracheostomy into the trachea and when the cuff is inflated the pharynx, nose and mouth are cut off from the respiratory tract and secretions which the patient is unable to swallow can no longer obstruct the airway, or gain entrance to the lungs. The rubber tube is attached via an expiratory valve to a breathing bag which is alternatively inflated and deflated by a small electric motor. If necessary oxygen can be added to the atmospheric air.

Frequent suction is needed to clear the mouth and pharynx of collecting saliva and mucus. Feeding is carried out by a fine oesophageal tube passed through the nose into the stomach.

Patients with paralysis involving the respiratory muscles, but not associated with the paralytic symptoms affecting the pharynx and muscles of swallowing, may be treated by a negative-positive pressure respirator of the Drinker or Both type. The paralysed patient is totally enclosed in a steel cabinet except for his head, which is supported on a headrest and small pillow. A sponge rubber collar fits round his neck making an air-tight seal. The rubber collar may be irritating to the skin, therefore washing with soap and water and careful drying must be done frequently. The use of powder on the skin is not advisable as it tends to cake. Pressure inside the cabinet is altered by an electrically driven air-pump attached at the foot end by a length of unkinkable rubber hose-pipe. Reducing the pressure in the cabinet causes inspiration; expiration is produced by slight positive pressure. The speed of the motor driving the pump can be varied, so allowing for adjustments in the respiratory rate. Should the electricity supply to the respirator fail for any reason a handle and lever can be used to operate the pump manually. The nurse responsible for the care of the patient must make sure that she knows how to attach the handle and work the pump should the necessity arise. Port-holes in the cabinet through which the nurse's arms can be inserted when attending to the patient, and a larger opening for a bedpan, are provided with rubber cuffs to form an air-tight seal when in use. The patient may be able to do without the respirator for a short time and if so the necessary nursing attention can be mainly given during the period that the patient is out of the cabinet. If treatment of a kind which cannot be satisfactorily given with the patient in the cabinet or in the short time that he is able to manage without the respirator is required, he can be kept breathing adequately by the temporary use of an anaesthetic type of breathing apparatus or a resuscitator.

The care of patients with bulbar and respiratory paralysis

requires uninterrupted nursing attention, and therefore a high ratio of nurses to patients, immediate availability of medical attention and often the services of a technician to maintain and adjust the apparatus. For these reasons it is usual to treat these patients in a special unit. Such 'respiratory units' often provide not only for the care of poliomyelitis patients but also for others requiring similar treatment for any cause.

Rehabilitation

The degree to which rehabilitation can restore the patient to normal activity is very variable. Some patients who have suffered severe attacks may remain almost totally paralysed and may even spend the rest of their lives in a respirator. For such patients great ingenuity and imagination are needed to make their existence as bearable as possible, and all the resources of occupational therapists, educational and social agencies will be needed.

It is quite often difficult to wean patients from dependence on a respirator. Halfway measures may be such things as a cuirass or a 'rocking bed'. The former is like a shell which fits over the patient's chest and exerts intermittent positive pressure but allows the patient a greater degree of mobility. The 'rocking bed' uses the weight of the abdominal organs in the diaphragm to aid respiration and is particularly useful for patients who find difficulty breathing at night.

Patients less severely crippled are likely to need physiotherapy for a long period and orthopaedic treatment in the form of braces and splints. In some cases surgery such as tendon transplantation, tenotomy or arthrodesis may be needed to correct a deformity, or to improve the stability of a limb and increase the effectiveness of the non-paralysed muscles.

As stated poliomyelitis is now rare in the U.K. However it is still endemic in many parts of the world. In Britain there are also many people who suffer from the effects of previous epidemics, some still being maintained by artificial respirators.

Meningococcal Meningitis (Cerebrospinal Fever, Spotted Fever)

Meningococcal meningitis or cerebrospinal fever, is a disease of low infectivity which does not run a very definite course. It usually attacks children and young adults and is called 'spotted fever' because of the characteristic rash, which is purpuric in type. Outbreaks are usually sporadic but sometimes occur in epidemics, overcrowding and poor hygienic conditions being predisposing causes.

The cause of the infection is *Neisseria meningitidis*, and the spread is by droplet infection, often from healthy nasopharyngeal carriers of the organism.

The incubation period is uncertain, probably 1 to 5 days, and the period of infectivity depends on the course of the illness, it will be short in those cases where the infection is rapidly and successfully treated by chemotherapy.

The onset is usually acute with fever, headache, irritability, stiffness of the neck and photophobia. Children frequently have convulsions at the onset and also may show an extreme degree of head retraction and stiffness. The petechial rash develops early in the illness, but is not always present.

The cerebrospinal fluid on lumbar puncture is found to be under pressure. It is often turbid and it contains an increased number of white blood cells.

Treatment

Sulphonamides remain the treatment of choice in meningococcal meningitis although, in the case of infants particularly, penicillin may be given at the same time. Sulphadiazine and sulphamerazine are two of the sulphonamides used. This antibacterial treatment is usually continued for one week.

Fluid intake for an adult should be at least 3 litres daily, and, if the patient is comatose, restless and uncooperative, most of this fluid may have to be given intravenously, or by an intragastric tube. An accurate record of fluid intake and output should be kept. If retention of urine occurs catheterization will be necessary. Drugs may be needed to combat restlessness and insomnia, e.g. barbiturates, paraldehyde. All the necessary nursing measures to protect the skin and to prevent pressure sores must be regularly carried out. Frequent care of the mouth is necessary to prevent the formation of sores and to keep the mouth moist. The eyelids tend to become sticky and will require bathing with boracic or saline lotion and the application of a light smear of petroleum jelly or a suitable ointment.

Before the introduction of chemotherapy meningococcal meningitis was particularly fatal in infants under 1 year and also not infrequently the acute phase passed into a more chronic form with adhesions which led to hydrocephalus. Blindness, deafness and spastic paralysis are other sequelae which are now fortunately much rarer.

Other Forms of Meningitis

Meningitis due to other organisms, e.g. pneumococci, streptococci or staphylococci, shows symptoms similar to those of meningococcal meningitis, and is treated by appropriate chemotherapy. Tuberculous meningitis is due to spread of

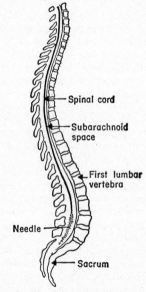

FIG. 46. Site for intrathecal injection.

infection from a tuberculous focus elsewhere in the body (see p. 62) and the onset is commonly more gradual than other types of meningitis. Streptomycin, para-aminosalicylic acid (PAS) and isoniazid are now used successfully in the treatment of this formerly fatal form of meningitis. Administration of streptomycin and either PAS or isoniazid is usually continued for about one year; streptomycin may be given intrathecally, i.e. into the subarachnoid space of the spinal cord, at the beginning of the illness in order to attain a sufficiently high concentration of the drug in the cerebrospinal fluid (Fig. 46).

The nurse must observe the patient for side effects such as deafness or vertigo to avoid permanent damage to the eighth cranial nerve.

Glandular Fever (Infective Mononucleosis)

Glandular fever is an infectious disease, probably caused by a virus, which most commonly affects children and young adults. It appears to have a low infectivity; epidemics are rare and most cases are sporadic.

The incubation period is probably about 12 days. The onset is usually sudden, with pyrexia, enlarged superficial glands of the neck, enlarged tonsils and sore throat. The fever may last for 2 weeks and sometimes relapses occur. Some enlargement of the spleen is common but is not present in all cases; sometimes a rash rather like rubella is seen on the trunk, arms and thighs. The diagnosis is confirmed by the examination of the blood revealing lymphocytosis with the presence of abnormal lymphocytes and by the appearance of antibodies in the blood serum which agglutinate the red cells of sheep's blood: this test is known as the Paul-Bunnell reaction. A negative reaction does not necessarily exclude glandular fever, but a positive agglutinin reaction is said to be a diagnostic of glandular fever.

Typhoid and Paratyphoid Fever (Enteric Fever)

Typhoid and paratyphoid fevers are caused by micro-organisms of the *Salmonella* group, *Salmonella typhosa* and *Salmonella paratyphosa* A, B and C. In this country the infection is usually due to *Salmonella typhosa* or *paratyphosa* B. In general paratyphoid fever is a milder disease than typhoid fever, but otherwise the course of the two is essentially similar.

Epidemics of typhoid fever are associated with poor hygienic conditions, such as contaminated water supplies, inadequate sanitation, and the presence of flies in large numbers. Smaller outbreaks are most commonly due to contamination of water, milk or other foods by excreta of a typhoid carrier. Shellfish grown in sewage-contaminated water have been the cause of some outbreaks. Most cases which occur on the U.K. are in people who have recently returned from countries where the disease is endemic.

Active immunization with TAB (typhoid and paratyphoid A and B) vaccine gives protection which is thought to last for about 2 years; after that time inoculation should be repeated whenever exposure to infection is a possible occurrence.

The incubation period is usually anywhere between 5 and 14 days. Infectivity lasts as long as the organisms are present in the stools and the urine of the patient, and the development of a chronic carrier state after recovery from the illness is always a possibility.

The typhoid bacteria when swallowed in food or water multiply in the lymphoid tissue (Peyer's patches) of the small intestine. Both bacteria and their toxins are absorbed into the blood-stream and a bacteraemia is present in the early days of the illness. The localized inflammation in the small intestine causes swelling followed by necrosis, sloughing and ulceration of the Peyer's patches. The mesenteric lymph glands and the spleen are enlarged. The gall-bladder may also be infected, and as a result of typhoid cholecystitis the patient may develop the chronic carrier state. Typhoid bacteria can invade the urinary tract, usually in the second week of the disease, and may cause pyelitis or cystitis. Later the patient may be found to be a urinary carrier of typhoid fever. Bronchitis almost invariably accompanies typhoid fever and secondary infection may lead to pneumonia. Typhoid abscesses may occur in bones; these develop very slowly and may not be discovered for some months or even years after recovery from the attack of typhoid fever. The pus in these abscesses contains typhoid bacteria.

The diagnosis of typhoid fever is made from the clinical picture, by finding the organisms in a blood culture and later in the stools, and by the presence of specific agglutinins in the blood, the Widal reaction test.

The onset of typhoid fever is gradual; the temperature rises slowly to about 39·4°C (103°F), while the pulse rate is relatively slow. Headache, often nose-bleeding, a dry cough and malaise accompany the fever and, although during the first few days the patient may remain up, by about the end of a week increasing illness and lassitude force him to remain in bed. Abdominal distension and constipation are more usual symptoms in the early stage than diarrhoea.

In the second week, the temperature remains high; the pulse may be found to have a double beat, the dicrotic pulse. The patient is apathetic but may be sleepless and confused at night. Abdominal discomfort is more marked and diarrhoea with the characteristic 'pea soup' stools is present in the majority of cases, together with the typhoid rash, which consists of crops of rose-coloured spots on the chest, abdomen and back. The mouth is dry with sordes tending to collect on the gums and teeth, and the tongue is furred and brown.

In the third week in severe cases the toxaemia increases and the 'typhoid state' may develop. The patient lies with his eyes open but not conscious of his surroundings; muttering, delirium, tremor and picking at the bedclothes complete the picture of a severely toxic state. Signs of pneumonia and of myocardial failure may be present. The output of urine falls and proteinuria (albuminuria) may be present; the stools are loose and frequent and incontinence of both urine and faeces is common. Two dangerous complications which are liable to occur at this stage are intestinal haemorrhage and perforation.

In milder infections and in cases treated with antibiotics this degree of toxaemia is not seen, and the patient is usually on the way to recovery in the third week. The temperature falls gradually and the abdominal symptoms, pain, distension and diarrhoea abate, and the stage of convalescence begins.

Treatment

The specific treatment is the oral administration of the antibiotic chloramphenicol. The dose depends on the age of the patient and also on the stage the illness has reached when the treatment is started; if severe toxic symptoms are already present large doses will be required. In all cases dosage of chloramphenicol must be adequate or relapses will occur. The administration of the drug is usually continued for about 3 weeks.

Although liability to complications is much reduced by successful chemotherapy, perforation of the small intestine, or haemorrhage from the ulcerated Peyer's patches and secondary pneumonia are still potential dangers in the third week of the illness. Perforation should be suspected if there is sudden abdominal pain, although it is possible that the patient who is comatose and toxic may make no complaint, and the recognition of this condition, which needs urgent surgical treatment, is dependent on the nurse's observation of a fall in temperature and a rising pulse rate. A similar change may denote a severe haemorrhage, in addition pallor is usually marked and blood in the form of copious tarry stools, often also containing bright blood, is passed per rectum. Immediate transfusion is frequently needed as a life-saving measure. Secondary pneumonia is treated with suitable antibiotics depending on the infecting organism.

A starch and opium enema or a starch and bismuth mixture may be ordered for the relief of diarrhoea. In cases where constipation is marked in the early stage aperients are avoided and enemas are not without danger, although if the patient is very uncomfortable a warm water enema may be given.

Nursing care is an essential part of the treatment of the patient suffering from typhoid fever, and includes all necessary measures to prevent the spread of infection (see p. 306).

The patient is nursed well supported by pillows in whichever positions he can rest with the greatest degree of comfort. If the patient is comatose or too ill to move himself a two-hourly changing of his position is necessary to prevent pressure sores and to help in the prevention of chest complication. Areas subject to pressure (heels, elbows, sacrum, shoulder blades and other bony prominences) need special attention. They should be kept clean and dry and the use of sheepskin pads may be beneficial.

If the patient is incontinent it is advisable to use a disposable 'incontinence' pad, which can be changed as required with little disturbance. The skin must be kept clean and protected by washing whenever necessary, careful drying and the application of a silicone barrier cream to the area of the buttocks and sacrum. Warm sponging once or twice a day helps to keep the temperature down and if carried out with care is soothing and refreshing. Continuous care is needed to keep the patient's mouth moist and clean; the measures suggested on pages 12 to 14 are suitable, in conjunction with an adequate fluid intake.

Diet. A low residue, moderately high joule diet is required, with sufficient protein and vitamins to provide for proper nutrition. Almost any food that the patient can be persuaded to take, provided that it contains no indigestible or bulky material, such as fruit, vegetables or tough meat or excess of fat, can be given. Fluid intake should be at least 2 litres in 24 hr. The basis of the diet in the acute stage is usually milk with the addition of eggs, glucose and additional protein in the form of Complan. Barley water, fruit juices and tea will help to augment the fluid intake. As the patient's condition improves a fuller, but still low-residue, diet can include steamed fish, chicken, milk pudding, bread-and-butter, sieved vegetables and fruit purée, gradually building a generous full diet without roughage. If abdominal distension and diarrhoea are marked and the urinary output falls, of if the patient cannot be persuaded to take sufficient nourishment and fluid, intravenous fluid may be needed. A record of fluid intake and output should be kept.

Control of Carriers

The unfortunate person who becomes a chronic typhoid carrier most commonly harbours the bacteria in his gall-bladder and excretes them in faeces. Occasionally the focus of infection is in the kidney and the organisms will then be passed with the urine. Carriers are probably responsible for most outbreaks of typhoid and paratyphoid fever in this country, and if measures cannot be taken to free them from infection then efforts must be directed towards ensuring that they do not spread the infection. In particular carriers should not take any part in the preparation and handling of food to be eaten by other people. Chloramphenicol will not cure the carrier state but where the bacteria are present in the gall-bladder the operation of cholecystectomy is usually successful.

Bacillary Dysentery

Although dysentery is a disease which is far more common in tropical and subtropical areas than in this country, outbreaks of bacillary dysentery occur from time to time. These are usually of a mild type caused by infection with a bacterium of the *Salmonella* group known as *Shigella sonnei*, or a similar organism, *Shigella flexneri*. More severe forms of the disease are due to yet another organism in this group, *Shigella shigae*, which is a frequent cause of epidemics in hot climates, particularly where hygienic conditions are unsatisfactory or where normal practice is disrupted, as for example by catastrophes such as hurricanes and earthquakes. Faecal contamination of water supplies and food and the agency of flies as vectors are the main means by which the infection is spread. Infants and children form a high proportion of the cases of dysentery occurring in this country, and at the other end of the scale outbreaks sometimes occur in communities of old people.

The incubation period is often short and may be only a few hours. The onset is sudden, with abdominal pain, frequent diarrhoea, mucus and usually blood in the stools, and a rise of temperature. In a mild case the symptoms abate in a few days; in more severe infections, the diarrhoea persists and may be accompanied by vomiting. The temperature remains high and the patient suffers from severe abdominal cramp. He also shows signs of dehydration with a dry mouth, dry inelastic skin and sunken eyes.

Treatment

Rest in bed and warmth, together with ample fluids by mouth in the form of water and tea are usually sufficient treatment in a mild attack. A sulphonamide preparation of the type which is poorly absorbed from the intestinal tract and therefore can exert a local bactericidal effect is often ordered; examples are sucienylsulphathiazole and phthalysulphathiazole (Thalzole) Morphine or codeine phosphate preparations may be prescribed for the relief of pain and diarrhoea.

Intravenous fluids may be needed in some cases, particularly for infants, in whom diarrhoea and vomiting can rapidly produce a dangerous state of dehydration and electrolyte imbalance.

Amoebic Dysentery

Amoebic dysentery is caused by a protozoon, *Entamoeba histolytica*. The infection is rarely encounted outside tropical or sub-tropical countries. The symptoms are similar to those of bacillary dysentery with abdominal pain and diarrhoea, but amoebic dysentery has a greater tendency to become chronic. Hepatitis and liver abscess are fairly common complications.

Emetine hydrochloride and metronidazole (Flogyl) are the drugs most commonly used in the treatment of this disease and it is given by intramuscular injection in doses of 30 to 60 mg daily for 5 to 10 days. Chloroquine may be prescribed as a supplementary treatment as this drug is effective in combating the hepatic infection. Antibiotics, such as tetracycline and paromomycin, may also be needed to treat any associated bacterial infection in the large intestine.

Food Poisoning

Food poisoning is caused by bacterial toxins which may contaminate food or by infection of the bowel by bacteria contained in the food. The organisms usually responsible are *Salmonella enteritidis* or other *Salmonella* organisms and *Staphylococcus aureus*, and they may have contaminated the food at any stage in its processing, preparation, cooking or distribution. Cooked foods which have been left and reheated are particularly dangerous. Outbreaks of food poisoning suggest that somewhere along the line from production to consumption proper hygienic measures are not being observed. The infecting organism is detected by bacteriological examination of the suspected food and the vomit and stools of the persons affected.

The onset of the illness is sudden with abdominal pain, vomiting, diarrhoea and usually a rise of temperature. Faintness and dizziness are often experienced, and in a severe attack the patient is quite prostrated. It is unusual, however, for the illness to last longer than 2 to 3 days, and recovery is commonly rapid, although the exhaustion and dehydration resulting from vomiting and diarrhoea may be serious in the very young and very old.

Treatment

Food is withheld and indeed the patient has no desire for food, but fluids such as water and weak tea should be given liberally as soon as these can be taken without vomiting. In severe cases intravenous fluid will be required.

An analgesic injection may be ordered for the relief of the abdominal pain. The stomach may be washed out to remove any remaining toxic material, although in most cases this will have already been achieved by the copious vomiting and diarrhoea.

One of the sulphonamide drugs which is not readily absorbed from the alimentary tract, such as sulphasuxidine, may be ordered. Once the acute vomiting and diarrhoea have ceased, rest, warmth and a generous fluid intake will usually complete the patient's recovery.

Botulism

A serious but fortunately rare form of food poisoning is known as botulism. The infecting organism is *Clostridium botulinum*, and it has been found in canned and bottled foods. The toxins produced by *Clostridium botulinum* seldom produce gastro-intestinal symptoms but affect the nervous system. Difficulty in speaking, swallowing and breathing are usually the first symptoms, and unless the specific antitoxin can be given immediately, death is likely to occur from respiratory failure.

Infantile Gastro-Enteritis

(Epidemic Infantile Diarrhoea)

Infantile gastro-enteritis is a form of gastro-intestinal infection which is liable to occur in infants, especially in those artificially fed, and was at one time epidemic in the summer months. The infection is often due to certain strains of *Escherichia coli*. There is usually a sudden onset with considerable fever, dry skin, and great thirst. Vomiting is not always present, but may be a late symptom. The stools are frequent and fluid, greenish in colour, slimy and offensive. Marked dehydration quickly develops. The infant's eyes are sunken, the fontanelle depressed and his skin dry and inelastic. In severe cases collapse occurs, the pulse is weak and thready, the skin is cold, the fontanelles are depressed and death may follow unless the appropriate treatment is given promptly. Although most cases recover, with appropriate treatment, relapses are not uncommon.

Preventive Treatment

Strict cleanliness in the preparation of an infant's feeds is the first step in preventing gastro-enteritis. If fresh milk is used it should be pasteurized and after delivery the bottles should be immediately stored in a refrigerator. Dried milk powder is frequently used in place of fresh milk for infant feeding; one of the reasons for this is that it is less easily contaminated during storage or in the process of making up the feeds.

In a paediatric ward feeds are prepared and sterilized in a milk kitchen. In the home utensils for preparing and giving feeds should be sterilized, and bottles and teats should be kept in covered containers in a solution of sodium hypochlorite (Milton). The solution must fill and cover the bottle, otherwise the bottle will float on the surface and not be disinfected. After use feeding bottles should be washed at once and boiled: precautions should be taken to keep flies away from milk, the utensils used for it, and the infant, as bacterial infection is easily spread by them. The use of feeding bottles in situations where effective cleaning and sterilization cannot be guaranteed is fraught with danger to the infant. For this reason bottle feeding is often discouraged and when breast milk has to be supplemented the mother is shown how to give food from a spoon and a cup. These can be more easily cleaned and kept clean than the bottle and teat.

An infant suffering from enteritis should be isolated from others, and the rules for isolation nursing, as set out on pages 307–311, should be carefully observed. All personal requirements should be kept entirely for his use; napkins should be of the 'disposable' type which are burnt when soiled.

Treatment

It is usual to give no food by mouth if the infant is vomiting; sterile water, half strength normal saline solution, or glucose and water 5 per cent (i.e. glucose 5 g to 100 ml of water) may be tried in small quantities, but may not be retained. The loss of water and electrolytes cannot be made good by oral fluids in any but very mild cases, and intravenous infusion, using sodium lactate or saline lactate, is usually begun without delay. A specimen of blood is required for assessment of the serum protein and of the nature of the electrolyte disturbance. These findings will decide which solution will be most effective and whether plasma protein loss needs replacement. A rectal swab is also sent to the laboratory for culture, although treatment with antibiotics, streptomycin or tetracycline, may be started without waiting for the results of the culture. Subcutaneous saline may be necessary if the infant's veins are collapsed.

Feeding is started very cautiously, and must be of a non-irritating nature without residue, e.g. whey, a weak solution of milk and water. Additional carbohydrate in the form of sugar and glucose may cause fermentation, but, if the infant will not take unsweetened feeds, saccharine may be used. If vomiting does not occur and if there is no increase in diarrhoea, the feeds can be gradually increased in quantity and strength, but this is entirely determined by the condition of the child; if there is any recurrence of symptoms a return must be made to the starting point. Constant care is needed and results are often disheartening.

The 'apple diet' is often satisfactory in those cases in which vomiting is absent and where the infant is more than 4-months of age. The pulp of 0·5 kg (1 lb) of cooked, sieved apples is mixed with 0·5 litre (1 pint) of normal saline solution, and 180 ml (6 fl oz) of freshly made weak tea, saccharine is added to sweeten it and the mixture is given with a spoon. It is usually taken well, the fluid is absorbed and the apple pulp excreted.

The skin of the buttocks and groins is prone to become sore from constant moisture and faecal contamination, and this can be prevented only by strict cleanliness and the application of a soothing and protective ointment such as zinc and castor oil. A square pinned round the infant in the usual way may be an additional source of irritation and in the acute stage of the illness it is better to place an absorbent pad under the buttocks. As the infant is limp and unlikely to move there is little risk of the bedding becoming soiled.

Tuberculosis

Tuberculosis is a disease resulting from infection with a bacterium. *Mycobacterium tuberculosis*, two types of which cause disease in human beings, the *human* type which is responsible for almost all cases of tuberculosis, and the *bovine* type which is now rare, owing to the measures taken to ensure safe milk supplies to the public; this type is the usual cause of tuberculous disease of the bones and joints.

Infection with *Mycobacterium tuberculosis* is widespread and, in large towns particularly, most people have been infected by the time they reach adult life, although comparatively few develop clinical signs of the disease. Infection most commonly occurs from inhaling the organisms from droplets or in dust. *M. tuberculosis* is able to withstand drying and therefore sputum infected with the organism, which is allowed to dry thus forming small particles which can be carried in the air, is a particular source of danger. Tuberculosis can also be contracted by swallowing the organisms, and this is the usual portal of entry for the bovine type, which can be found in milk from tuberculous cows. Infection by the bovine type has been largely prevented by ensuring that milk supplies are not contaminated, either by eradicating tuberculosis in milk herds or by heat treatment of the milk, which kills the bacteria. In this country both methods are practised, and the majority of the milk supply either comes from tubercle-free cows or is pasteurized. Control of airborne infection is more difficult, but better housing with less overcrowding, and education of the tuberculous patient and the general public in proper hygienic habits, particularly in relation to coughing and spitting, are measures that have played their part in the decreasing incidence of tuberculosis. Furthermore, since the undiagnosed and undetected tuberculous case is a greater danger in the community than the known tuberculous patient, the detection of early signs of pulmonary tuberculosis by such means as mass radiography helps to control infection. Most of the cases of tuberculosis seen in the U.K. are now in people who are recent immigrants.

In the majority of cases tuberculosis is a chronic inflammatory disease. Before the advent of successful chemotherapy patients suffering from lung tuberculosis might spend many months or even years in a sanatorium, and children with tuberculous disease of the bones and joints often remained in a special hospital for the greater part of their childhood days. The aim of treatment in the main was to provide a good environment with fresh air, good nutrition in order to build up resistance to the bacteria and to provide gradual rehabilitation. These principles are still followed, but the duration and severity of the illness can now be reduced by the use of chemotherapeutic drugs, streptomycin, isoniazid and para-aminosalicylic acid (PAS). These drugs provide the weapon that was lacking for so long, a bactericide which can destroy *M. tuberculosis* in the living tissues.

In the great majority of cases of tuberculous infection the primary focus is in the lung (see p. 62) and from this primary focus infection can spread either directly or through the blood-stream, and therefore almost any organ or tissue in the body can become affected. In addition tuberculosis can occur as a general infection, miliary tuberculosis, often associated with tuberculous meningitis; tuberculous inflammation of the peritoneum, of the kidneys and of skin are other examples. Pulmonary tuberculosis is the commonest form, and this is described in Chapter 3.

The chemotherapeutic agents now available are also effective against such formerly fatal forms of the disease as generalized (miliary) tuberculosis and tuberculous meningitis.

Venereal diseases, of which gonorrhoea and syphilis are the most important, are so named because they are usually, though not invariably, acquired through sexual intercourse. They are diseases of considerable social importance for several reasons; they produce serious and disabling effects which have repercussions on the next generation, gonorrhoea can be a cause of sterility, and syphilis in the pregnant woman is a possible cause of abortion, still birth, or congenital defects in the infant. The knowledge that these diseases are usually sexually acquired has given them a particular stigma which often prevents medical advice from being sought at an early stage. They are also diseases whose incidence rises sharply when normal family and social life is disturbed by unpleasant and disrupting influences, such as occur in times of war. One of the problems of the 'permissive society' has been the great upsurge in the incidence of venereal disease.

Gonorrhoea

Gonorrhoea is caused by a diplococcus, *Neisseria gonorrhoea*, which attacks the mucous membrane of the urethra, the genito-urinary tract and the glands related to them. In the female gonorrhoeal infection often begins as an inflammation of the urethra, there is burning pain on micturition, and a purulent discharge. However, in many cases there are no obvious symptoms and the disease can only be discovered by contact tracing'. Local abscesses may form in Bartholin's and other glands, and infection may spread to the endometrium and Fallopian tubes. Gonorrhoea in the male begins as an acute urethritis with pain on micturition and a purulent discharge, while the prostate gland and seminal vesicle may become the sites of chronic infection. General symptoms, fever and malaise may arise if the gonococcus enters the blood-stream and this blood-borne infection may reach the joints, causing a septic arthritis. Infection may be spread by the fingers to the eyes and cause purulent conjunctivitis and sometimes eventual blindness, if care is not taken to wash the hands thoroughly after contact with the discharge. A gonorrhoeal vaginal discharge in the mother may infect the infant's eyes during the passage down the vaginal canal at birth causing acute inflammation and possible permanent damage.

Treatment

Chemotherapy is successful in most cases, either sulphonamides, penicillin or other antibiotics. Penicillin is the drug most commonly used, although there is evidence that some strains of the organism have developed penicillin resistance.

Syphilis

Syphilis is caused by a corkscrew-shaped micro-organism, *Treponema pallidum*, and is most commonly acquired through sexual intercourse, but extra-genital infection can occur from inoculation with the treponeme, as for example on the lip through kissing. A pregnant woman suffering from syphilis can pass the infection to the fetus, and if the infant so infected is born alive signs of the disease may be apparent shortly after birth or may appear at some later date. This type of infection is known as congenital syphilis.

The incubation period is usually about 4 weeks, and the first symptoms are localized, the primary stage of the illness. An ulcer, the primary sore or chancre, appears at the site of infection, which is commonly the external genital organs. There is a hard ulcerated patch about the size of a shilling at the site of infection. The infection travels by the lymph stream to the nearest glands, which enlarge but do not suppurate and are not painful. The sore heals, but is followed in about 3 weeks by the secondary stage.

The organism is now circulating freely in the blood-stream, and this state is the most infectious. The blood test for syphilis, the Wassermann reaction, is now positive. General symptoms include pyrexia, loss of appetite, lassitude and headache, sore throat and pains in the joints. Ulcerations can be seen in the mouth, on the tongue, uvula and tonsils, these are long silver grey ulcers, 'snail-track' ulcers. General enlargement of lymph glands is common.

The rash, which is typical in secondary syphilis, appears on the face, limbs and trunk. In its early stage the rash shows as dusky red spots, a macular rash; later this fades and a papular rash with raised coppery spots replaces the macular stage. Occasionally this is followed by pustules and lesions resembling psoriasis; large crusted scabs known as 'rupia' are sometimes seen.

Other skin manifestations are condylomata, papillomatous wart-like growths, greyish in colour and moist, which appear around the anal and vulval areas, axillae and under the breasts.

The symptoms of secondary syphilis if untreated may last as long as 2 years, but eventually they subside, to be followed at an interval which may be as long as 15 or even 20 years by the tertiary stage.

In the tertiary stage chronic inflammatory changes may be present in any organ or tissue of the body. Painless swellings, gummata, which break down to form ulcers, occur in skin, muscle or bones and can also be found in the stomach, liver, spleen and other internal organs. Inflammatory eye conditions such as iritis and keratitis and inflammation of the aorta and the aortic valve of the heart are sometimes syphilitic in origin. Aortitis may lead to the formation of an aortic aneurysm.

Neurosyphilis, affecting the brain and spinal cord, is a still later manifestation of the damage caused by the *Treponema pallidum*. The neurosyphilitic conditions, dementia paralytica and tabes dorsalis, are described in Chapter 12.

The manifestations of congenital syphilis are somewhat similar to those seen in the secondary and tertiary stages of the acquired disease. The infant shows the skin and mucous surface lesions shortly after birth and often fails to gain weight satisfactorily.

Inflammation of the nasal mucous membrane, rhinitis, causes a chronic discharge, 'snuffles', and destruction of the bony framework of the nose produces the deformity known as 'saddle nose'. Sores at the angles of the mouth produce radiating scars. Later, after the second definition, uneven and notched teeth, Hutchinsonian teeth, syphilitic deposits in the periosteum of the tibia, causing sabre-shaped deformities, and the presence of iritis and interstitial keratitis are characteristics of congenital syphilis. The nervous system is also not infrequently involved; damage to the eighth cranial nerves causes deafness and any of the late manifestations of acquired syphilis can occur in congenital syphilis.

Treatment

For many years the form of chemotherapy used in the treatment of syphilis was organic arsenic combined with bismuth. Penicillin is now the usual drug, although other antibiotics such as the tetracyclines may be used for patients with a sensitivity to penicillin. The earlier the treatment is given the greater the prospect of successful avoidance of the dangers of tertiary and late syphilitic manifestations. Even when the patient has developed neurosyphilis, improvement can be expected from the administration of penicillin. Penicillin for pregnant women suffering from syphilis is essential in order to protect the fetus from the results of the mother's infection. The infant after birth needs careful and repeated examinations for any signs of congenital syphilis, and if such are detected should receive immediate treatment.

In all cases of venereal disease efforts are made to trace the source of the infection and other persons to whom it may have been passed. This 'contact tracing' is carried out in an attempt to control the spread of what can become a serious disease.

15
Psychological aspects of illness and mental disorders

THOSE who know anything of either the legendary or recorded history of mankind will know that from time to time great leaders and thinkers have arisen who have stressed the importance of the ordinary man, the rights of the individual and the responsibility of man for man. Often, after a time, these teachings have become forgotten or ignored, but have left behind such witnesses as the Ten Commandments, Magna Carta, Habeas Corpus and the Declaration of Human Rights.

Nursing, both as a profession and as a vocation, is dedicated to the individual. During the passage of the first half of the twentieth century the social conscience of the nation has developed even faster than it did during the second half of the previous century, partly due no doubt to the impact of two world wars. The practical outcome of the general desire to see every man, woman and child afforded opportunities for education, for useful and satisfying employment and to ensure that no one should suffer unnecessary ill health are seen in the development of the Welfare State and the National Health Service.

Along with this has grown an awareness that if we are to understand the individual we must study him in relation to his niche in the community, and not attempt to separate him from his environment. It has also become increasingly realized that the physical and psychological components of the total personality cannot be divided, and that harmony must exist between these spheres for the ideal development of the individual into an integrated healthy maturity. The word psyche means soul and reference to the psychological aspects of the individual embraces both mental and emotional processes, the emotions being the primitive driving force of existence.

'Health' is not easy to define, but, as was mentioned in the 'Introduction' (p. 6), the World Health Organisation sums it up as 'a state of complete physical, mental and social well-being'. Concerning the unity of the physical and psychological aspects, it is now recognized that disturbance, although primarily in one sphere, will certainly produce repercussions, to a greater or lesser degree, in the other, and if this disturbance is sufficiently severe, whether primarily physical or primarily mental, the patient's adaptation to his environment will suffer.

Even before birth the young of a species is affected by abnormal changes in the environment; babies are born with inherited physical and mental attributes. Heredity is moulded as the baby grows by the nature of his environment and its response to his activity. The most important single factor during the early formative years is the mother–child relationship. If the baby is loved and wanted then the first secure foundation is established.

The personality is moulded further by other contacts and by experiences and thus character develops. It is obvious that surroundings will have the greatest effect in the early, malleable period of life. Breathing, feeding and excreting in that order are the first events to impinge on the consciousness of the new life and the quality and warmth of parental care, housing and the atmosphere of family life are therefore all important. Feelings of love, trust and security can develop where loving care and nurture, emotional stability and a suitable dwelling allow for a happy home. If on the other hand feeding is deficient or casual, or the home is overcrowded, dirty and noisy, or petting and scolding succeed each other quite unpredictably and irrationally, or sleep is insufficient, neither mental nor physical growth can proceed normally. Digestive upsets, irritability, bouts of screaming, restlessness, sleeplessness and other physical or mental signs will clearly indicate that all is not well. These conditions can of course occur at any stage in life and will lead eventually to disaster if not put right. Any thoughtful and observant person can adapt this description to somewhat similar situations which might supervene at any age, perhaps due to loss of parents, a broken marriage and so on, but the effect, though parallel, will always be greatest in the most formative years of life.

Throughout life mental and emotional states are expressed by the body in terms of behaviour. Stance and expression, both visible phenomena, give clear indications of the prevailing mental and emotional climate; think, for example, of the drooping shoulder, the down-turned mouth and the slouching gait. They are as easy to read as the buoyant step and the ready smile.

The interaction of mental and physical processes is often illustrated to the full during ill health. For example, a patient in a delirious state shows a memory disturbance, is confused or disorientated, and this mental upset is due primarily to the somatic (*soma* = body) condition which is responsible for the delirium. This, in fact, is a physical disturbance producing marked repercussions in the mental sphere. Conversely, there is the tense and worrying individual who has bottled up anxiety over a period of time until it is expressed as an organic symptom such as a duodenal ulcer, or some other somatic complaint, and this is an example of the psychological basis to physical illness. The psychosomatic approach in medicine considers the effect of pathological conditions on the whole patient, mind and body, though the manifestations of the disease may be mainly physical or mainly mental.

Although mental and physical illnesses are so often closely associated, up to the present time patients with mental disorders are treated in psychiatric hospitals or units, and those whose symptoms are mainly physical are treated in general hospitals. The Mental Health Act, 1959, abolishes the special designation of mental hospitals and makes provision for the treatment of patients in any suitable type of hospital. The comprehensive hospital of the future will meet all the needs of the community in that area. The care of the old, the care and treatment of the mentally sick and of patients suffering from acute medical and surgical conditions will thus progress within one medical centre. Patients whose psychiatric illness needs continued treatment and support will in the future be helped by a variety of agencies outside the hospital, and it is hoped that the problem of chronicity may be largely avoided. This changing concept of the care of mentally disordered patients is accepted as a progressive and essential step, although practical difficulties must necessarily control the rate at which the provisions of the Mental Health Act can be put into practice.

Although the outmoded practice of certification of mental patients no longer exists, the aim being that the treatment of psychiatric illness should be organized as informally as the treatment of physical illness, certain compulsory measures are available and can be brought into action at medical level, if and when necessary. The accent is on informality, however disturbed the patient may be, but in some instances, with the patient's and relatives' best interests at heart, such measures are utilized. The most commonly invoked Sections of the Act in such cases are Section 29 which provides for compulsory admission for observation for a period not exceeding 72 hours, and Section 25 which permits such admission for a period not exceeding 28 days.

Concerning nursing in these two spheres, the gap between mental nursing and general nursing is slowly but surely being bridged, each group recognizing that while special skills are needed in different types of illness, nursing care in any situation is based on meeting the total needs of the patient. It is the special province of the psychiatric nurse to care for emotionally disturbed people, and her main skill lies in understanding and handling patients whose illness is reflected in abnormal or difficult behaviour.

Built around this central skill are additional skills that the nurse needs to develop in order to appreciate and to meet the recreational, occupational, rehabilitation and spiritual needs of the patient. Thus the establishment of a successful nurse–patient relationship is the main 'therapeutic tool'. She also needs to be skilled in carrying out an ever increasing number of practical and psychotherapeutic nursing procedures. The nurse in the general hospital is primarily concerned in the care of the physically sick, but she too must bear in mind the 'wholeness of the individual', and therefore she needs to be an expert in human relationships, with an ability to recognize and meet the differing emotional needs of each of her patients. To help her in acquiring these skills she should have some knowledge of the social factors which produce emotional, physical and mental problems. The student nurse is given a good idea of the normal physical development as she studies anatomy and physiology, hygiene and dietetics, she gains some realization of the social background of her patients as she visits with community nurses, and has contact with social service departments. She learns to think about human behaviour in her psychology classes, and she can pursue this subject by further reading and in practical application in discussing the care and management of her patients with ward sisters and tutors. Some knowledge of the present concepts of mental disorders and their main features is highly desirable as a part of every nurse's training, and it is hoped that the following brief introduction to psychological medicine will stimulate the student's interest in this important group of disorders.

A BRIEF INTRODUCTION TO PSYCHIATRY

Confusion is often apparent regarding the meaning of psychiatry and psychology and of the work of specialists associated with these spheres.

Psychiatry or psychological medicine is that branch of medicine whose special province is the study, prevention and treatment of all types of mental illness however produced. A psychiatrist is a medical doctor who has proceeded to specialize in psychological medicine and who is taking or who has taken a special post-graduate qualification in this sphere.

Psychology is the systematic study of thinking, feeling and behaviour. A psychologist is usually not medically qualified but is a specialist who has completed a university course in the science of psychology. He may subsequently have selected a special field, such as educational, social, industrial or clinical psychology.

Approach to Diagnosis

Within the field of psychiatry there are two main divisions, namely mental handicap and mental illness.

Mental Handicap

This is an arrested development of the mind, and the condition is variable, ranging from a level of intelligence only slightly below average to a state of severe intellectual impairment defined as 'subnormal' or 'severely subnormal'. Severely subnormal patients may have multiple disabilities, handicapped patients may suffer from psychopathic disorders. Such individuals may be considered as mentally incomplete rather than psychologically ill and, therefore, the main problem lies in the educational and social spheres. Medical and nursing participation is vital, however, and medical research is active within this area of psychiatry.

Mental Illness

Classification of the various mental illnesses presents problems. Diagnostic categories are essentially an attempt to group our knowledge in an orderly manner, but the present-day tendency is not to label a patient but to establish a multifactorial diagnosis, that is to say an attempt to estimate the type of personality involved from past history, present investigations and observations; then to consider the circumstances, if any, which might have precipitated the illness and this leads to a diagnosis of the process along which the patient is reacting. This process is seen at a certain stage when the patient is admitted to hospital or seeks medical advice. For example Mrs. Brown, basically an over-worrying, anxiety-prone person, has recently had excessive home problems; in addition she has been physically undermined by an attack of influenza and now has developed an anxiety state with some depressive features.

The necessity for flexibility in the approach to diagnosis having been established, it should next be mentioned that mental illness tends to fall within one of three groups. These terms really describe the severity of the patient's reaction: (1) The neuroses or psychoneuroses, and (2) The psychoses, (3) Disorders of personality.

The term *psychoneuroses* includes those illnesses in which the patient is unhappy, full of causeless but incessant anxiety, indecisive, assailed with doubts and fears, and such symptoms may encroach on the time and energy of the sufferer so that living is hampered, the effort becomes intolerable, and a breakdown occurs. Yet these patients remain in touch with reality, their basic personality is preserved and to the uninitiated they do not appear to be mentally ill. So often the mistaken idea is held that these patients are voluntarily putting on these symptoms and that they should 'snap out of it' and 'pull themselves together'. This is synonymous with advising a patient with a fractured femur to 'pull his fracture together'. Psychoneurotic patients need medical and nursing help, and if prompt and efficient measures of treatment are initiated there is every possibility that the sufferer may recover sufficiently to resume his former life.

The psychoses are those conditions in which the patient is more severely disturbed. The psychoses may be functional, in which case the basic cause is improperly known, or resulting from some organic process or drugs. Whatever the underlying causative factors, however, contact with reality tends to be severed, in most instances such patients are obviously suffering from mental disorder, and their appearance, behaviour and conversation may reflect a grave disturbance of personality.

The Psychoneuroses

The psychoneuroses include such illnesses as the anxiety state, psychosomatic illness, hysterical neurosis, obsessional compulsive neurosis and neurotic or reactive depression.

Anxiety state. Pathological anxiety is a state in which morbid and prolonged fear colours the individual's entire horizon and is so severe and persistent as to prevent him from carrying on his normal daily life. Sometimes this fear is displaced on to one or more objects, sometimes it is loose and floating. For instance the patient may say that he is constantly apprehensive and fearful because of attacks of precordial pain and tachycardia and during these episodes he feels that he will die. Reassurance that the symptoms are the result of, and not the cause of, his fears will satisfy him temporarily. On the other hand he may state that anxiety and panic are perpetual, that everything seems a threat to him, but that he can see no apparent reason for these fears. In addition to the mental symptoms, anxiety has physical concomitants, for the persistent emotion of fear produces a physiological response in the body; thus the sympathetic nervous system is over-active and physical symptoms such as palpitation, breathlessness, tremor, sweating, nausea and occasionally parasympathetic symptoms, such as diarrhoea or frequency of micturition, are part of the total picture. As previously indicated, the patient often pins his symptom of fear on to one or more of the resultant physical repercussions.

Psychosomatic illness. In all physical illnesses, psychological factors should be borne in mind for, as has already been stated, no illness is ever completely physical or completely mental, these two spheres being inevitably interlinked. However, there are certain physical disorders which in the past have come under the aegis of general rather than psychological medicine, but which nowadays are known to merit a joint approach. Psychosomatic illness, therefore, may be considered as a physical expression of underlying anxiety, frustration or anger. It is common knowledge that worry may predispose to ulcers, hypertension and other such conditions. Underlying frustration and fear readily contribute to syndromes such as migraine, while suppressed anger and tension are emotions which are often in the background of disorders, such as asthma and certain skin diseases. For instance 'Mr X', who never lost his temper, who disliked showing anger and irritability, had lived for some years under the cloud of a nagging wife. This he had accepted on the surface with meekness, but basically his anger was constantly roused. This underlying emotional trauma was eventually expressed as a skin lesion, and so psychiatric as well as medical treatment was necessary in order to reverse the condition.

Hysterical neurosis. This is a psychological reaction in which symptoms of either physical or mental illness are unconsciously produced or prolonged by the individual for his real or imaginary benefit. Hysterical symptoms might be considered as a defence against anxiety, for painful mental experiences associated with underlying conflict are translated into functional symptoms as described above, and this conversion of anxiety brings peace to the individual who appears outwardly calm and unworried. However, the control of tension in this pathological manner demands a high price, for the resultant symptoms prevent the patient from living a normal and happy life. It is important to remember that in hysterical illnesses the symptoms are unconsciously produced, for if the patient is fully aware of their adoption, the condition approaches the level of malingering. Hysteria is a very difficult illness to understand, and therefore a brief description of a case may be helpful.

'Miss X', a patient aged 19, had always been a spoilt dependent girl owing to having a domineering and over-protective mother. She was due to attend for an important interview and, if successful, her career would take her abroad. This proved a conflict situation, for the patient wanted to progress in life but the pull of the mother made separation unthinkable. To succeed in the interview and leave home therefore would be intolerable, but the disgrace of failure would be equally so. Miss X became apprehensive, irritable, worried, with feelings of nausea, but on the morning of her interview these anxiety symptoms were translated into a hysterical symptom, and the girl awoke no longer worried, and in fact with a placid demeanour—but she had lost her voice (hysterical aphonia). By this symptom both aspects of her basic conflict were pathologically satisfied. Psychiatric treatment was obviously essential so that she could be helped to resolve her underlying difficulties and thus be happy and well, rather than unworried, martyred, but sick.

Obsessional compulsive neurosis. An obsessional neurosis is a disorder in which the person is occupied with compulsive thoughts, images, inclinations or acts, and this to such a degree that his adaptation to the environment is hampered. Compulsive experiences are resented by the individual who recognizes them as morbid, pointless and irrational, but is unable to deny their intrusion on his time and energy without help. Thus the patient may be absorbed in repeated handwashing, in repeated patterns of thought, in repeated obsessional activity such as checking, re-checking, excessive tidiness and so forth; these compulsive symptoms take up so much of the individual's time that they seriously interfere with his normal occupation and activities.

Neurotic (or reactive) depression. This illness is characterized by a variably depressed mood occurring as a personal reaction to conflicts or situations of stress, e.g. bereavement, financial catastrophe or an unhappy love affair. The patient's reaction to the conflict or stress reaches pathological *intensity* but features of retardation, agitation, delusional thinking and hallucinations are always absent. Self-pity, social withdrawal and apathy are usually present and the person's normal sleep pattern and appetite tend to be disrupted.

Often the patient can be distracted from his worries and unhappy thoughts and at such times transiently present as being 'their usual self'.

The Psychoses

The Affective Illness (Disorders of Feeling)

These include mania and depression, and the main abnormality is one of mood. Thus the patient is either sad, hopeless, agitated, in a state of total misery, or on the other hand is elated, euphoric and exuberant.

Depression or **melancholia**, is a feeling experienced by most people at times, but when it exceeds its apparent cause in intensity and duration, such as the loss of a near relative, or when it occurs in the absence of any apparent cause, then a pathological level of depression has been reached and the patient is ill. His mood is one of gloom and hopelessness, he is convinced that life for him is finished, his interest and initiative are inhibited, he cannot 'feel' affection as he normally would for his family, and usually is assailed with ideas of self-blame and guilt. These may become so intolerable and his self-hatred may reach such a level that all aggression turns inwards, resulting in an attempt at self-destruction. In severely depressed patients homicidal acts are not uncommon, for the patient feels that he has ruined his loved ones, infected them in some desperate way and that he must spare them a continued existence in such a horrific life. Motor activity in depressive states varies, for in some instances the melancholic patient is in a state of physical retardation, which is reflected in a mask-like expression, slow movements and monosyllabic speech, while another depressed patient may have an anguished expression, restless movements, wringing of hands and repetitive patterns of speech.

Mania. Manic reactions are often associated with depression, as in manic depressive psychosis. The patient in a state of mania becomes over-active, over-talkative, restless, has grandiose ideas and attempts to overcome underlying feelings of insecurity and tensions by dominating the environment and severing contact with reality in a manic flight. Sometimes the meaning of this flight seems to be a 'holiday from gloom', an involuntary means of escaping from underlying feelings of depression.

Schizophrenic Reactions

This is a large group of illnesses, the fundamental feature being a loss of contact with reality. Patients suffering from typical schizophrenic states show:

(1) A disorder of thinking in which thought becomes disconnected.

(2) A disorder of emotion, which presents as an affective apathy, instability or inappropriateness.

   (3) Hallucinations which are usually the perception of the patient's own thoughts projected as voices and coming from the external environment.

   (4) A disorder of behaviour which is often bizarre, impulsive and incomprehensible to the observer.

There is an overall tendency to withdraw from reality into fantasy; in some instances the withdrawal is complete and the patient is inaccessible, while in others the patient may appear superficially in contact, but may actually be concealing a considerable degree of mental disturbance.

Organic Reactions

The organic mental illnesses include those in which the psychiatric symptoms are a response to physical trauma, catastrophe or disease. This group is a large one, and the symptoms produced vary considerably according to the site and degree of the lesion involved. Broadly speaking there are two main presenting syndromes:

   (1) The patient may be in a state of confusion or delirium which may be acute or subacute. In most instances this is a reversible state if appropriate treatment is initiated.

   (2) The patient may be in a state of dementia, and thus there is a progressive reduction in intellectual ability and emotional control, accompanied with deterioration of the personality generally. The process of dementia may be stemmed or arrested, but the condition is not reversible.

Organic states include:

   (1) Brain injury.

   (2) Disorders of circulation.

   (3) Intoxications: these may be exogenous such as alcohol, barbiturates, bromide, or endogenous such as puerperal toxic states.

   (4) Deficiency syndromes.

   (5) Epilepsy.

   (6) Inflammatory or infectious states such as syphilis, encephalitis and meningitis.

(7) Degenerative states such as senile dementia.
(8) Congenital or hereditary states such as Huntington's chorea, congenital hydrocephalus.
(9) Cerebral tumour, including metastases from malignant growths in another part of the body.
(10) Endocrine disorders.

Psychopathic Personality

This is a basic and persistent character disorder which has its foundations very early in the individual's life. The person is unreliable with defective moral judgment, prone to impulsive, imprudent and inconsiderate acts. There is an inability to profit from experience, to look ahead and assess future results of present actions, to adapt or fit into community life, or to make a lasting emotional relationship. This last factor makes treatment a problem, for in order to help the patient a psycho-therapeutic relationship must be formed between the psychiatrist and the patient. As a rule the history of psychopathic patients shows abnormal conduct from an early age, for instance truancy from school, minor offences, possibly commitment to an approved school or institution. These people do not learn from experience and are not amenable to normal corrective measures. Very often there is evidence of a disturbed home background, desertion by one or both parents, and in some cases no home at all. Occasionally there is no such unfavourable background, and the psychopathic personality may appear in an otherwise average home setting as the 'black sheep' of the family. Abnormalities in the electro-encephalogram of these individuals are often apparent, and these are similar to the graphs of a child. Some people, therefore, hold the view that this illness is organically promoted, but others believe it to be due to early environmental traumata particularly associated with the mother–child relationship during the initial stages of emotional development.

Generally there is no single element responsible for a person's breakdown, the causes being many and varied. In certain disorders, notably the neurotic reactions, it would appear that factors involved are mainly psychogenic; for instance where emotional maturity has been hampered through early traumatic experiences, the scene may be set, particularly if heredity is poor, for a future breakdown if life proves sufficiently stressful. On the other hand, as previously illustrated, there are mental disorders in which the main cause is basic organic disease, i.e. general paralysis of the insane or senile dementia. In schizophrenia and manic-depressive illness the full cause is as yet unknown.

It is as well to remember that psychiatric diagnoses may not be mutually exclusive. It is possible to encounter a patient suffering a psychotic illness, for example, and who also exhibits obsessional traits in his personality or behaviour. Similarly, often there is no clear distinction between elation and depression in a manic–depressive psychosis. Thus one can encounter an almost simultaneous 'mixed mood state', i.e. the patient exhibits elated behaviour whilst their topics of conversation are of a depressive nature.

TREATMENT OF PSYCHIATRIC DISORDERS

Treatment is decided after careful assessment of each individual patient, and after due consideration of all the factors involved in his particular illness hence the subject cannot be dealt with in a short outline such as this, which is only an introduction to psychiatry. In general it may be said that there are three main approaches in treatment, namely psychological, which includes the various forms of psychotherapy, physical, treatment, and social rehabilitation. Psychological treatment may be carried out individually, or the patient may be treated in a group. There is a growing use of behaviour therapy in the treatment of patients with certain phobias, such as obsessional phobias.

Physical treatment includes the use of tranquillizing drugs, anti-depressive drugs, electroplexy and modified insulin therapy. Insulin coma, widely used in the past in the treatment of schizophrenic illness, has now been replaced by modern tranquillizing drugs. In certain cases the operation of leucotomy, i.e. dividing some of the nerve fibres in the frontal lobe of the brain, may be performed, usually for the relief of intractable tension accompanied by anxiety and depression.

Social Prophylaxis

Mention should be made of the growing provision of preventive measures in the community, for example the child guidance service and the provision for treatment of adolescent disorders, more consultative clinics for outpatients, and community centres designed to help patients in the early stages of mental illness and so possibly prevent hospitalization. The attention which is now being given to the inclusion of more instruction and realistic teaching of psychology and psychiatric disorders in the curriculum of both doctors and nurses should promote a better understanding of mental illnesses and earlier detection of their onset.

Supportive Measures

This is an era when as far as possible it is thought better for psychiatric patients to receive community or domiciliary treatment and, if hospitalization is necessary, this should be as brief as is compatible with the patient's recovery. Further community resources for a continuity of therapy, or continued support if this is necessary, form part of the developing pattern. Psychiatric day hospitals and night hospitals, after-care day centres, hostels, sheltered workshops, and industrial and social centres from which domicilliary services can be organized, are growing throughout the country and are all designed to meet contemporary needs and to provide treatment outside the hospital wherever possible. One of the most important advances in supportive treatment is the changing attitude of the general public, so that mental illness comes to be accepted not as something to be turned away from in fear and horror, but as an illness in which the patient needs understanding, kindness and help just as much as he would if suffering from rheumatism or asthma.

DRUG DEPENDENCY

It has often been said that we are a 'nation of pill swallowers' and that the sale of pills, potions and powders is rising rapidly. However undesirable this may be it is not the problem implied by drug dependency or addiction. This is characterized by an overwhelming need to obtain and take the drug in ever increasing doses, and to develop physical and psychological symptoms if the source of supply is cut off.

It is probably true to say that there have always been a few drug addicts, most of whom were introduced to the drug medicinally or had easy access, e.g. doctors, nurses or pharmacists. Now the problem is greatly increased both in number and by the fact that the age level is now amongst the younger age groups, teenagers and even school children. Some of these may take the drug initially just for the experience; because their friends do and because they have been told it provides 'kicks'. Some may stop before it is too late, others find to their distress that they are 'hooked' and unable to stop the habit. Many of these addicts may have a personality defect shown by instability, irresponsibility, poor school or employment records. Others have a disturbed social background such as a broken home, but some may be of high intelligence and from secure social backgrounds, yet get caught in the sub-culture of the drug taken perhaps as a result of friends.

There tends to be a progression in drug taking, often the addict starting by smoking cannabis (pot, weed, hash, hemp to give but a few of its synonyms) in a 'reefer' cigarette, this gives a pleasurable sensation. The 'pep pills' (amphetamine barbiturate derivatives) may be taken to abolish tiredness and to increase energy. From this point he may seek bigger thrills and try narcotic or 'hard' drugs such as heroin, cocaine, morphine and pethidine. These drugs are usually given by injection and so begins the habit of 'mainlining' i.e. injecting into a vein. This itself provides almost a religious ecstasy as the individual prepares the syringe, watches the blood rush into it and eventually administers the drug, and many addicts admit they get pleasure from the procedure. However, the life now becomes centred around the ever increasing need for a 'fix' from weekly, to daily, to few hourly. Money has to be obtained to get the drug and may result in criminal activity. Infection frequently develops from the use of dirty syringes and needles and as little money is available for food and these people are undernourished, death may result from septicaemia or viral hepatitis. Ordinary daily activities such as working for a living are completely impossible and the personality further deteriorates, the only interest being in the obtaining of the drug. If the drug is unobtainable then withdrawal symptoms develop. These include watery eyes, itching and running nose, abdominal cramps, nausea, vomiting and shivering. These symptoms can be relieved by administering the drug or substitute methadone which is, however, itself addictive if used in excess.

Such individuals may seek treatment themselves but more often they reach hospitals because of some other condition such as infection, or they may be ordered to have treatment when sentenced by a court because of criminal activity.

Since 1968 treatment centres have been set up throughout the country—mainly in large cities such as London, Birmingham and Manchester, and certain doctors have been licensed by the Home Office to prescribe heroin or cocaine for addicts, it being an offence for other doctors to do so other than in a medical emergency. (Heroin can still be prescribed for the relief of pain in terminal malignant conditions.) However, in many towns there are no such treatment centres and addicts may be treated in general or psychiatric hospitals.

One of the main problems is that few drug addicts appear to want to be rid of their addiction and it is this that makes their treatment so difficult. Often they will not co-operate while in hospital and many of those apparently cured relapse soon after returning to their old environment. This in itself is not surprising, as all their friends may still be addicts and make the drug easily available to them and after-care tends to be spasmodic.

Because of this it would appear that the most effective way to treat the growing addiction problem in the world is by prevention, rather than cure. In this the nurse may help as an educator of her own peer group, and by realizing that her access to drugs may make her peculiarly at risk herself.

While caring for such patients there should be firmness yet sympathy and a realization that these patients are ill both in mind and body despite their often brash and colourful exterior. There should be an absence of censure from the nurse's dealings with the patients and an attempt to demonstrate that they are considered worthwhile members of the community. Many of them feel unwanted and unloved, and have commencd taking drugs for this very reason, therefore, any treatment must be aimed at giving them some form of self-respect and security.

Methods of treatment vary and may include psychotherapy,

group therapy and aversion therapy, along with the attempt to withdraw the drug in a gradual manner. If withdrawal is accomplished an intensive programme of rehabilitation is required and many need to leave hospital for the security of a hostel as a half-way house before being able to face life on their own.

Appendix

SI Units*

The internationally agreed version of the metric system is known as the Système International d'Unités, or SI for short. Its use will ensure that all quantities expressed in metric units will be stated in the same manner in all disciplines. Metric units have already been introduced into numerous aspects of the Health Service such as the dispensing of drugs. It is now intended to extend their use, particularly for reporting the results of laboratory tests.

The units for commonly occurring standard measurements are shown in the following table.

Quantity	Unit	Symbol
Length	metre	m
Mass	kilogram	kg
Time	second	s
Temperature	degree Celsius	°C
Volume	litre	l

Four particular points should be noted:
  (1) For multiples or fractions of mass (weight) the prefixes or symbols are added to the word gram or the symbol 'g'.
  (2) Pressure measurements by sphygmomanometer will continue for the time being to be expressed in mm of mercury, i.e. the height of a column of mercury measured in millimetres. Blood gas measurements will use the SI unit of pressure—the Pascal (Pa). Industry is likely to use the bar where high pressures are involved, e.g. in gas cylinders. 1 bar = 100 kPa = 14·5 psi.
  (3) The unit for temperature—the degree Celsius—is identical in value to the degree Centigrade.
  (4) There is an additional SI unit—the mole—which is the measure of the amount of substance present. For substances of defined chemical composition and known structure it is recommended that amount of substance concentration is used. (For molecules this is obtained by dividing the mass concentration [in

* The section on SI Units has been taken from the DHSS leaflet *SI Units are Simply Metric Units* with permission of the Controller of Her Majesty's Stationery Office.

grams per litre] by the molecular weight). It can be applied to any defined particle such as ion, atom, molecule or radical, but the nature of the particle must be specified.

Multiple Units

The method of expression of multiples or fractions is already familiar in many instances, e.g. kilometre, centimetre, millimetre, millilitre, microgram. The following table uses the metre as the basic unit to demonstrate how this system works:

Prefix + metre	Symbol	Length in metres
kilo-metre	km	1000
centi-metre	cm	0·01
milli-metre	mm	0·001
micro-metre	μm	0·000 001

How to Use SI Units

A unit can be expressed either by writing its name in full (e.g. gram), giving the appropriate prefix if necessary (e.g. milligram), or by putting the symbol for the prefix in front of the symbol for the basic unit (e.g. mg). Care is needed to ensure that the symbols are accurate and that capital letters and small letters are properly differentiated: e.g. M is the symbol for mega; m is the symbol for milli. The difference is a thousand million—and that could be crucial!

Drugs

(1) These have been used in metric quantities for some years, e.g. millilitres (ml), milligrams (mg). Errors are most likely to occur with milligrams and micrograms. In handwriting or where typewriters are not fitted with the symbol 'μ' (micro) any word using this prefix, e.g. microgram, should be written out in full. It is recommended that no abbreviation should be used for 'microgram' when prescribing or labelling medicine.

A MILLIGRAM IS A THOUSAND MICROGRAMS

If in doubt about dosage consult a senior colleague, the prescriber or a pharmacist.

(2) The mole will replace the milliequivalent for certain constituents of intravenous fluids. However, a number of substances used in these fluids do not have a defined chemical composition and will continue to be stated using mass concentration (e.g. g/1 mg/1).

Laboratory Report

Some results will appear strange at first but your laboratory should state the normal ranges when the report is sent. If in doubt about interpretation you should consult a senior colleague or the laboratory originating the report. If you receive a laboratory report over the phone it should be written down with particular care and checked by reading back.

Dietetics

SI units of weight (milligram, gram) and fluid volume (millilitre, litre) have been used in nutrition and dietetics for many years. (1 lb = 453·6 g; 1 oz = 28·35 g; 1 fluid ounce = 28·41 ml).

However, until now the energy value of food has been expressed in kilocalories (kcalne). The SI units are the kilojoule (kJ) and the megajoule (MJ).

1000 kJ = 1 MJ.

To convert kcal to kJ and MJ:
1 kcal   = 4·2 kJ
1000 kcal = 4200 kJ
             = 4·2 MJ

To calculate the energy value of food:
1 gram protein yields approximately 4 kcal   = 17 kJ
1 gram carbohydrate yields approximately 3·8 kcal = 16 kJ
1 gram fat yields approximately 9 kcal   = 38 kJ

You may have already appreciated that indices can be used for a statement of values instead of a cumbersome series of noughts. The full table of prefixes, symbols and values can therefore be expressed as follows:

Prefix	Symbol		Value
tera	T	10^{12}	1 000 000 000 000
giga	G	10^{9}	1 000 000 000
mega	M	10^{6}	1 000 000
kilo	k	10^{3}	1000
hecto	h	10^{2}	100
deca	da	10^{1}	10
deci	d	10^{-1}	0·1
centi	c	10^{-2}	0·01
milli	m	10^{-3}	0·001
micro	μ	10^{-6}	0·000 001
nano	n	10^{-9}	0·000 000 001
pico	p	10^{-12}	0·000 000 000 001
femto	f	10^{-15}	0·000 000 000 000 001
atto	a	10^{-18}	0·000 000 000 000 000 001

Note: $10^{-1} = 0·1 = 1/10$; $10^{-2} = 0·01 = 1/100$; $10^{-3} = 0·001 = 1/1000$ etc.

The SI system permits the use of indices and many people in laboratories and similar establishments will find them extremely useful. However, anyone using indices should not only fully understand the mathematics themselves, they should also be certain that the colleagues with whom they are communicating understand them too.
INDICES SHOULD NOT BE USED WHEN STATING DOSES

APPROXIMATE EQUIVALENT DOSES IN THE METRIC AND IMPERIAL (APOTHECARIES') SYSTEMS*

WEIGHTS

Grams	Grains	Milligrams	Grains
10	150	45	$\frac{3}{4}$
8	120	35	$\frac{3}{5}$
6	90	30	$\frac{1}{2}$
5	75	25	$\frac{2}{5}$
4	60	20	$\frac{1}{3}$
3	45	15	$\frac{1}{4}$
2·6	40	12	$\frac{1}{5}$
2	30	10	$\frac{1}{6}$
1·6	25	8	$\frac{1}{8}$
1·3	20	6	$\frac{1}{10}$
1	15	5	$\frac{1}{12}$
0·8	12	4	$\frac{1}{16}$
0·6	10	3	$\frac{1}{20}$
0·5	8	2·5	$\frac{1}{24}$
		2	$\frac{1}{30}$
		1·5	$\frac{1}{40}$

Milligrams	Grains	Milligrams	Grains
		1·2	$\frac{1}{50}$
400	7	1	$\frac{1}{60}$
300	5	0·8	$\frac{1}{80}$
250	4	0·6	$\frac{1}{100}$
200	$3\frac{1}{2}$	0·5	$\frac{1}{120}$
150	$2\frac{1}{2}$	0·4	$\frac{1}{160}$
120	2	0·3	$\frac{1}{200}$
100	$1\frac{2}{3}$	0·25	$\frac{1}{240}$
80	$1\frac{1}{3}$	0·2	$\frac{1}{300}$
75	$1\frac{1}{4}$	0·15	$\frac{1}{400}$
60	1	0·12	$\frac{1}{500}$

* These tables may be used for the direct transference of doses from one system to the other. Multiples of these equivalents must not be used, since in multiplying, the error of the approximation might be raised to a significant figure.

FLUID MEASURES

Millilitres	Minims	Millilitres	Minims
10	150	0·8	12
8	120	0·6	10
6	90	0·5	8
5	75	0·4	6
4	60	0·3	5
3	45	0·25	4
2·6	40	0·2	3
2	30	0·15	$2\frac{1}{2}$
1·6	25	0·12	2
1·3	20	0·1	$1\frac{1}{2}$
1	15		

```
1 fluid ounce  = approximately 30 ml
1 fluid drachm = approximately  4 ml
15 minims      = approximately  1 ml
```

ACCURATE EQUIVALENTS

Mass

1 kilogram (kg)	= 15 432 grains
	or 35·274 ounces
	or 2·2046 pounds
1 gram (g)	= 15·432 grains
1 milligram (mg)	= 0·015432 grain

1 pound (avoirdupois) (lb)	= 453·59 grams
1 ounce (avoirdupois) (oz)	= 28·35 grams
1 grain	= 64·799 milligrams

Capacity

1 litre (l)	= 1·7598 pints
1 millilitre (ml)	= 16·894 minims
1 litre (l)	= 0·0353 cubic foot
1 litre (l)	= 0·22 gallon

1 pint (pt)	= 568·25 millilitres
	or 0·56825 litre
1 fluid ounce (fl oz)	= 28·412 millilitres
1 fluid drachm (fl dr)	= 3·5515 millilitres
1 minim (or min)	= 0·059192 millilitre

Length

1 metre (m)	= 39·370 inches (in)
1 decimetre (dm)	= 3·9370 inches
1 centimetre (cm)	= 0·39370 inch
1 millimetre (mm)	= 0·039370 inch
1 micron (μm)	= 0·000039370 inch

1 in	= 25·400 mm

CELSIUS (CENTIGRADE) AND FAHRENHEIT EQUIVALENTS

Celsius Fahrenheit $°F = (°C × \frac{9}{5}) + 32$				Fahrenheit Celsius $°C = (°F − 32) × \frac{5}{9}$					
°C	°F	°C	°F	°F	°C	°F	°C	°F	°C
−50	−58·0	49	120·2	−50	−46·7	99	37·2	157	69·4
−40	−40·0	50	122·0	−40	−40·0	100	37·7	158	70·0
−35	−31·0	51	123·8	−35	−37·2	101	38·3	159	70·5
−30	−22·0	52	125·6	−30	−34·4	102	38·8	160	71·1
−25	−13·0	53	127·4	−25	−31·7	103	39·4	161	71·6
−20	−4·0	54	129·2	−20	−28·9	104	40·0	162	72·2
−15	+5·0	55	131·0	−15	−26·6	105	40·5	163	72·7
−10	14·0	56	132·8	−10	−23·3	106	41·1	164	73·3
−5	23·0	57	134·6	−5	−20·6	107	41·6	165	73·8
0	32·0	58	136·4	0	−17·7	108	42·3	166	74·4
−1	33·8	59	138·2	−1	−17·2	109	42·7	167	75·0
2	35·6	60	140·0	5	−15·0	110	43·3	168	75·5
3	37·4	61	141·8	10	−12·2	111	43·8	169	76·1
4	39·2	62	143·6	15	−9·4	112	44·4	170	76·6
5	41·0	63	145·4	20	−6·6	113	45·0	171	77·2
6	42·8	64	147·2	25	−3·8	114	45·5	172	77·7
7	44·6	65	149·0	30	−1·1	115	46·1	173	78·3
8	46·4	66	150·8	31	−0·5	116	46·6	174	78·8
9	48·2	67	152·6	32	0	117	47·2	175	79·4
10	50·0	68	154·4	33	+0·5	118	47·7	176	80·0
11	51·8	69	156·2	34	1·1	119	48·3	177	80·5
12	53·6	70	158·9	35	1·6	120	48·8	178	81·1
13	55·4	71	159·8	36	2·2	121	49·4	179	81·6
14	57·2	72	161·6	37	2·7	122	50·0	180	82·2
15	59·0	73	163·4	38	3·3	123	50·5	181	82·7
16	60·8	74	165·2	39	3·8	124	41·1	182	83·3
17	62·6	75	167·0	40	4·4	125	51·6	183	83·8
18	64·4	76	168·8	41	5·0	126	42·2	184	84·4
19	66·2	77	170·6	42	5·5	127	52·7	185	85·0
20	68·0	78	172·4	43	6·1	128	53·3	186	85·5
21	69·8	79	174·2	44	6·6	129	53·8	187	86·1
22	71·6	80	176·0	45	7·2	130	54·4	188	86·6
23	73·4	81	177·8	46	7·7	131	55·0	189	87·2
24	75·2	82	179·6	47	8·3	132	55·5	190	87·7
25	77·0	83	181·4	48	8·8	133	56·1	191	88·3
26	78·8	84	183·2	49	9·4	134	56·6	192	88·8
27	80·6	85	185·0	50	10·0	135	57·2	193	89·4
28	82·4	86	186·8	55	12·7	136	57·7	194	90·0
29	84·2	87	188·6	60	15·5	137	58·3	195	90·5
30	86·0	88	190·4	65	18·3	138	58·8	196	91·1
31	87·8	89	192·2	70	21·1	139	59·4	197	91·6
32	89·6	90	194·0	75	23·8	140	60·0	198	92·2
33	91·4	91	195·8	80	26·6	141	60·5	199	92·7
34	93·2	92	197·6	85	29·4	142	61·1	200	93·3
35	95·0	93	199·4	86	30·0	143	61·6	201	93·8
36	96·8	94	201·2	87	30·5	144	62·2	202	94·4
37	98·6	95	203·0	88	31·0	145	62·7	203	95·0
38	100·4	96	204·8	89	31·6	146	63·3	204	95·5
39	102·2	97	206·6	90	32·2	147	63·8	205	96·1
40	104·0	98	208·4	91	32·7	148	64·4	206	96·6
41	105·8	99	210·2	92	33·3	149	65·0	207	97·2
42	107·6	100	212·0	93	33·8	150	65·5	208	97·7
43	109·4	101	213·8	94	34·4	151	66·1	209	98·3
44	111·2	102	215·6	95	35·0	152	66·6	210	98·8
45	113·0	103	217·4	96	35·5	153	67·2	211	99·4
46	114·8	104	219·2	97	36·1	154	67·7	212	100·0
47	116·6	105	221·0	98	36·6	155	68·3	213	100·5
48	118·4	106	222·8	98·6	37·0	156	68·8	214	101·1

Index